Advance Praise for *Cycle of Lives*

"This is a big, audacious book about a big, audacious disease. It's as if David is shining a light into all the dark crevices and saying, 'We see you, cancer, and you're not going to bring us to our knees.'"

—**Jennie Nash**, author of *The Victoria's Secret Catalog Never Stops Coming and Other Lessons I Learned From Breast Cancer*

"Cancer advocacy means something different to each person. David has chosen to take his 'cancer club membership' to paper and penned this must-read book that stands apart from the pack as one of the most authentic, compelling, inspirational, and passionate works of non-fiction around."

—**Matthew Zachary**, leader; speaker; disruptor; and founder of the adolescent and young adult cancer organization, Stupid Cancer

"With luminous clarity, Richman's open-hearted interviews with real people facing cancer across ages and circumstances reveal the simple truths that unite us all."

—**Dan Shapiro**, PhD, psychologist, speaker, author; Vice Dean for Faculty and Administrative Affairs, Garner James Cline Professor of Humanities in Medicine, Penn State College of Medicine

"This remarkably insightful book is beautifully written. David reveals the multitude of emotions that cancer patients experience, through vivid, relatable story-telling. This is medical narrative writing at its best!"

—Ann Marie Beddoe MD MPH, gynecologic oncologist;
director of Global Woman's Health at Mount Sinai Medical Center
NY; co-founder of The Women Global Cancer Initiative

"The emotional side effects of cancer often go undetected, but because of David's book, I am now more aware of and have a different perspective of peoples' experiences. I am a better patient advocate because of the stories shared in this book."

—Gail Johnson, head patient coordinator, Valley Health System,
Mount Sinai Comprehensive Cancer Care

"The narrative around cancer tends to be told by people who've had exclusively triumphant—and often remarkably similar—trajectories. But cancer is a complex array of diseases, and as David Richman demonstrates through his extraordinary cross-country bike journey, every experience of it is unique. This is a big-hearted book, full of love and grit, one that shows there is no "typical" cancer story and invites us all to a deeper, more empathetic conversation around illness, grief, and survivorship."

—Mary Elizabeth Williams, author,
speaker, stage-4 melanoma survivor

Cycle
of
Lives

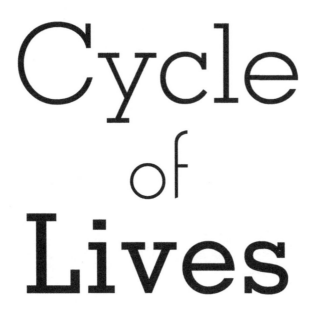

15 People's Stories, 5,000 Miles, *and a*
Journey Through *the* Emotional Chaos *of* Cancer

DAVID RICHMAN

RIVER GROVE
BOOKS

This book is a memoir reflecting the author's present recollections of experiences over time. Its story and its words are the author's alone. Some details and characteristics may be changed, some events may be compressed, and some dialogue may be recreated.

Published by River Grove Books
Austin, TX
www.rivergrovebooks.com

Copyright ©2020 David Richman

Distributed by River Grove Books

Design and composition by Greenleaf Book Group
Cover design by Greenleaf Book Group
Cover images used under license from
©Shutterstock.com/Have a nice day Photo

Publisher's Cataloging-in-Publication data is available.

Print ISBN: 978-1-63299-299-4

eBook ISBN: 978-1-63299-300-7

First Edition

Contents

Foreword: H. Lee Moffitt

I know cancer. I have looked it in the eye. I have rallied the troops to fight back. And, I have seen an army assemble.

In the 1970s and early 1980s, I was a member of the Florida House of Representatives. During those years when I served in the legislature and as Speaker of the House, I lost several dear friends to cancer: Joseph Lumia, Judy Barnett, George Edgecomb, to name a few. After going through my own battle with cancer and knowing of too many friends and colleagues who continued to face this relentless disease, I realized there was a great need for a research-based cancer center in Florida. Once committed to taking action, I knew one of my most important works in life was to do everything I could to contribute to the care and cure of those afflicted with cancer and end this beast. Enough was enough.

I was able to secure seventy million dollars from the legislature, which came primarily from the state of Florida's cigarette tax, for construction of a cancer center. In October of 1986, three years after its groundbreaking, The H. Lee Moffitt Cancer Center & Research Institute officially opened. Since then, I have been humbled to stand with countless brave and hopeful cancer survivors, the brightest researchers and doctors, caring families and loved ones, and so many more who have found themselves, by choice or by fate, in the midst of fighting this disease. Today, Moffitt Cancer Center, consistently ranked in the top ten nationally recognized cancer hospitals and the only National Cancer Institute–designated Comprehensive Cancer Center based in Florida, is not only dedicated to treating cancer patients, but just as importantly, we are tirelessly dedicated to research in hopes of finding a cure.

I met David Richman and learned of his book on bringing together the many emotional aspects of the cancer experience through a mutual friend. Karen was going through her second battle with cancer; first, she beat thyroid cancer, and then she encountered triple negative breast cancer—all before she was 40. During her recovery, Karen and I had the opportunity to walk the halls of the state legislature together, the same halls where I had served more than thirty years before. I thought of old friends, how impactful cancer had been in our lives, and how much Moffitt Cancer Center had grown. Together, Karen and I met with the governor to discuss the cancer center, our goals, our needs, our impact on the community, and our dedication to serving those afflicted with cancer. I noticed right away that Karen had the same drive as me to fight the battle; I have come to know that once affected, so many good people join our army and engage in this mission to do what we can to make a difference.

This book describes the emotional aspects of the cancer experience, as told from different viewpoints, those of survivors, of caretakers, of doctors. The stories contained within will touch you with their humanity, trueness, and insight into the human experience. This book will help you understand the deep emotional trauma that cancer can cause, while showing you the optimism, hope, and courage that so many bring to their experience.

When I walk through Moffitt Cancer Center, I see cancer in its most in-your-face way, and I am witness to the battles that are being waged. I see the doctors and nurses and technicians and researchers who are fighting every day for our patients. I see the emotion, the dedication, the compassion, and the unity of purpose that defines the Moffitt culture, and I am inspired and hopeful.

When I look back on how far we have come in the fight against cancer and when I attempt to measure the ways in which Moffitt Cancer Center has touched so many families and patients with cancer, I know the battle will be won. If cancer has touched your life or the life of a loved one or friend, or if cancer has inspired in you a calling to dedicate your life to fighting back, this book will open your eyes to the emotional journeys we all find ourselves facing.

—**H. Lee Moffitt,** founder and namesake of Moffitt Cancer Center

Foreword: Dr. Douglas Letson

F or twenty-six years, I have embraced my purpose in life: to contribute to the prevention and cure of cancer. To prepare for fulfillment of my purpose in life, I devoted fifteen years to medical education and postgraduate training in outstanding institutions such as Harvard Medical School, under the auspices of experts in orthopedic oncology. As an academic orthopedic surgical oncologist, I have had the opportunity to contribute to the vast array of impressive advances in cancer care that, while not always curative, are significantly improving survival time and quality of life. Accelerated advances in cancer care are essential to save more and more lives and reduce the burden of cancer on many more patients, families, and communities.

In 2020 in the US alone, we expect to see "1,806,590 new cancer cases and 606,520 cancer deaths." Between 1991 and 2017, the cancer death rate fell continuously, resulting in "an overall decline of 29% that translates into an estimated 2.9 million fewer cancer deaths than would have occurred if peak rates had persisted."[1] Increased survival is a testament to the critical function of research in creating preventive, curative, and quality-of-life advances. Consider, however, that a 29 percent decline in overall deaths took twenty-six years. Is that an acceptable length of time for saving more lives? No. We need to accelerate advances that increase survival and quality of life at a much faster pace than in the past, and recent indicators are encouraging.

We have seen phenomenal advances for patients with blood and solid tumor cancers in just the last four years, and we need to sustain the momentum. One of the most effective ways to fuel that momentum is to support cancer research, which is predominantly housed in NCI-designated academic oncology institutions throughout the US. These institutions accommodate multidisciplinary teams composed of the best and brightest experts in the field of cancer research, and they are the clinical scientists who have led many recent advances. They are the source of hope for all of us, regardless of our connection to cancer, so aptly nicknamed "The Queen of Emotional Chaos" by the author.

We are all touched by cancer. As dedicated academic oncologists, we marshal our best resources to heal our patients. When our best efforts fail and we lose a patient, we grieve, yet we keep going because we want to be there for other patients, many of whom we will be able to heal. Doctors are not immune to cancer. We get cancer. Our beloved family members and friends get cancer. We know firsthand that a diagnosis of cancer is chaotically life-altering. Indeed, cancer, the Queen of Chaos, injects high doses of fear, anxiety, and uncertainty into the life of the patient, the caregiver, and the patient's family. Many patients and their families experience the burden of economic hardship, role strain, physical and mental exhaustion, anger, depression, and even feelings of guilt and self-recrimination.

I was inexpressibly honored to be asked to write the foreword for this book about the cancer experience. The book will enlighten people about the burden of cancer, and it will inspire people to share their personal experience. Just as important, it underscores the need to fund cancer research, which is the lifeblood of progress in saving more lives and preserving the stability of more families and communities.[1]

—**G. Douglas Letson, MD;** Executive Vice President, Physician-in-Chief, and
President of Moffitt Medical Group at Moffitt Cancer Center

---

1   Siegel RL, Miller KD, Jamal A. Cancer Statistics: 2020. CA CANCER J CLIN 2020;70:7–30

Preface and Acknowledgments

....

When I was seven or eight years old, my parents hosted a summertime pool party of epic proportions. The front and back yards were lined with oil-filled Tiki lamps. Next to the ping-pong table, a wading pool full of ice overflowed with Foster's beer cans. The stereo console had been moved outside, along with a stack of records that spun loudly with the sounds of the time. The deck around our large pool was soaked from the splashing and sloshing of drunken, volleyball-playing adults. A bartender wearing a pink and yellow Aloha shirt laughed with the guests as he poured red and orange and blue drinks into tall wooden glasses that held huge slices of pineapples, limes, and lemons, along with cherries stabbed by plastic toothpicks molded in the shapes of mermaids and monkeys. And the people—there were so many people, apparently friends of my parents, most of whom I had never seen before, nor saw again after that night.

In what seemed an endless stream of incoming characters, I took stock: There were a dozen loud, happy, beer-drinking Australian men who worked for my dad, a man and woman who came all the way from Hawaii, a bikini-wearing publisher and her much-younger boyfriend who flew in from New York, and so many more. The entire day and night I relished the flow of unique and interesting characters who came and went as if they had popped off the pages of a book to take a swim, down a few drinks, smoke their pipes and cigarettes, sway in movement to the music, and exchange animated and interesting conversation with all the other characters in our backyard before heading back to their intended paths.

The memories from that night are so vivid, not just because the scenes were a veritable kaleidoscope of strange and unusual colors and sounds, but because the flow and the energy, and the easy, endless laughs and intoxicated joy of the night stood in such stark contrast to the subdued, colorless, anxiety-filled days and nights of my youth. I didn't know why those people came or where they came from, but it didn't matter; my bedroom window afforded me a viewpoint that night that my mind has never forgotten.

In one of the few memories I have of my mom showing any softness in life, at one point late into the evening, instead of coming in to yell at me for still being awake, she came into my room, wrapped her arm around my shoulders and gently urged me to go sleep, saying that by my doing so, I wasn't going to miss anything. After getting into my bed and pretending to prepare for sleep, I crept back to the window and wondered at all I watched for what seemed hours more. Many, many nights after, I dreamed that I would peek through that window and find a scene that might even faintly resemble that one remarkable and lively night.

Sometimes it takes time to process what I observe, sometimes I observe things that immediately tattoo themselves onto my mind's eye. Regardless, it seems I've often found myself pondering the world as if viewing things through a window, like life is an endless collection of scenes taking place while I watch from a solitary vantage point rather than from within the spectacle itself.

As I set out to write this book, I brought a lifetime's practice of willful observation to help guide my style and intent. As a result, I hope to have brought interesting, moving stories to the reader—*as told through the reflections of the book participants*—even though I was only an after-the-fact observer of their exceptional and gripping narratives.

Throughout the book, I've attempted to shed light on the emotional journeys of the participants, on the circumstances and feelings that crafted how they dealt with the traumas they encountered. If I've been at all successful in that endeavor, then, like me, you'll be able to appreciate the profoundness of their experiences, and you'll be moved to try to better understand the emotions of the people around you who might be going through traumas of their own. My hope is that we can all become better-equipped interactive participants in their journeys, motivated to ask more questions and offer deeper levels of support, rather than quietly observe from afar.

If I were given ten thousand pages to put down the thoughts about what I learned during the journey of my *Cycle of Lives* book project, both about myself and about others, I'd probably need more paper, but I can easily list the few people without whom I would have never been able to undertake and complete such a massive endeavor.

Believing in yourself is a type of fuel that can drive you to the ends of the earth, but having someone believe in you more than you believe in yourself can power you to the edge of the universe. My wife has shown her belief in me in many ways. She was the support crew who flew across the country and back several times along my ride, and she drove hundreds of miles a day for weeks and weeks, trudging back and forth along my route to provide food, water, supplies, first aid, and most importantly, to act as a caretaker, nurse, and psychologist to my tattered body and mind. She was a thoughtful test-reader and a tough editor, who often gave me powerful insight into my shortcomings as a writer and storyteller in her attempts to push me to do better. She pressed me when I needed pressing, and she gave me the space to find my way through the muck when I wanted to be left alone to try to figure my shit out. And she's done those things and more while running her law practice, providing direction and counsel to my kids, mentoring at-risk youth, and balancing all the tugs on her time each day. Clearly, I married up.

Fortunately, my kids, David and Danielle, have chosen to match my desire to keep them close to me with their willingness to be included in all aspects of my life—and include me in theirs—and it's been that way since they could string together a sentence. Together, we've been through undeniably rough times and many more gloriously rewarding times, and I expect we will do so always, together, sometimes at each other's throats, more often having each other's backs completely and without question. Danielle drove to pick me up countless times as I squeezed a training ride along the route to one of her golf tournaments or a family outing, and barely complained about how sweaty and stinky I was. David rode with me the first few days of the ride, on very little training, which was uplifting and inspirational, another reminder that once you set out to do something, nothing besides *you* can stop you. Thanks to you both for always being there on this life journey with me.

Before, during, and after this project, many people have shaped and guided me, having a profound effect on how I view the world. In particular to several larger-than-life influences, if I haven't told you enough, I'm doing so now: Chad Zdenek and the entire extended Zdenek clan, Mag Black-Scott, Jonathan Varenchik, Jerry Padilla, Dave Fuehrer, Juan and Diep, Andrew Williams and his mom and brothers, John Simmons, and all of the people who've spent time with me and my family, sharing your lives and making great memories, thank you.

I wish to especially thank Jennie Nash for believing in me and working so hard to shape this book into one that mirrors my intended vision. She's a great writer, but her skills and passion as an editor were indispensable.

The entire team at Greenleaf has been professional and passionate, and I hope to publish many books with them in the years ahead. In particular, I'll be forever grateful to Amanda Hughes for taking a deep and personal approach to her editing process. I don't know how to measure the quality of my own book, but I do know that the book is multiples better having been in her caring and competent hands.

I'd like to give a special thank you to the *Cycle of Lives* participants. Their courage through adversity and their openness to discuss things with me that they had mostly not shared before continues to swirl inside of me, penetrating my heart and mind, leaving me with a sense of their own unique beauty and meaningfulness.

Many companies supported me on the ride, including Co-Motion Cycles, IHG Hotels and Resorts, Doc's Skin Care, POC Sports, Kask, Marriott International, Hammer Nutrition, Voltaic Systems, Blue Lizard, Holiday Inns, Mobile Illumination, Lizard Skins, Red Roof Inns, Best Western, Saltstick, and more. And to all of the people who made donations and contributions— especially those along the ride who had no idea who I was or what I was doing until we met in passing—thank you for your generosity and support.

Lastly, I want to thank my sister, June. We talked a lot and about many things light and heavy, but it wasn't nearly enough. Your life was too short, but the impact on those you encountered was everlasting.

Me

Relationship to cancer: Never had it

Age: Fifty-five

Family status: Newly married with twenty-one-year-old twins

Location: Southern California

First encounter with cancer: Forty years old. My sister, June, was diagnosed with brain cancer.

Cancer summary: June fought cancer for four years and then succumbed in May of 2007, at the age of forty-six.

Treatment specifics: June endured multiple surgeries, chemotherapy, and radiation therapy.

Community involvement: Most every year, I organize some type of event in June's memory, combining athletic endurance with fundraising for cancer research and care. In 2016, I went searching for answers to the emotional issues related to cancer on an almost five-thousand-mile bike ride from California to Florida and then up to New York. I met face-to-face with the people whose stories are in this book, many of whom I'd been speaking with for years. Along the ride, I reached out to people to find out how they got through the trauma of cancer, how they made sense of it, and how their lives were affected during and after. Their collective experience is contained in this book. It is the culmination of my search for answers to the question of why no one talks about the full spectrum of emotions that come with their cancer journey. This is my effort to start those conversations.

Strongest positive emotion during cancer experience: Gratitude

Strongest negative emotion during cancer experience: Sorrow

It's All About the Bike

··

A softball-sized spot deep in the middle of my lower-right back churned out a sharp, radiating pain. My upper body felt immune to any relief my awkward stretching could offer. My ass was chafed and near bleeding from saddle sores that had crept up overnight, announcing their arrival like the blaring horns of battle—only this battle was one fought while seated. I could find no comfort on any part of my top-of-the-line Brooks bicycle seat. I looked down at the nose of the seat, made by those British masters of leathercraft who'd been fitting cyclists the world over for almost 150 years, and cursed the seat and its makers for the frauds they were.

My legs were heavy and burning. My stomach had shut down, as if it were full of hardened cement. The thought of trying to down a little water to stave off dehydration made me swim with nausea. I was sunburned, and my eyelids begged for a reprieve. The outside of both my little toes were squeezed so hard against my new Shimano shoes (damn frauds too) that I entertained the idea of cutting a hole in the sides for some glorious release from the pain.

Here I was, almost six hundred miles into a five-thousand-mile cross-country bike ride, one I was doing for all kinds of good and altruistic reasons related to cancer and my sister, but I couldn't have cared less about any of it. I found a side road adjacent to the highway and hobbled off the bike, thinking I would sleep for a few minutes. Sleep would make all those pains disappear. As the deep heat of the September Arizona asphalt sizzled the sweat off the back of my arms and legs, I asked myself, *What the hell are you doing this for?*

There were many answers, but truthfully, the more painful reasons wouldn't appear until deep into my journey. Pedaling hard day after day in one-hundred-plus-degree heat along endless stretches of highway, there was nothing to do other than crank the gears: the fourteen literal ones housed inside the German-engineered Rohloff Internal Hub on my rear wheel, and the innumerable ones housed inside my Richman-engineered mind. Deep and prolonged pain has a way of clarifying the murky things we tuck away in the corners of our minds; self-inflicted pain doubly so.

Why Bike Five Thousand Miles?

Sure, I was a bit crazy, but that wasn't why I biked five thousand miles. I wanted to do something significant to support a cause I believed in, but that wasn't why either. A big part of my "why" was this book and the people who shared their stories with me, but there was still much more. The answer—the true, personal meaning behind this whole project—started to become clear to me on that brutal day outside of Payson, Arizona, as I lay just off the side of the road, struggling to find the will to get back up after a twenty-minute nap and climb back on my bike to begin riding again. The real answers always came back to my sister.

June died a couple of months after her forty-sixth birthday. She left behind a husband and two kids who loved her, a collection of in-laws who called her their own, friends and coworkers who admired and relied on her, and a couple lost and lonely family members—one of whom was proud to call her his sister. June had brain cancer, but the type of cancer that took her is irrelevant. She's gone. What matters is she died too young: She didn't live to see her dreams come true, she didn't get to see her kids grow up, she didn't get to grow old with her husband, and she wasn't given the chance to feel the blessings and heartbreaks a lady who grows old earns the right to feel.

The five-thousand-mile cross-country bike ride, which I came to call Cycle of Lives, was the latest adventure I had undertaken in her honor and the deepest by far, not just because it was a long ride but because the experience brought me to a point where I could face all the questions and feel all the emotions I had about losing her. The ride brought me to that point because I had decided to ride in search of those answers, those feelings. I sought them out. I planned my route to bring me face-to-face with all these people who had been touched by cancer—doctors, mothers, patients, caregivers, survivors, sons, daughters, and brothers like me. Throughout this journey, together we've thought about the unthinkable, discussed the undiscussable, and discovered answers to the questions about our trauma experiences that we thought were unanswerable.

The Seeds of the Journey

The seeds for this journey were planted eight years prior, as I slowly made my way around one of the three hundred or so laps I ran at the local high school track during an American Cancer Society twenty-four-hour Relay For Life fundraising event. June had died a few days before the event, and although she couldn't keep her promise to camp out and watch all the people that day, I wanted to keep mine and stay on the track for the whole event.

That first relay was a gut-wrenching early summer's day. I spent hours watching many loved ones show their support for friends and family in the midst of fighting all types and stages of cancer. I witnessed the brave, the frightened, and the stunned-into-numbness. I watched young and old alike walking for their cause if they had the strength or, if not, sitting quietly along the trackside camping areas, trying to lend the support of their presence. I saw wide-ranging interactions between people dealing with genuine trauma—all the silence, hugs, tears, and whispers.

I'd like to say that I talked to more than a few people that day, but I can't. I was preoccupied with my own inner workings. Even if I hadn't been, I witnessed things I couldn't process or understand, let alone explore by talking to others. I was there on the track and also not there, at times aware of myself and other people and at times distracted. I was either stuck in my own head or hypnotized by the other people, all of whom appeared to be deep within their own internal sanctums. I could sense that everyone there was, at times, stuck in the same fog as me. We were all present together, but we were navigating so much more than laps around a track.

Every year for the next ten years, I would either participate in a Relay For Life event or organize another epic physical challenge to raise funds for cancer research in my sister's memory. I was on a quest, but physical accomplishments were never going to get me where I needed to go. I began to realize that I needed to face the very emotions everyone on that Relay For Life track was working so hard to avoid.

The Queen of Emotional Chaos

What makes cancer such a maddening disease is its complexity. Scientific advancement has given many people an opportunity to live longer with cancer, and often be cured of it, but cancer is still shrouded in a blanket of mystery. Doctors still work in a world made up of odds—the same treatment applied to the same kind of cancer under similar conditions can have vastly different outcomes. Many people fight off the disease and go on to live healthy, cancer-free lives for many decades, *but we still don't always know why.*

There are many definitive truths involved in cancer research, care, and treatment. After testing, we might know that specific drugs work or don't work in certain instances. We may even know what the predicted outcome might be when comparing one surgical approach to another, but doctors do not have the luxury of working in absolutes. Absolutes may offer more peace than unknowns, but there are not many absolutes in cancer. Instead, there is a stream of endless unknowns, creating a chaotic and unpredictable environment for the feelings of anyone faced with a challenge like cancer.

In his marvelous manuscript on the history of cancer, Siddhartha Mukherjee called cancer the "emperor of all maladies," but cancer is also the queen of emotional chaos. Zooming out enough to contemplate that chaos in its many different forms is a necessary step in understanding the emotional and psychological aspects of an experience with cancer.

Cancer hits most people like a shovel right in the face. It's hard, swift, disorienting, and instantly debilitating. Cancer is an ominous, otherworldly thing—part disease, part curse. Cancer is as scary as it is overbearing. Once hit in the face with cancer, most people can do little more than triage—identify the immediate needs and administer whatever care is available. If the cancer diagnosis is yours, then this often means choosing a caregiver, identifying treatment protocols, making serious lifestyle changes, inquiring about employment continuation, finding a way to meet your family's needs, addressing any financial concerns about your treatment or ability to work, and dealing with the many other tasks that demand consideration in the instantaneous, cancer-centered reality that sets in immediately after diagnosis. If you're not the patient but instead a caregiver, researcher, or loved one, the list of items to tackle might look different, but it is often no shorter or less intense.

Most people, whether they are a caregiver or the receiver, don't have the time or resources to take a deep breath and calm down for long enough to address the deeper emotional side effects and psychological repercussions of their new reality. They endure major surgery, debilitating treatment protocols, overwhelming exhaustion, physical weakness, severe pain, financial stress, loss of control, fear of mortality, abandonment, death, grief, guilt, and more.

My experience has shown that cancer usually crashes into one's life with a sort of primitive, metal-to-flesh force, and people don't often jump right into unpacking the vast array of emotion the experience evokes for them— sometimes they never do. Since I first recognized the common thread binding people touched by cancer—the tendency *not* to examine, discuss, or even acknowledge the emotional side of their experience—my goal has been to shine a light on the things we've all kept buried, in the hopes that people might better understand what they and their loved ones went through.

I'm not a researcher or psychologist. I'm not a therapist or counselor. I am, in fact, a professional in the financial services business, an amateur endurance athlete, and an author. But I was called to do this work, and I've spent more than four years finding people who would share their stories with me and planning a bike ride to go and meet as many of them as I possibly could.

I believe that if we can enhance our understanding of the full spectrum of emotions and feelings associated with cancer, then we can better process what we and the people we love may be going through. If we understand these feelings, we can better relate to ourselves and each other as we navigate the harsh, overwhelming realities wrought by this horrible disease.

Choosing My Participants

The most important aspect of the Cycle of Lives project was not the bike ride itself—that part was an epic logistical undertaking, a formidable physical test of endurance, and a way to raise some money for charity. The most important aspect for me was the stories. I wanted to bring a diverse collection of personal accounts together in one place to give the reader a chance to "meet" diverse and interesting people, to capture the broadest range of emotions and experiences about cancer possible, and to tell the story of the cancer experience from multiple angles. Most books about cancer are told from one person's perspective. For mine, I felt that to get the best mix of personal stories, I would need to take into account the following four principles:

1. AGE

I felt it was necessary to share stories from people whose cancer experience came both early and late in life, and at other points in between. I wanted stories from people who'd encountered cancer as children, people whose fertility concerns were at the forefront of their minds while undergoing treatment, and people who were entering their golden years when their diagnosis came.

Additionally, I wanted to explore people's feelings both while they were battling cancer and as they reflected back on their experience years later. I wanted to talk to people whose encounters with cancer were brief and those whose entire lives were affected.

2. TYPES OF CANCER

I think a book examining fifteen different people's experiences with one particular type of cancer would be interesting, but for my own book, I wanted the depth of experience represented to be spread out among different cancers. Even though the word *cancer* elicits some common feelings regardless of type or treatment, the fact remains that people dealing with brain cancer have a different experience from those dealing with breast cancer, lymphoma, prostate cancer, or any other type.

3. SEVERITY OF CANCER

I also thought it was vital to seek out stories from people whose experience spanned various stages of cancer. Being given a diagnosis of cancer of any stage almost always evokes a host of existential questions that people have no choice but to grapple with—the questions becoming deeper and more existential the higher the number of the stage diagnosed. Facing these questions is a painful, beautiful, and unavoidable consequence of being alive.

4. RANGE OF EMOTION

The most essential part of the Cycle of Lives project is my effort to understand the full spectrum of emotions invoked by cancer. To this end, I used Dr. Robert Plutchik's widely accepted model of The Wheel of Emotion as a framework. The short version of Dr. Plutchik's theory is that we all have the same basic emotions and thus the same subconscious emotional responses to the traumas we experience. Dr. Plutchik poses that there are only eight basic emotions, and they exist as opposites. For example, sadness is the opposite of joy, and fear is the opposite of anger.

But it's necessary to understand the difference between what we call "emotions" and the similar but distinct concepts of feelings, moods, and passions. If you accept the premise that we all have the same basic *emotions*, you can then explore the reactions, feelings, moods, and sentiments that result from those basic, fundamental emotions we all share. We can't change the emotions we experience, but we can change the way we *deal* with our emotions, the way we view the world and the people around us.

To capture the widest range of emotions possible, I sought out interesting, communicative, emotionally intelligent, inspiring, and relatable people who experienced feelings along such a broad spectrum that they often even encompassed opposing viewpoints.

Convincing People to Talk

Since this book is about the emotions related to cancer, it was vital that the participants allowed me a special pass into their thoughts and feelings. I knew I'd be asking a lot of them, so I needed people who would let me explore the hidden truth of their experiences. How were they made up inside? What made them make one choice over another? How were they equipped to deal with the traumas they encountered—or not? How did they come to terms with the difficulties they didn't dare talk about with anyone? Those types of questions could only be answered if the participants were willing to share the most private and intimate details of their experiences with me.

Our ability to form relationships is often limited by our preconceived notions about others. But people are like icebergs—most of them is hidden away beneath the surface. If we don't try to understand what's down there, if we squeeze our eyes shut and plug our ears, if we close our minds and hearts to the things we can't see, then we will never be able to make sense of it all. I think that deep down inside we are all trying to uncover the meaning of life, evaluate our experiences, and see the human condition for what it is so we can gain perspective on ourselves.

One of the reasons that makes every story in this book unique is that each one proves that we are not always the people others think we are. We may not even be the people *we* think we are. In truth, we are, each of us, much more than the people we appear to be. Some of the book participants were quick to open up and some were not. Some ended up not being able to talk at all. They wanted to but found that they simply couldn't.

On long training rides, I spent hours thinking about my talks with the different book participants. I contemplated the more layered thoughts and tried to understand what made these remarkable people think the way they did about things. With my mind largely uncluttered during a multi-hour bike ride each day, I found that I could often solve little problems or develop strategies for future discussions with my book participants. Pedaling for hours and hours also helped me work through the confusion that came hand in hand with some of the heavier issues my book participants shared with me.

If we're being honest, what's really exceptional about anyone? It's an intriguing question to contemplate when evaluating the impact one person might have on others. After all, don't we all yearn to discover the rarity in others? To be moved by the extraordinary in a largely mundane world? Almost every one of my book participants considers themselves unexceptional. Sure, they might have to admit that some facets of their story, once properly examined, might seem breathtaking for a minute, but it's fascinating how unmoved they are by their own unimaginably profound journeys. What has come to seem normal to them is anything but, and that's where the magic of the Cycle of Lives stories lies—in the beautiful and haunting truths revealed to us by otherwise ordinary people.

Midmorning Day One

I'd set out on my five-thousand-mile, six-week bike ride to accomplish a number of goals. I wanted to meet the participants of this book in person after spending so much time on the phone with them. I also looked forward to finding diverse people along the way who could help me understand the emotional journey of cancer. I wanted to test myself physically, emotionally, and mentally. Finally, I hoped to find answers to some of the more unsettled issues in my life. One of those issues revolved around my sister's family, and taking off on my bike on day one, I started to feel the discomfort of it as I headed up the coast of the Pacific Ocean. My destination was the UCLA Jonsson Comprehensive Cancer Center, some twenty miles from my home in Manhattan Beach, California.

The staff at the Jonsson Comprehensive Cancer Center took extraordinary care of June. As a cancer board subject, she received enhanced medical attention for both curative and palliative concerns. It didn't hurt that June's charisma also drew special attention. Even when stricken with terminal brain cancer and being cared for by others, she engaged people with her charm, genuineness, and authenticity. June drew out the best in people because she offered absolute safety and warmth to everybody she came into contact with.

I intended to take a few photos and shake some hands once I was at the center, even though the people who'd actually taken care of June were no longer on staff. I'd helped the center with many fundraising events over the years, so I wanted to show some appreciation for an organization that had touched thousands of lives, as well as pay my respects for their long-ago efforts to aid and comfort my dying sister.

As I pedaled up the Strand—a miles-long bike path that winds along the Pacific Ocean from Palos Verdes to Malibu—I continued to think about the immenseness and solitude of my endeavor. Other than my kids and my fiancée, no family were involved in my life at any level. I was only hours into my journey, and already it felt lonelier than I had expected.

As I'd done for my endurance and fundraising events in previous years, I attempted to create some buzz for the Cycle of Lives project. I'd been fortunate to have the support and involvement of friends, coworkers past and present, supporters of my prior events, their referrals, and more. These advocates stepped up for every event each year by supplying financial donations or spreading the word in their own circles of influence, and even to media outlets. Their loyalty and generosity motivates me and serves as a touching reminder that June's memory is being kept alive by these events. The Cycle of Lives fundraiser was higher profile than any of my previous efforts had been, and the chatter around the event was at a constant elevated level.

But there was one group of people I didn't hear from. In fact, in all the years of doing fundraising events, I had never heard from them: June's family and friends and our small extended family. This reality was made all the more painful by the electric support I was already receiving for the Cycle of Lives project.

When June died, she left behind a large family that she, her husband, and their kids had been extremely close with. She'd also kept a diverse circle of friends who had been a big part of her pre- and postdiagnosis life. These "Junebuggies," as they were known, had never been shy about showing their adoration for June. So where had they all gone?

As I biked closer to the Jonsson Center, I engaged in a two-sided argument with myself.

So what? People move on. Get over it. Everyone deals with grief in their own way and then rides off into their own future.

Yeah, but to hear from no one? I reasoned with myself. *Not* one *person from my family or especially from her family—not one of her friends? Nobody ever offered support or even just reached out to stay in contact.*

Be serious. The more years go by, the more people forget.

A few years before, after completing my fifth annual fundraising event in June's memory, my exasperation got the better of me. I had written a letter to a couple of June's family members. I urged them that if they wished to refuse to provide any support, to at least offer me some peace and let me know they were aware of my efforts—to offer me some small gesture of recognition for my efforts to pay tribute to someone they held so dear.

I received no response. Not "Thank you," not "Leave us alone," not a word that could offer clarity or understanding. These were the same people I'd sat down for Thanksgiving and Christmas dinners with. I saw them at the hospital when June's kids were born. They were the same people who'd walked the track at the Relay For Life, who were at June's side as she was sick and dying.

There's a fine line between doing good out of an earnest desire to help people and doing good for attention. I sometimes struggle with the fact that I need to bring attention to my fundraising projects in order for them to have an impact on people. I'm just not comfortable imposing myself on others by asking for money and other help. So I decided that allowing June's family's radio silence to get under my skin was counterintuitive. Was I being self-centered by looking for their approval or attention? If I was doing these events for the sake of others, what did it matter what *some* people thought?

Everybody deals with things the best they can, I told myself.

Sure, but in all these years, not one single word *from these people?*

I doubted I'd ever feel resolution about that internal struggle. It tormented me as I pedaled to and then from the Jonsson Comprehensive Cancer Center on day one of my ride.

After a quick photo op at the center, I biked to meet with Bobby in Westwood just blocks away. He was the first book participant on my itinerary. As I pedaled to our agreed-upon breakfast spot, I reflected on how different my experience with family was from Bobby's. Each year, he directs one of the largest Relay For Life events in California. His motivation comes from Brandi, the wife he lost to cancer many years ago. Bobby, now remarried, and his wife, Kirsten, are committed to raising funds and awareness for cancer care and research each year to keep Brandi's legacy alive. Bobby's efforts keep Brandi's family and friends connected each year in an important and lasting way, which I witnessed when I first met Bobby, months before the ride, during his Relay For Life event.

I longed for a parallel reality where I could've reminisced with even one of June's family members or friends, where I could've smiled with and hugged and cried with just a single person—someone who'd been close to my sister. But no such reality existed for me, and it would eat at me during my journey across the country.

As I rolled up to the restaurant, however, the hollowness and desolation inside me was swept away by Bobby Newquist's big, warm smile.

Bobby

Relationship to cancer: Caregiver and advocate

Age: Forty-six

Family status: Married with no children

Location: Southern California

First encounter with cancer: Thirty-five years old

Cancer summary: Bobby's wife, Brandi, was diagnosed with stage II breast cancer at thirty-five. The cancer returned and metastasized in an aggressive fashion. She died at forty.

Treatment specifics: Brandi was diagnosed with breast cancer, which metastasized to her lymph nodes, lungs, bones, brain, and kidneys. She tested positive for the BRCA1 gene and underwent radiation therapy, chemotherapy, a double mastectomy, a double oophorectomy, lymph node removal, and various other procedures to extend her life and manage her pain.

Community involvement: Brandi and Bobby were active advocates for the American Cancer Society. Bobby and his current wife, Kirsten, remain active and direct a successful Relay For Life event each year, fundraising for the American Cancer Society in Brandi's memory.

Strongest positive emotion during cancer experience: Humility

Strongest negative emotion during cancer experience: Anger

How we met: I was out with friends one evening about a year before the bike ride. A bunch of guys had decided to get together for drinks to celebrate someone's birthday. After a couple of beers, the stories were flowing.

A few of us present that night had taken a vacation to Mexico together seven years before for the purposes of an endurance event I had organized to raise money for cancer care and research. It was an eighty-five-mile solo run along busy Highway 307 that began on a sticky, ninety-degree day in late June. The run took me more than twenty-two hours to complete and tested me both mentally and physically. The few buddies who'd come with me on that trip ran by my side and cheered me on.

That night we met for drinks, the group who'd gone with me to Mexico reminisced about the crazier memories from our ten days there. Afterward, one of my friends pulled me aside.

"You should talk to Bobby about your cancer book," he said and nodded his head toward the one guy present I didn't know. Bobby had a broad, genuine smile. He looked cheery and confident but not in a forced way. He had a comfortable, understated aura about him. I approached him, and within minutes we were deep in conversation. Over the next year, Bobby told me his cancer story.

A New Pair of Glasses

B obby sat in the lobby of his lawyer's office. It had been another late night, and he was still trying to shake off the fog. When you've had more drinks than hours of sleep, the math works against you. Bobby liked his lawyer. Roger was one of the few people he could be around without bracing for impact. Bobby could be just Bobby, not some twisted-up, stressed-out, defensive version of himself. When Bobby was shown into the office, he saw Roger wasn't waiting at the small round side table where they always sat, but over on the large, tufted-leather sofa on the opposite side of the room.

"Wanna chat?" Roger asked.

Bobby smiled. "On or off the clock?"

"Off, of course," Roger said with genuine concern. "How you doing? You okay?"

The pounding in Bobby's head increased. *How the hell do you think I'm doing?*

He was only a few years past thirty, but his life already felt as if it were coming apart at the seams. He was being sued in the wake of his friend and business partner's death. He was going through a second divorce. His patent design business was struggling, he was completely broke, and bankruptcy loomed on the horizon. His dad's heart was wearing down. He didn't know which friends he could trust. As if that weren't enough, Bobby had begun hanging out in some pretty rough spots at night.

"I'm fine, I guess," Bobby said.

"I know you're going through a lot."

Ain't that the truth, brother.

Bobby shrugged. "Hey, nobody's giving me a medal for 'Toughest Life Ever.'"

"Talk to me," Roger said. "What's going on?"

Bobby let out a deep sigh and sunk deeper into the sofa. After a short pause, he answered. Letting his guard down, he described the despondency he felt, how he struggled to stay positive. He didn't go into too much detail about his failings, because who wants to describe the full scope of their bad behavior? But he did touch on the more painful events that were affecting his life.

"You can't go around getting in fights, Bobby."

Bobby nodded. *So that's what this is about*, he thought. The onslaught of dark times had brought out equally dark things in Bobby. He felt he was ruined, financially and otherwise, so he began to act as if he had nothing left to lose. Hard times had come *hard*, and Bobby wanted to fight back against what was happening to him. He knew he could climb into his own head and engage in a mental boxing match against it all, but even when he did, he left the scuffle needing more. He could only find satisfaction in the primitive pleasure that a flesh-to-flesh punch can sometimes bring.

"I'm like that gunslinger in the movie *Shane*," Bobby said. "I'll take it and take it, but if you hit me, if you purposely try to harm me—you'll unleash a monster." Bobby gestured toward the stack of papers he needed to sign. "It's getting to the point that I can't take it anymore. You see how ruined I am. Everything's ruined."

"I understand," Roger said. "It seems that way."

It is *that way*, Bobby thought. No matter how much he tried to hold on to his optimism and confidence, they were disappearing. In the past, he'd never thought of himself as a failure. Bad times were usually no match for his competence and drive, but everything in his life had become an exercise in failure.

"Look. I've been doing this a long time, Bobby. It will all pass. Really," Roger said. "I mean, you're a bright guy. You're young. You have plenty of sand in the hourglass. I know it seems like a lot right now, but you'll get through it all."

That's easy for you to say. Try living my life for a day.

"Maybe," Bobby said. "But it sure doesn't look like it from where I'm sitting."

"Bobby, trust me. The sun's coming up tomorrow."

Bobby closed his eyes. He wanted to cry and scream, anything to get away from the pain and difficulty and bullshit. He wanted to believe Roger, but he didn't.

"I appreciate the thought," Bobby said. It was a lie.

A few weeks later, Bobby got a phone call that would prove his lawyer right.

• • •

Spending late nights drinking whiskey and looking for fights helped Bobby cope with his situation, but music is what gave him a less destructive way of releasing his daily accumulated stresses. In particular, dark, heavy rap music offered Bobby the reprieve from life he needed to keep things together.

The night he got the phone call that would change his life, Bobby was blasting "Lose Yourself" by Eminem and loudly singing along.

As Bobby hunched over his drafting board, immersed in the lyrics of the song and the lines of his drawing, the phone rang, causing him to turn down the one thing that drowned out all the dark noise in his head.

"Bobby here," he answered.

"Bobby? It's Christine."

He hadn't talked with his ex-wife's friend since the split, so he was wary about what she might want from him.

Although Bobby's two marriages failed in part due to his wives' bad behavior—the first was addicted to drugs, the second cheated with one of his best friends—he accepted his share of the blame. If it took two people to make a relationship work, then it took two to let it fail. Bobby was aware that he could've earned the label of "world's worst communicator," both in terms of his self-awareness and his communication with others. Bobby didn't speak about his failures, about all the bad things that were going on in his life. He didn't talk about thoughts and feelings in general. His stoic attitude and deftness at avoiding interpersonal connection left him alone to wallow in the tumult that came his way. Since Bobby kept his pain behind closed doors, to outsiders like Christine, he probably appeared unaffected.

"I know this is really awkward," Christine said. "I mean, I know the divorce isn't final yet, but there's someone I think you should meet. She's a friend of mine, and honestly I think she might be someone you'd like."

"Someone he might like" was the last thing Bobby wanted. He was losing faith in the goodness of others and in his ability to direct his life as he desired. He was barely able to sift through the rubble of his destroyed life—let alone think of introducing anybody into it.

"I don't think so," he told her.

"Well, I think you would really be perfect for each other," Christine insisted. "She's leaving to move back home to Missouri soon—*real* soon. What could it hurt?"

He demurred a few more times, but she persisted. Bobby thought it was pointless. He was in no place to think about dating. But Christine was a decent person, and she wouldn't have called unless she had put some thought into it. After a while, Bobby relented. After all, maybe it was time for him to try lighting the darkness in a healthier way for one night.

Meeting Brandi

A few nights later, Bobby met Brandi at a small Italian restaurant for dinner. He arrived with enough emotional baggage for a world tour, but Bobby hid it under the table as he sat waiting for her to arrive. He was determined to be his best self. What did he have to lose?

When she finally came through the door, his face flushed with hot blood. She was stunning. Long, dark, loose curls flowed down her back. Her shoulders were that special blend of feminine—soft, smooth, and strong. She scanned the tables, and Bobby stood. She burst into a huge smile that crinkled her piercing eyes, holding Bobby in place with an intense and deep look. Her smile was a lavish, beautiful, swath of white. Bobby felt paralyzed by her undeniable aura of self-confidence.

If she isn't Brandi, this is going to be awkward as hell, Bobby thought.

She must have read his mind, because she nodded her head in recognition and walked over to his table.

Bobby had always been a certain type of guy around women. He was confident and felt comfortable being himself, partly because he felt he hadn't met his intellectual match before and partly because he wasn't looking for emotional intimacy. Bobby didn't feel rattled around beautiful women. He liked acting as if he was in charge and was always a little showy about his masculinity. He liked being—or at least pretending to be—in control of everything. He knew these things about himself, so despite two failed marriages, he expected himself to be the same Bobby that night as he always was—but Brandi just plain disarmed him.

Why won't your legs move? Take a deep breath and sit back down, Bobby.

As they sat down, Bobby tried to understand why he felt so flustered. He was dizzy from the electricity. He focused on Brandi's face as his mind raced to make sense of the sparks flying fast and furious between them.

"So, *you're* Bobby?" she asked. She had a sly look in her eye, as if she easily saw something he wasn't even slightly aware of.

He'd come to dinner intending to hide all the bullshit in his life from his date, but after one look from Brandi, none of it felt important enough to conceal anymore. They started talking, in a crisp, clear, real way—a way Bobby wasn't used to. They didn't stop talking the whole night. All the while, Bobby felt as though everything in his life except Brandi was fuzzy and out of focus. It was as if he'd put on a new pair of glasses and could see clearly for the first time. From the first minute of that odd, newfound clarity, Bobby felt something special was happening.

Depending on how and when he'd measure his life after that night, it became both a dream come true and worse than he could ever imagine. But regardless of what came next, for that night and many afterward, fate had at long last tipped the scales in Bobby's favor, and his experiences would serve to show him all the good life had to offer, not just the grimness.

Brandi

As coincidence would have it, Brandi grew up in the same town where Bobby's favorite rapper, Eminem, was born: St. Joseph, Missouri, a small town along the Missouri River in the northwest part of the state. Brandi's mom and dad divorced after having a couple of kids; both remarried partners who already had children of their own, and then had more children with their new partners.

For long stretches in her formative years, Brandi lived with just her mother and sister. Brandi was particularly close to her mother—a strong woman who taught her daughters to believe they could accomplish anything they wanted. Her mother was her confidante and mentor. She guided and supported Brandi the way only the person who knows you better than anybody else can. As a result, Brandi strove for success at every opportunity. Her confidence was organic and true, and it permeated every aspect of her life. She tested out of high school and entered college as a psychology major just before her seventeenth birthday. By twenty, she had graduated and began working at a support center, dreaming of the life she would make for herself close to her mom and friends in the place she knew best.

But those dreams were not to be. When Brandi was in her early twenties, her mother died of ovarian cancer. Suddenly, Brandi was very alone. Her anchor was gone, and she would have to face life untethered moving forward, unable to go to the person who had helped her hold it all together all her life. Brandi decided to move away from Missouri. She ended up in Southern California, far from the home that had ceased to exist for her once her mom died.

Living on her own in a way she'd never imagined, Brandi attempted to establish new roots. Although she didn't practice psychology, she used her schooling in the career she found after arriving in California. Brandi became an insurance adjuster specializing in disaster claims. She thrived in her field and felt fulfilled getting to do what she enjoyed best: interacting with people in a purposeful way. She loved being able to help people who were going through shockingly difficult times. By combining her desire to succeed with the opportunity to apply her drive to something she enjoyed doing, positive things happened. She earned a good income, she bought a home, and she was living very comfortably. But she had no one to share her success with.

The nature of Brandi's job often took her on flights to the East Coast,

away from her home in Los Angeles. Flying across the country, over the center of the states where her first home had been, never failed to inspire painful
emotions. She'd had some boyfriends in California, but ten years had gone
by, and she wasn't married. She had friends, but they were scattered, and they
weren't the ones she'd known since childhood. Near the end of 2002, Brandi
decided that she was going to move back to Missouri right after the New Year.
She thought doing so would bring her the kind of success in her personal life
that she already enjoyed in her work life. Brandi hadn't planned on everything
changing just weeks before moving day.

Coming Together

Neither Bobby nor Brandi felt they had room in their lives for a new relationship, but they both felt a connection to each other they had never felt before.
After their first date came a second and a third. In those first two weeks,
they saw each other probably ten times. Their connection was fast, it was substantial, and most surprising of all for Bobby, it began to tie them together
emotionally in a way neither had ever dreamed would happen.

Although on their first date they had talked about the fact that Brandi was
preparing to move, they didn't broach the subject the next few times they saw
each other. Bobby was sure it lurked in the back of Brandi's mind the way it
did in his, but they avoided talking about it. They did talk about Bobby's problems, however. The person Bobby had been just a few days before wouldn't
have let anybody see what was really going on in his life, but it was clear that
things with him and Brandi were different.

Bobby knew he couldn't have hidden anything from her if he wanted to.
She'd have seen right through him. She was *smart*, and it allowed him to shed
all the tension and doubt he felt about showing his true self. Brandi was able
to slice through Bobby's crap—all his unimportant, false posturing and bom-
bastic airs. She asked Bobby direct and intuitive questions, and she only cared
to know the *real* answers.

He understood right away that Brandi was in a league of her own. She
appeared in many ways to be more evolved than he was. At the very least she
was his match, especially on an intellectual level. She also had a comfortable

confidence that was instantly calming and alluring. It both complemented his own self-assuredness and provided him with the security he needed to allow himself to be human.

Must be those glasses.

So, Bobby went back to dealing with his divorce, his lawsuit, and the financial issues he was embroiled in. But now he did so openly, without feeling alone, for the first time ever. He didn't feel that he had to act a certain way. He didn't need a false front to hide behind. He could just *be*.

While he was still navigating those murkiest of times in his life, Bobby developed a mantra of sorts, a kind of self-talk he used to combat the constant bad news: *You don't know how much you can handle until you're forced to handle more than you think you can. That other shit was nothing. You can handle this. Bring it on.*

But after spending time with Brandi, he had a new way of looking at the world. He knew the kind of bring-it-on thinking he'd been doing before was self-delusion. Brandi touched in him some hidden reserve of hopefulness, and he found that he wanted to believe in it, to cling to it. They had only known each other for days. Bobby marveled at how feelings as strong as these could manifest so soon, feelings that crushed his unhealthy bravado, that showed him hope instead of despair. Nothing but the deepest part of his spirit could understand.

All of the pressures that had made Bobby feel as if he was in one of those industrial metal crushers just weeks before ceased to hold the same weight. The issues were there; they just didn't feel as overwhelming. They had all been overshadowed by one problem: This one-in-a-million person had just entered his life, and he was about to lose her. Everything else became inconsequential.

Bobby decided to take a chance and offered up a plan. It was a few days before Christmas, and Brandi was half-packed for her big move. "How about we go to Missouri for New Year's?" he asked. "We'll fly out, I'll meet your friends and family, and then we can drive back together—alone in a car for three or four days."

"You mean a test?" she asked.

"Yes. We'll either end up hating each other, in which case you can finish packing, or . . ." He trailed off, leaving the rest unsaid.

"Or?" Brandi asked, that same sly smile from their first date beautifully slicing his heart. She wouldn't let him off the hook.

"Or maybe you'll just decide you don't want to move back."

• • •

Two things happened on the drive back from Missouri. First off, Brandi never stopped talking. He didn't hesitate to try to match her engagement and energy, but it was difficult to keep pace with her right away. Bobby had never been used to deep conversations, where someone asked insightful questions and then listened to the answers. Not only did Brandi listen, but she did it purposefully, logically, and in a way that forced Bobby to quickly get comfortable showing her his real self. Her charm was undeniably seductive, and she led him to talk about things he'd never felt safe sharing with anybody, ever.

Secondly, by the time they returned to Los Angeles, Bobby and Brandi knew they were in love. That particular complication made things a little awkward at first. Brandi had to unwind her plans to move to Missouri. Bobby was still encumbered with the various battles going on in his life. They both felt they should keep their budding romance quiet from their respective Los Angeles circles. How could they explain to others what they didn't yet understand themselves? This was especially true in light of his pending divorce and Brandi having told her friends she was moving. While they decided to keep things under wraps with other people, they dove headfirst into the deep end with each other. The hope kindling inside of Bobby flamed into belief, and as the days ticked by, the limitations on their feelings melted away in the face of their growing bond.

Still, life wasn't all tea and roses. Bobby was dealing with heavy things, and he knew he wasn't going to transform from a disaster into his best self without bumps in the road. He wasn't always easy to be around, regardless of the hope and love they'd ignited. Bobby had been dancing around his relationship to rage for a couple of years, and his temper could flare without much provocation. But he was determined to improve and soon found that Brandi was in for the hard work.

Not only was Brandi there for the more challenging aspects of Bobby's life, but she also taught him to find and nourish the worthier side of himself.

Bobby knew how to punch guys and bang his head to loud music and scream at the world. But before Brandi, he didn't know how to step out of the dark shadow of who he wanted to be but wasn't. Brandi helped him shine a light inside to cast those shadows away. With her, he never wanted to hide. And in that brightness they found together, Bobby flourished.

The next several months flew by. Spring approached and love was in the air—the open air. They stopped hiding their relationship and were free to talk about the future. Despite whoever they'd been before they met, neither hesitated to begin planning for a future together. They just *knew* in a way that seemed almost too perfect.

Then came April third.

The First Cancer Diagnosis

Brandi had a thing for remembering dates. In fact, she had a thing for remembering *everything*. Bobby had described her to his friends as having an "almost photographic memory." He said "almost" because nobody would have believed how photographic a memory she actually had. Without hesitation, she could tell you what happened on any random day in the recent or long-ago past. April third became a date she would have liked to have been able to forget.

A couple of days before that inauspicious date, Brandi was lying in bed and mentioned that a particular spot on her breast was sore. She and Bobby checked, and they both felt a small lump. It made Brandi cringe when touched. Even though her mom had died of ovarian cancer, Brandi hadn't ever considered the potential problems genetics could pose—the BRCA1 gene was not as well understood at that time. But by 2003, there was enough public awareness about genetic predisposition that Brandi didn't want to take any chances given her family history.

The following day, Brandi went to her doctor's office. They confirmed the lump and administered a mammogram and an ultrasound. Once they determined that Brandi had a solid mass, they went in for a biopsy.

That night was rough. Bobby could tell that Brandi had the same rock in her gut that he did. They were told they'd have to wait a day or two for results. Bobby didn't want to go to work the next day, but Brandi urged him to.

"Either way, we'll deal with it," she told him. "You might as well keep your mind on other things for now."

Every time the phone rang that day, Bobby jumped. Finally, it was Brandi. "It's cancer," she said.

There couldn't have been two worse words in the entire world. Bobby ran to the car and raced home. When he got there, Brandi was on the couch, her arms wrapped around her legs. Her eyes were a little red, but she still had that Brandi smile. They held each other, not saying anything for a long time.

"Maybe *we* shouldn't deal with this," she told him, breaking the silence. "You didn't sign up for this. It's too much for anybody."

Like the first time he saw her in that restaurant a few months prior, Bobby's mind was on fire. But instead of the millions of thoughts that ran through his brain then, now he had only one. It was pure. It was true. He had another one of the "seeing things in focus for the first time" times, and the clarity was otherworldly.

"We'll get through it all *together*," he said. "End of story and never to be brought up again." He believed they'd punch cancer in the face as one and then move forward past it.

Although it sometimes felt like a huge leap of faith to have such strong feelings, Bobby knew they deserved each other. That made it easier to concentrate on moving forward in life together. This diagnosis was the first giant step on their path, and another manifested itself almost immediately. Brandi was thirty-five and unsure of what the treatment plan might do to her fertility in the future. She and Bobby talked about it, and even though they had known each other for such a short time, they both decided it was a good idea to think of their future together and harvest her eggs.

Sometimes you just gotta jump and not look down; just trust it.

The lumpectomy was successful, and Brandi's tumor was removed with healthy margins. Sentinel lymph node mapping and a biopsy followed, revealing no cancerous cells. Four cycles of chemotherapy and almost three dozen radiation treatments later, they finally began to allow themselves to believe they could move on with their lives. By the holiday season—one year after they first met—they were off the cancer roller-coaster ride. Brandi's beautiful hair came back, and she came back from the weakness, the nonstop vomiting, the confusion and blurriness that veinfuls of therapeutic poison brings. She came back from it all. Surgery, chemotherapy, and radiation weren't easy, but they had taken Brandi's treatment regimen in stride. They weren't going to let breast cancer stop them; they had bigger plans for their lives.

Soon thereafter, the business lawsuit was behind Bobby, he'd escaped filing bankruptcy, and his divorce was a distant memory. With all that and the cancer behind them, he and Brandi could again put their sole focus on their relationship.

Before her cancer diagnosis, they had spent virtually every minute together, and the subsequent eight months had been the same. Some of the most intense and exploratory conversations between them had happened while Brandi was in the chemo chair. They had revealed themselves to each other and become inseparable. They both talked about how they had found what they wanted. They inspired each other to be their best selves, for themselves and each other.

A few months later, Bobby decided to take Brandi to Las Vegas to celebrate being one year out from cancer. Knowing how she was with dates, he wanted her to have a better memory of April third. So, on April third of 2004, one year to the day after her diagnosis, Bobby asked Brandi to marry him. She accepted, flashing her bright smile as always.

2002 had ended with them meeting. 2003 had been about her cancer and Bobby's messes. 2004 was going to be about getting married and beginning their life journey together. But life has a way of reminding you who's in control—and it's not you.

The Second Cancer Diagnosis

Only a few weeks after accepting Bobby's marriage proposal, Brandi's doctor explained to her and Bobby that a routine checkup had revealed an enlarged lymph node. The doctors performed surgery on Brandi to remove it, and the results came back cancerous.

Baptism by fire, Bobby thought. *But the sun will come up one day, right? And maybe burn you right up.*

Her doctors surmised that the cancerous node must have been missed from the first cancer surgery—unfortunately, a not uncommon occurrence. Bobby

and Brandi ran into a lot more unfortunately not uncommon occurrences—
the lack of bedside manner, the inconsistent pain-management procedures,
the tests that could have been performed sooner. Bobby's frustration over
their medical experience was also not uncommon. But the incompetence was
maddening, and the other irritations they encountered were more common-
place among cancer patients than they could have imagined. Bobby wasn't
bitter—Brandi would never allow him to be—but he had become a little
hardened and sardonic in dealing with Brandi's caregivers, especially when
she wasn't looking.

They quickly learned that they needed to do their own research. It was
incumbent upon them to find out as much as they could. They came to learn
why doctors say they *practice* medicine. It turned out to be more of an art
than the hard science they'd wanted to believe it was. Not all her doctors were
subpar, of course, and the care Brandi received wasn't bad on the whole, but
certain experiences were unbelievably troubling. They found most caregivers
tried to do the right thing, but that didn't lessen the helplessness that Bobby
and Brandi felt, often because of those same professionals.

Doctors just don't know shit about what's going on, Bobby thought. *You talk to
one and they tell you one thing, and then you talk to another who tells you something
totally different—and they're all just as certain about what they think.*

There are some things that people know, and then there are some things
that people just *know*. Brandi and Bobby just *knew* they belonged together.
But Bobby had become so accustomed to beating himself up for the bad things
that happened in his life that he had a few momentary lapses in confidence.
He once apologized to Brandi because they hadn't met sooner.

"We go through things when we go through them. If we'd met earlier in
life, you wouldn't be the Bobby I know and love," she told him.

"Yeah, but I just wish I didn't have so much crap in my past."

"So I should feel bad too?" Brandi asked. "I should be sorry about cancer? I
should feel guilty and uncertain about the way things are for us now?"

"Of course not," he said.

Bobby thought he knew a lot, but Brandi taught him about the important stuff—love, life, togetherness. He learned from her that they should look
at each day as a fresh start and that each start was a new part of their story.

Cancer or no cancer, a beautiful new chapter had begun in their lives, one they were going to write together.

Planning for the wedding was made more difficult by Brandi's second cancer diagnosis. They weren't in any particular rush to get married, but they weren't going to wait too long, either. Prior to the news, they discussed going away alone, combining a destination wedding and honeymoon, and then returning to start a family. They balanced that option with more traditional ones, but neither was keen on wrangling family and friends for a big spectacle. Their relationship had been mostly private until then, and that's the way they preferred it. Only the people closest to them understood the uniqueness of the circumstances they were dealing with. But the cancer forced them to look at everything in a different light.

They could have waited to see how things went with her treatment, but they were going to have to go through more chemotherapy and radiation, and Brandi just wouldn't have thought about getting married without hair. At the time, Brandi was almost back to her normal self. She was strong and energetic, her sense of taste and smell had come back, and she had *all* her hair. But they knew it was going to be a rough road ahead, and she wouldn't feel better for a long while. They knew they needed to keep the reserve tank filled, but more than that, they felt they were going to beat the cancer. They had done it before.

Bobby had found a beautiful place in St. Maarten for a ceremony and honeymoon, and they were married on July twenty-first, 2004, at sunset on a picturesque beach. The solitude of their union wrapped them in a veil of love that shielded them from the rest of the world but also humbled them and made them feel at peace with the world. For three weeks, they savored each day of their trip for what it was and because of what awaited them at home. They ate exquisite food every night because they knew Brandi's sense of taste would soon disappear. She dressed up every night because she knew soon she would wear only sweats. She did her hair in elaborate styles because soon she would have no use for a hairbrush. She wore makeup and they stayed up late at night, some-times until the sun came up, because they knew she would be wiped of energy every day, all day, when they returned.

It wasn't hard for Bobby not to think too much about what was going to happen when they got back. After all, their time away was perfect. Although her diagnosis and pending treatment lurked in the background, they didn't really talk about it. Instead, Bobby relished Brandi talking endlessly about anything and everything noncancer.

When the honeymoon ended, the chemotherapy began. Brandi had twelve treatments over a four-month period. They endured the side effects they had known to expect were coming when they were still on their honeymoon. But what they hadn't expected turned out to be far worse.

BRCA1

When you're walking in the alley behind some bar and someone punches you, it hurts like hell. It knocks the wind out of you and messes with your sense of reason. But when you know the punch is coming—even if it still hurts like hell—you can at least brace for it.

Brandi's chemo was the punch they knew was coming. But her experience with the BRCA1 test was like walking down the street completely unaware of the blow coming to knock you out.

Today, things might've gone a lot differently for Brandi and Bobby. In the world of cancer care and treatment, things are fluid. What was untreatable twenty years ago is curable today. Knowledge that seems obvious now wasn't in the collective consciousness ten years ago. The entire medical community's approach to certain cancers can change in just a matter of years.

Most things aren't all bad or all good. A lot depends on perspective, and even in the direst of times, Brandi and Bobby tried to look past the bad on their cancer journey. Of course, they were angry and desperate. They felt cheated. But mostly they were scared. Brandi's natural inclination was to try to focus attention on the positives. When testing told her that she carried the BRCA1 gene, she said to Bobby, "At least we know what we are dealing with now. That's a good thing."

"You're right," he replied. "At least we know."

Once they knew what they were dealing with, they could try to brace for impact, but it was hard. It was inconceivably hard. They didn't think test-ing positive for the BRCA1 gene was a death sentence for Brandi, because there were always ways to fight it, and people did survive. But they also knew they'd have to tap every ounce of courage and energy they had to beat it. They did more research, talked to a lot of professionals, and agreed with the doctors who urged taking an aggressive approach to dealing with the realities of Brandi's prognosis.

In 2005, two years after they met and five months after they married, Brandi underwent fourteen hours of surgery to try to get ahead of the cancer that was attempting to overtake her body. The doctors removed both breasts and both ovaries: a bilateral mastectomy and a bilateral oophorectomy. During the same surgery, she had a transverse rectus abdominis myocutaneous (TRAM) flap breast-reconstruction procedure. No matter what, they had decided to try to look forward, and reconstructive breast surgery meant that they could think of tomorrows.

They talked about the future as often as seemed reasonable, and their future included having kids one day. But as Brandi was being prepared for the grueling procedures she would undergo, Bobby hesitated to express too much on the subject to her. On one hand, he desperately wanted to support Brandi's belief that they'd overcome her cancer. On the other hand, the sobering reality was that he couldn't let himself think too hard about a future that had little chance of unfolding, if they were to believe the odds they had been told.

After her surgery, when Bobby was finally allowed to see Brandi, he was led into the recovery room by medical staff. They had told him that her body had gone through a lot during surgery, in hopes of managing his expectations. But they hadn't come close to preparing him for what he saw.

Fighting to make sense of what he was seeing, Bobby searched for his wife in the person who lay on the bed. It took a moment, but eventually she appeared. Brandi was swollen from head to toe in a way that defies possibility. It was unimaginable that a human body could transform itself in so short a time. The shock passed almost as instantly as the recognition took ahold of him, and Bobby reached to hold Brandi's limp hand. He felt a rush of emotions—fear, confusion, isolation, and helplessness. They overtook every hopeful, positive, happy, peaceful feeling he'd ever had.

Bobby held her hand as she awoke from the anesthesia. As he watched her struggle to open her eyes, which appeared to take every ounce of fortitude she had, Bobby felt ashamed. He'd been so angry for so many tiny, insignificant things that had happened in his life. Looking at Brandi then, he couldn't make sense of those things. Nothing in life was or could ever be as painful as watching her struggle to open her eyes.

He was thankful for just one thing: There was no way Brandi was aware enough to sense his desperation and anguish. He allowed himself to feel weak in that moment and allowed the suffering to show. Sometimes his despondency had come in the form of something as simple as a heavy sigh, or in tears that gushed from both sides of both eyes, or in his body caving in around his heart, but as he watched her then, it came in the way he needed to draw all the strength he could find and send it down to his legs—otherwise, he'd have fallen in a heap of misery and heartache. Even a stranger could have read it on his face at that moment, let alone the woman who knew him better than anyone in the world—if she'd been the tiniest bit herself.

Not even Shane could've kept an unemotional face all the time. Not even him.

Accepting Dying and Death

"After I die, you have to go to counseling," Brandi said. "I want you to promise me now."

"How can I promise you that?" Bobby asked.

"Because I'm asking you to," she said and pierced his soul with a deep look as only she could do.

"I won't think about you dying."

They stared at each other without saying anything. Bobby knew she didn't want to press him too hard. He knew she was as sensitive about the idea of him moving on after her death as he was. But, still, like always, she wasn't going to let him off the hook. He relented.

"Okay. I'll go, but it might not happen for a very long time," he said, the optimistic words betrayed by his disheartened tone.

"And you'll go for at least three months?"

"Yes. I'll go for at least three months."

She stared deeply into his eyes.

"I promise," he said. "Really, I promise."

After her surgeries, the doctors threw everything they could at Brandi, and there were a few moments of hope, but ultimately they had to face the reality that Brandi was not going to survive. Within months of the mastectomy and oophorectomy, the cancer had metastasized to her lungs. Once that happened, there was no possible scenario in which she could be expected to live very long.

Brandi and Bobby continued to communicate the way they always had, allowing openness and truth to rule their thoughts. Now their communication took on a more determined and urgent quality. Bobby understood there was a finite amount of time Brandi had to reconcile as much as she could for herself and for him. He didn't so much give in to her in relenting as he gave in to their painful reality. Bobby promised her he'd go to three months of therapy after she died, and he wasn't lying, but even though he knew she was going to die, he didn't want to give up believing that she might live.

When the cancer advanced to her lungs, the level of pain Brandi felt became surreal. Much of the next several months were spent in vain on the impossible task of managing her pain. The doctors did their best to make her comfortable, but success rarely meant that Brandi's pain lessened. Instead, success was measured by how unaware of the pain they could make her feel while still allowing her to be any semblance of the Brandi she'd been before.

When Bobby and Brandi weren't dealing with the cancer and its immediate effects on her body, they chose to deal with the inevitability of her death. This meant that they talked about everything imaginable—finances, friends, counseling, and the Relay For Life she'd found and become a part of. They talked about Bobby's career, the house they had remodeled together, and how he needed to resist disappearing into either one once she was gone. Brandi made him promise to move on and swear he wouldn't stay in a negative place.

He sometimes tried to push back on her directives, embarrassed and ashamed to admit he would move on. Ultimately, he came to realize that she had accepted her death and the reality that the world and all the people she loved would go on without her. Brandi could have made dying about her, but she made her dying about Bobby living on.

"I'm not ecstatic that you're at your best, you know," she told him one day. "Some other girl is going to get the benefit of all my hard work."

"Won't happen."

"Come on, Bobby. You need to be in a relationship. I mean, nobody could've ever measured up to me, we both know that, but someone in the future will—if you let them. Please allow that to happen. Don't let all my hard work go to waste."

Nothing was left unsaid between them. Everything had closure or resolution—except for one thing. Bobby knew Brandi didn't want to die any more than he wanted to let her go. But they both had to do the thing they wanted least. They were draining liters of fluids from her lungs. The cancer had spread to her brain, her bones, her kidneys, and who knew where else by then. She was ingesting more pain medication than anyone could comprehend, but Bobby knew she didn't want to find out what it felt like to die, so they gave her more. One day her wish was granted. She never had to feel it.

• • •

When Bobby spoke at Brandi's funeral, he did so through tears of reflection rather than tears of shock. There was nothing shocking about Brandi's death. It hadn't come suddenly or unexpectedly. He didn't have thoughts about his loss and his grief so much as he had thoughts about how he was going to *move on* from his loss and his grief. He and Brandi had come to terms with her death, and although his insides felt shredded, he couldn't deny that he also experienced a sense of tranquility—even peace—at her death. Her pain, her suffering, it was all done.

Bobby drew some small amount of comfort in knowing that the torture she endured—the torture *they* endured—was over now. But it was only a small amount of comfort. In the end, he was overwhelmed with gratitude that he and Brandi had met each other. Even if their time together had lasted for only a few blinks of an eye in the physical world, Bobby knew that what they had together transcended any measurable time. Their relationship had permanency because it had allowed them to witness and enjoy the best that life could offer in the time they'd had together.

In the days following Brandi's death, Bobby's emotions flared up. He was raw. He was desolate. But he was determined not to become a martyr. He'd promised Brandi that each minute of every day he would continue to be the best self that she had brought out in him, that he would use it to guide him forward and remain open to what the world might still hold. As a result, he tried to balance his own anguish with the promises he'd made to Brandi—something much easier to do when he had his old friend, loud music. He drowned himself in hard beats and angry lyrics, shouting along to songs that allowed him to purge some of the agony.

Four weeks after Brandi's funeral, Bobby got a call from his mom.

"I know it's too much, Bobby," she said. "I'm sorry to call you with this."

"Dad?"

"I wish it wasn't. He's gone."

Because his dad had lived with chronic issues stemming from a bad heart, Bobby knew his dad's death wasn't a surprise. The months previous had seen his dad in and out of the hospital. While Bobby and Brandi had been immersed in the final struggles of their battle, his dad had been fighting his own. When Bobby got the call from his mother, he immediately experienced more release from the pain of loss and the wretchedness of death.

That damn hourglass . . . the sands are always flowing.

• • •

When Bobby and his sister were young, their parents took them on all sorts of road trips across the country. Bobby and his sister would sit in the rear-facing seat of the station wagon, staring into distant headlights, each plugged into their Sony Walkman in search of escape from the confines of the cramped car. It was their reprieve, the thing that held them together from one national park to another, from the Pacific to the Atlantic and back again, from one roadside diner to the next.

Then his dad gave Bobby a C. W. McCall cassette called *Wilderness*. He must have listened to the tape a million times during those endless stretches of summer. One of the songs, "Aurora Borealis," touched Bobby in a way no other ever had. In the song, the narrator talks about being the last person awake on a camping trip and how, mesmerized by the endless starlit sky, he stayed up all night and watched the morning star rise as he reflected on life and the eternity of memories. Although Bobby couldn't have predicted it as a young boy, when he said goodbye to his dad, he found comfort in the knowledge that he could keep their memories alive forever. He vowed to do just that for both his dad and Brandi.

Moving Forward

Bobby was able to purge the heaviest feelings of sorrow and agony within months of losing Brandi. After all, he'd grieved over losing Brandi long before she died. He hadn't suppressed his grief in the slightest. Instead, he'd dealt with it in the most painstakingly open, healthy, and accepting manner possible. He knew if Brandi were looking down on him, she'd understand that.

Hell, she created it. She made it so my moving on was a requirement of her eternal peace.

How could he fail to move on when he had promised Brandi he would? But the puppy-dog eyes, the sad gazes that came from others rankled. They were simply being kind, but they didn't understand the depths of his acceptance; they hadn't been there late at night as he'd grappled with an enlightened angel who understood, and elevated him to understand, that it was all right to forge ahead. It was *essential* to forge ahead. They just didn't get that Brandi's death was something that she herself had refused to allow to rule Bobby's existence. In return, Bobby wouldn't allow *Brandi's* life to be defined by her death, plain and simple.

Kirsten

Bobby had dated Kirsten in high school but hadn't thought about or heard from her in twenty years when she sent him some kind words of condolence after Brandi's death. Bobby hadn't always been kind to girls back when he last knew Kirsten, and as he read her note, he was reminded of how their relationship had ended.

You must be going through things you never believed you would, Kirsten's email read. *And I can't say I understand what it must be like, but I'm sorry for the loss you must feel. You can never know all the people who care about you, but if you did, you'd find that there's someone halfway across the country who remembers you and how amazing you are and feels for what you must be going through. If you ever need a friend, I'm one. Kirsten.*

"Look, I'm not a good guy," Bobby had told her back when they were both teenagers. "I'm, like, a really bad guy. You don't deserve me, trust me. We shouldn't see each other because I don't want to treat you badly."

Normally, when breaking up with a girl, Bobby would lie and make something up, anything to avoid being honest about his feelings. But with Kirsten, he just felt she was too nice—no, too *fine*—of a person for him to be involved with. He couldn't bring himself to lie when he ended their brief relationship.

A couple of weeks after receiving Kirsten's email, Bobby decided to jump on a plane and get away from everything. Her new home state of Ohio seemed as good a getaway as any, and he called Kirsten to ask if she'd like to get together for lunch. They met and found themselves talking about everything, including what he and Brandi had been through, what he was still going through, a seven-year failed marriage that Kirsten was mostly over, their careers, and the ups and downs of their lives since high school. Over the several weeks that followed, they continued their conversation over the phone nearly every day. Bobby even made his way to Ohio again so they could spend some more time face-to-face.

And Kirsten had been right: It *was* nice to have a friend to talk to. When Bobby was on the phone with Kirsten, when he visited her in Ohio, he was free to be okay instead of lost in his grief. He didn't need to worry about who might see him spending time with a woman and judge him or furrow their brows and ask him again how he was doing.

How do you think I'm doing? My wife *died*, he would think when faced with this particular brand of concern. *I might never be okay with that, but I'm doing fine now. I know you care, but your sympathy is not helping.*

As the months passed, Bobby lived two lives. In the first, he was at home, closing the books on all the medical bills and insurance claims. When he wasn't doing those things, he worked, saw the therapist he promised Brandi he'd see, and spent time with his mom. He also grieved. He cried. He screamed away to loud rap music. He wrote in his journal. This first life was a heavy and draining one. Bobby knew it was a necessary part of whatever process he needed to go through so he could move forward with his life. In his second life, he'd visit Ohio and be with Kirsten. They'd go out to dinner, laugh, stay up late talking or sometimes crying about the trials and rewards life had offered—and might offer in the future. The second life was less heavy and more fulfilling. Bobby was grateful, because it helped him with so much of what he still needed to get through.

Over time, Bobby's two parallel lives began to edge closer and closer to merging into one. To their shock, Bobby and Kirsten found themselves in love.

Kirsten was the kind of smart, communicative partner he longed for—much like what he had found in Brandi. But Kirsten was also uniquely herself—a confident, serene, accepting force who was able to balance putting the past into perspective with keeping the future in full view. With her help, Bobby allowed his heart to open once again, and using the tools he'd gained through his time with Brandi, he began a fresh, new, exciting chapter in his life.

Bobby's Epilogue

When I met Bobby, he and Kirsten had been married for seven years. He talked about how fortunate he felt to have reconnected with Kirsten when he had, since he was now as happy as he could hope to be. Had he and Kirsten picked back up at any other time in his life, Bobby wouldn't have been the same Bobby, the one he'd become through his relationship with Brandi.

"I do feel a little guilty sometimes about how perfect my life is," he said. "And it wouldn't be if Kirsten weren't the exact person she is, or if Brandi hadn't taught me so much. Look, there's no way I'll ever feel unhurt about what Brandi and I went through. It was the most horrible, tragic, sad, excruciating thing to go through. If she hadn't died, we'd be married, probably with kids, and I know we'd have a fantastic life together. But that didn't happen. She died. I can't go back and change that, and there's no way I'd change my life now."

Bobby and Kirsten keep Brandi's memory alive through the Relay For Life event they organize in her honor. Bobby's life is rich and full. He speaks of only one regret: "C. W. McCall. I never did tell Brandi about it. I just forgot. But 'Aurora Borealis' meant so much to me. I wish I'd remembered to tell her. I listen to it a few times a year and remember Brandi, Dad, and the other people who have gone. I think about how they live on forever in the memories they created. I wish Brandi knew that I do that."

Afternoon Day One

With a belly full of pancakes, eggs, toast, hash browns, bacon, and juice—you can eat endlessly when you're burning five-thousand-plus calories per day—I rode away from my breakfast with Bobby physically satiated. But I was still deprived emotionally. I had been reminded of how fortunate Bobby was to find an outlet for his grief. He could share the pain and powerlessness of watching someone he loved so much die a horrible and tragic death, and so he was able to reconcile some of his anguish and heartbreak. Bobby's experiences with Brandi weren't locked away, eating at him, leaving a void that became darker and more foreboding to explore. His wounds were out in the open—raw, bare, and exhibited for others to see. Because he was able to cry and laugh and mourn and remember, he was able to receive love and support and understanding and compassion. Bobby found peace, and in that peace, he was able to be fully present for the rest of the life he had yet to live.

As I pedaled toward my next stop, I knew that I enjoyed none of Bobby's peace when it came to losing June. In part, I had no way to fill that hollowness. I had cried and smiled and mourned and remembered *alone.* There were no mutual friends or family to turn to who could share my feeling of loss. People could offer their condolences for what happened, but they couldn't help me fill the void inside. No new day's light shone on my experiences and memories.

As I neared the hospital where my next book participant, Jen, worked as a pediatric oncology nurse, I turned my thoughts to all the people with whom I could share this epic journey ahead of me. I was, after all, at least able to sift through countless memories of my sister. By contrast, Jen had very few memories left of the person she lost to cancer.

When I pulled up to Children's Hospital of Los Angeles, I was struck with the thought that Jen and I had an oddly parallel road ahead. I was excited about the cross-country journey ahead of me, but it was one that I hoped would help me learn from a hundred painful memories from my experience losing June that still felt like a confusing and hurtful exercise in loneliness and isolation. Jen, on the other hand, was excited about the future that lay ahead of her, because she was just beginning to build the foundation for a lifetime of memories, all enriched by the lessons she'd already learned from her past.

Jen

Relationship to cancer: Caregiver, medical professional

Age: Twenty-six

Family status: Married with no children

Location: Los Angeles, California

First encounter with cancer: Six years old

Cancer summary: Jen's father was diagnosed with non-Hodgkin's lymphoma when she was six years old, and he died just nine months later. Moved by the experience, Jen entered nursing school and was quickly drawn to oncology.

Treatment specifics: Jen's father had stage IV non-Hodgkin's lymphoma and home hospice care.

Community involvement: Jen is a pediatric oncology nurse at Children's Hospital of Los Angeles.

Strongest positive emotion during cancer experience: Acceptance

Strongest negative emotion during cancer experience: Sadness

How we met: Jen was introduced to me by a work friend. When I told this friend about the Cycle of Lives project, she immediately said, "I've got the most incredible person for you to talk to."

"The *most* incredible?" I chided.

"Without a doubt. She's my son's fiancée. Her story is pretty tragic, but she's the most lighthearted, giving, grounded young woman ever. Trust me, you need to talk to her."

At first, Jen was reluctant to tell me her story. She was in the middle of obtaining additional nursing credentials, her fiancé was studying for the California bar exam, and they were planning their upcoming wedding. "Besides, I'm not sure what anybody could learn from my experiences," Jen said. "They're pretty personal to what I went through."

I convinced her to schedule a few talks, and she came to tell me her story, which extends far beyond the experience of losing a parent to cancer. Jen's story is about the impact each of us can have on one another, and how the scope of that impact can be measured in innumerable ways, both the explainable and the unexplainable.

A Mile in Her Shoes

Wheel of Fortune

Jen's dad started getting sick a few months before first grade ended, when she was six and her brother was ten. Jen knew her dad was sick, but it was hard for her to know *how* sick. Neither her mom nor her dad told her too much. She was sometimes allowed to be in the room and close to him, and sometimes she wasn't. Jen thought that it wasn't the same kind of sick as a cold—it was maybe more like the flu, which she had one time, but his flu didn't want to go away.

It was also confusing because her dad didn't *look* sick, not at first. He looked well enough to play Candyland and Trouble, like they sometimes did, or play in the backyard, wrestling and tumbling around with her and her brother, which they used to do a lot, though not anymore.

When her dad went to see doctors that summer, Jen and her brother often went with him and waited while he was being seen by the doctors. After, they went to a restaurant and ate hot dogs and french fries and milkshakes. They went on the swings at the park and drove places to see things like schools they'd go to when they got older and places that reminded her dad of things they had done together. Whatever kind of sick he was, it didn't seem so bad.

Things changed a lot when her dad stopped going to work. She didn't go with him to the doctor's office, and they stopped driving with him to the park or anywhere else, because he didn't leave the house. Jen didn't mind, because she liked being one of her dad's nurses. She liked helping the real nurses who came to the house to take care of him. When summer ended, she wasn't sure she wanted to go back to school. She was excited to start second grade, make new friends, and meet her teacher, but she didn't want to stop taking care of her dad. Her mom promised she could still help the nurses after school.

Jen didn't understand much that was going on, but she knew her dad was getting sicker, because by Thanksgiving he almost always stayed in his room. After that, people started coming by. They were family members and people like Uncle Tony and Aunt Kathy—who her mom said weren't *actually* family but were sort of the best kind of family—and other friends and some people she didn't know. All of them were very serious and talked with quiet voices. They cried with her mom and hugged Jen and her brother hard and long when they left.

When her dad didn't feel so sick, Jen would go into his room alone after dinner before bedtime. One night, her dad said he was feeling better. She asked her mom if she could watch television with him, and her mom told her it was a great idea. They put on *Wheel of Fortune*, and her dad drifted in and out of sleep while they watched. Jen had just taken her bath and was curled up next to him in her pajamas, wet hair and all. She sat in the small sofa chair pushed up alongside the bed, close enough that she could stand up and fluff her dad's pillows. He always told her how much he liked her to fluff his pillows. Sometimes she'd hit the top of the pillow with one hand and the side with her other hand, whacking the pillow so hard that it bounced her dad's head forward, and he laughed deep and loud. Other times, she just softly patted the top of the pillow, making sure not to bother his sleep.

"You want your pillow fixed, Daddy?" she asked him that night.

"Nah, I'm good, Nurse Jen," he said and smiled at her. He'd never called her that before, and she felt so happy and proud that he thought she was so important that he would call her *Nurse* Jen.

"*A Streetcar Named Desire*," Jen's dad blurted out. Jen looked at the television. She knew how to read—in fact, she was probably the best reader in the whole second-grade class—but she had no idea what was secretly spelled out on the white boxes the pretty lady tapped when the people playing the game guessed the letters.

"It's *A Streetcar Named Desire*, I'm telling you. It's right there," her dad said.

"*I'd like to buy a vowel. May I have an o please?*" a woman's voice said from the television. Jen looked at her dad to gauge his response.

"No!" he cried. "Oh my God, Nurse Jen. Can you believe this? It's like the best movie ever. It's so easy. Am I right?"

"Yes, Daddy," she said.

"*No o's! Spin again . . . five hundred dollars,*" came the host's voice.

"*I'd like a d, please.*"

"*Yes! There are two d's!*"

"*I'd like to solve the puzzle,*" the contestant said finally. "*Is it A Streetcar Named Desire?*"

"Of course it is!" Jen's dad laughed. "Didn't I tell you, Nurse Jen? One day we're going on that show, and we'll teach them a thing or two about puzzles, okay?"

"Yeah! Yes, Daddy. Can we?"

"We'll try, Nurse Jen. We'll try."

Jen bounced up and down in the sofa chair, laughing and twisting her head from side to side as little droplets of water from her hair sprayed on her dad. He smiled at her.

• • •

Jen's best friend was called Kimi. Kimi's mom sometimes picked her and Jen up from school, and they'd go to Kimi's house to have hot chocolate, color in books, and watch television. But when she was out of school for Christmas break, Jen stayed home. Sometimes she had playdates with her friends, and sometimes her mom took her and her brother to McDonald's and then the park. Mostly they stayed home and were quiet and got hugged too long and too hard too often by the people who came by to talk softly with her mom.

After Christmas was over and Jen was back in school, nurses were at the house all the time. Jen would sneak in to see her dad before breakfast, and the older nurse would smile and wave her in to pat her dad's pillow. He slept most of the time. After school, or after she went to Kimi's house after school, Jen would ask her mom if she could go visit her dad. The younger nurse was there later in the day, and she'd smile and ask Jen to help sometimes.

"Can you see if your dad wants a straw for his 7-Up?" the nurse asked one day.

Jen climbed on the sofa chair and leaned over to whisper in her dad's ear. "Do you, Daddy? Do you want a straw?"

"That would be so nice, Nurse Jen. Yes. That would help me so much," her dad whispered. "Did you have fun at school?"

"I guess. My teacher made us come up with words to rhyme. Like with the word *cat* or, um . . . *bear*."

"Did you do good?"

"Yes, really good. I wrote *care*, for you. Can I help you come up with words on the spinning wheel show tonight?"

"That would be wonderful, Nurse Jen."

A couple of nights later, even though it was a school night, Jen's mom said Jen should go to Kimi's for a sleepover. Her brother didn't have to go to a friend's house for a sleepover, but she did. She didn't like it because she didn't want to miss playing a game or watching television with her dad. Before she went to Kimi's house, Jen went to say goodbye to him. He was breathing very soft and sleeping, so she patted his pillow lightly. He moved a little and Jen froze, but he smiled, even with his eyes closed. She was happy she hadn't woken him.

The next day, Jen and Kimi didn't go to school. They stayed at Kimi's house and played. When Jen went home after lunch that day, there were some people at the house, and the door to her mom and dad's room was closed. Her mom cried and hugged her really hard and really long. She told Jen the nurses were gone and that they had all taken such good care of her dad. She told her that the nurses had been so grateful for her help. Finally, she told Jen that her dad was not going to be sick anymore.

Seeds Grow

After her dad died, Jen didn't know what to think or how to act. She was sad a lot, especially at nighttime, but she still went to school, did her homework, took baths, played with friends, and had dinner with her mom and her brother. Her mom cried a lot, which sometimes made her and her brother cry too. The house felt smaller, because Jen didn't go in her mom's room like she used to when it was her mom *and* dad's room. Her mom didn't go in there much either. She slept on the couch most nights.

People always came by the house with food to eat and groceries. They helped do the laundry, mow the lawn, and clean the house. Sometimes they stayed a long time just talking to her mom. Jen liked that, because her mom looked happier when there were people over. Jen didn't always understand everything everyone talked about, but she and her brother were allowed to hear everything. In fact, her mom seemed even happier when she and her brother were involved in the conversations, especially when Jen and her brother talked about school, friends, and things they liked.

When second grade ended and summer came, more people came, and sometimes they came from far away. She liked Uncle Tony and Aunt Kathy the best. They were her favorites, and they seemed like her mom's favorites too. They told a lot of stories back and forth to each other, again and again. They laughed, and sometimes they cried, and sometimes they did both at the same time.

Third grade came and went, and so did fourth grade and fifth grade. Over that time, Jen got used to people being at the house. They didn't bring food or groceries as much, because her mom liked going to the grocery store and cooking food. They also didn't do laundry, mow the lawn, or clean the house, because Jen and her brother did those things more and more. They didn't mind helping their mom, and she told them how much she appreciated the help. Most of the time everyone was happy. Her mom was always saying to people how lucky and blessed she was and how proud she was of her kids. Jen could see she meant it.

As the years passed, Jen and her brother played sports and made more friends. Her mom drove her and her brother and all their friends to practices, took them to lunch after games, and invited them to the house. All their friends liked Jen's mom. She could tell. Her mom made her friends laugh and talked with them in a way that they said their own parents didn't. She listened to what they were saying and cared about what they wanted to do.

When she was in sixth grade, Jen's middle school had a tree-planting ceremony. Uncle Tony and Aunt Kathy came up to help, and a lot of the people who'd come to their house for years came to help too. Many trees were planted by many people that day, and the school made a special place in between the school and the park that her dad had always taken them to for Jen's family to plant a tree for her dad. A lot of people cried that day, too, but like always, there was more talking and telling stories and remembering things about her dad. Jen noticed there was much less crying, and the crying seemed different from what she remembered from a few years prior. It wasn't as dramatic as before; it seemed somehow less painful, but still sad.

• • •

When she was in the seventh grade, Jen's school went on a field trip to a hospital. It was the first time she'd been in a hospital. She remembered a little of what it was like at her house when the nurses were there to take care of her dad, but she hadn't known what being in a hospital was like, and she loved it. She ran the entire way home from school that day. She told her mom all about the field trip and how they learned about accepting patients into the hospital, what critical care meant, and how many different specialties of medicine and different types of nurses and doctors there were. She told her mom how she wanted to be a nurse, not just because her dad would have liked it but because she wanted to help care for people, to make their time in the hospital not as bad or scary for them.

The night of the field trip, Jen and her brother and her mom watched *Wheel of Fortune* after dinner. Jen remembered that watching that show had always been kind of awkward in the past, but that night as it played in the background, they talked about her dad, and it wasn't awkward anymore. Talking about things made her feel safe and comfortable, and Jen could see that her mom liked when she and her brother talked about their dad. After the show ended, they called Tony and Kathy. They were all on speaker together, and everyone told a story. Tony and Kathy talked about working at the Secret Service with Jen's dad, her mom talked about how they met bumping into each other in the hallway in high school, her brother talked about a fishing trip he took with his dad, and Jen talked about the field trip and about how her dad had called her Nurse Jen. She even remembered the name of the movie her dad screamed at the television when she was young.

She told them all she could remember about what she called the "*A Streetcar Named Desire* night," and it felt good to be so close to her family that night, to know her brother had happy memories of their dad, that her mom could talk about their dad without sounding so sad, and that Tony and Kathy were a part of it too.

• • •

When Jen and Kimi were sophomores, Kimi's dad suffered a severe stroke. Kimi turned to Jen and her mom for help putting things into perspective, to help make sense of it all. Jen felt for Kimi and understood some of her fears. Kimi told Jen she didn't know how to wrap her mind around what it would be like to lose her dad.

Jen didn't compare her own pain and loss to her friends', and she didn't mind that her friends showed sympathy for her or sought out sympathy for their own issues. She felt she understood what her mom meant when she said she was grateful for all she'd been through—even if she wished she hadn't had to endure some of it. Jen saw that her mom had carried such a varied and difficult burden but had still managed to mentor her, teach her to appreciate life, and show her how to feel gratitude and a sense of obligation to help others. Her mom showed Jen how it's healthy to open up and share your pain with people who love and care about you. How you should allow people to help you deal with the difficulties that life sometimes brings.

When Jen contemplated the different choices about where to apply for college, she talked to her mom about the options and asked for her advice. It was a crazy, magical time, and the energy among her friends was through the roof. More than a few times during her senior year, Jen had four or five friends over, and they all asked her mom for her thoughts about where they were thinking of applying. Jen loved those times. She admired her mom and was very close to her, so to see how close her friends had become to her mom was something very special.

Jen was a little nervous about applying to schools that were far away from her family, but her mom supported her desire to go to a top college known to have a quality nursing program, whether it was far away from home or not.

• • •

UCLA was a four-hour drive from home. After talking with her mom many times to make sure she was settled about being left alone in the house, securing promises from Tony and Kathy that they'd visit mom even more than they already did, and making sure her brother thought it was a good idea, Jen accepted UCLA's offer.

After Jen's high school graduation ceremony, her mom, her brother, Tony, Kathy, Kimi, Kimi's mom, and a few other friends went to their special tree, the one they planted years before. They didn't stay long, because they were having a short party at their house before Jen and all her friends went out to celebrate. They took some pictures, and everyone hugged her and her mom really hard and really long when they both started crying. Everyone started to laugh about the fact that they were all crying.

"I feel like he's been watching over us the whole time," Jen told the group as she rubbed the tree's trunk and looked up into its expansive branches.

Jen understood that her family had missed out on so much because of her dad's early death, but she didn't know any different. It had been that way her whole life. Losing him had been tougher on her brother, because he'd been older. And, of course, in a tiny nine-month window, her mom had lost her best friend, her husband, and her soulmate. Jen knew Mom wouldn't ever fully recover from that. Jen didn't feel that her dad dying was a tragedy that left a gaping wound that would define her. Instead, the tragedy left a significant mark on her life that couldn't be touched, measured, or covered up. Jen knew the mark would never shrink or disappear but that everything else would expand around and outward from it. The mark would always be there, but time would allow for such things as gratitude and perspective and love to grow out of it.

A few short months later, she was on her way to college. Jen and her mom talked the entire drive down to UCLA. Jen was nervous and excited, the unrest hitting her from multiple directions, but by the time they got to Westwood, her anxieties had been calmed. Her mom seemed to always know what to say and how to say it, particularly when Jen needed advice or attention the most.

The hug Jen and her mom shared before her mom drove off the next day was the longest, hardest hug Jen had ever shared with anyone in her whole life. The tears that streamed down her cheeks as she stood watching her mom drive off were both the saddest and happiest she'd ever known.

Blossoms Form

Jen promised herself she'd talk to at least five people during orientation. She knew she'd make a lot of friends in the nursing program and at the dorms, but she wanted a diverse group of people to interact with. Since orientation was for all students, Jen knew it was a good place to start meeting people. She ended up talking to far more than five people that day, but none were as memorable as Matt.

Incoming college freshman have two topics to use as icebreakers: where they're from and what they're going to study. The people Jen spoke to at orientation all knew where they were from, but when Jen shared that she was studying to become a maternity nurse, she learned that only a few other people seemed to feel a similar absolute certainty about their career goals. Then she met Matt, who declared without hesitation that he was at UCLA to become a trial attorney. He'd wanted to be one since he was five or six.

Jen saw Matt a few days later when they both were wandering their dorm hallways. He stopped to say hello, and she asked him how classes had started for him, jokingly asking if he was ready for the bar exam yet. He told her he was getting close, but the late nights of studying were hard on him, and he might need to go see a nurse. Did she know anybody she could refer him to? They became instant friends.

Freshman year zoomed by, and Jen spent her summer back home with her mom. Jen loved talking about all the details that she hadn't shared with her mom during their almost daily phone calls throughout the year. Kimi and other friends who were back home for the summer all got together many times to eat dinner, watch movies, go on hikes, and even have a picnic under her dad's tree. Summer was perfect, and her second year of college brought with it a new sweetness. That year, she and Matt started dating. Their friendship had grown, and they had spent enough time together in enough different settings that it seemed safe and natural to see if there was more between them. Jen told Matt that her own parents had met in the hallway of their high school, and that when she bumped into Matt the year before while walking the hallways, a spark went off inside of her. She said she felt they were meant to meet that way.

That same year, Jen also began clinical rotations. Jen had her sights set on a specialty in labor and delivery. When she saw babies being born, the care that went into the neonatal intensive care unit, and the love and joy that permeated the labor and delivery ward, she was content with her decision. Jen didn't dread much about her college experience, but knowing she'd have to do a rotation in the oncology unit gave her apprehension. She felt as though she was at peace with all she'd gone through as a child, but she also knew that you never know how you're going to handle things until you're facing them head on. On the eve of her oncology rotation, she called her mom.

"I don't know if I can do it, Mom."

"I know, darling, but you're strong and so capable. You've always been able to handle so much, smiling the whole time. Try to smile, and I'll bet it won't be as bad as you think. If it is, it'll be for just a short time. There are a lot of expecting moms who are going to need your help."

The first day of her oncology rotation was in the pediatric oncology unit. The moment she entered the floor, Jen's heart raced, her mind clouded over, and her stomach jumped up into her throat. She felt as if she'd held her breath the entire day. For eight hours, Jen endured standing by bedsides, watching and learning as little kids recuperated from radiation, prepared for surgery, and were subjected to various treatments. She learned about some of the different types of chemotherapy being administered to children, from babies all the way up to teenagers, who were lined up in multiple rows of chemo chairs. She saw doctors and nurses and patient-support advocates counseling family members. She saw, too, children's drawings on the walls, games being played, tears flowing, and laughs being shared. Through it all, her head spun as she thought about her dad, her loss, the way he'd called her Nurse Jen, and all the plans she had for her life.

When Jen got back to her dorm that night, she was exhausted—emotionally, physically, and spiritually. All she wanted to do was call her mom. "Mom?" she asked and began to cry.

"How are you, honey? I've been waiting for the phone to ring. Are you okay?"

"Yeah, Mom. But I've made a big decision," Jen said. "I don't know how I *couldn't* work in pediatric oncology. I don't know, it's just . . . well, I'm sure it's what I'm meant to do."

Jen and her mom talked for another few minutes until Jen was too tired to keep talking. They did it again the next day, and the day after that.

Junior and senior years flew by, and Matt and Jen's relationship continued to blossom. After graduating with her nursing degree, Jen was offered a position in the pediatric oncology unit at Children's Hospital of Los Angeles. She accepted without hesitation. Matt graduated with a degree in political science and started law school at UCLA. The following year, Matt proposed. Two years later, they married at a winery near Jen's home. Uncle Tony gave Jen away and danced the first dance with her. There were many long hugs, many kisses, and all kinds of tears that day. And Jen knew her dad was watching over it all.

Jen's Epilogue

I was fortunate to spend quite some time on the phone with Jen before I felt that I understood the essential moments and emotions of her experience with cancer. When I asked about her ability to go through life absent a chip on her shoulder—a chip that few people would blame her for—she hesitated to explain and was almost self-effacing in her response. Jen wasn't happy and well-adjusted in a calculated way; she just *was* those things at her core—because of nature, nurture, or both.

Jen was grateful her mom had given her an environment where she could communicate without fear and explore her emotions without self-consciousness, to share her ups and openly deal with her downs. Though Jen acknowledged that, all things considered, she'd had a remarkable childhood and was embarking on the life she'd always envisioned for herself—finding true love and pursuing her passion for nursing—there were still down days. She just didn't let those days define who she was or what she wanted to get out of life.

I was impressed by Jen's love of pediatric oncology. She told me she was certain she'd work in that field her whole life.

"Do you ever get personal with a patient or their family?" I asked once.

"You mean tell them what I've gone through?"

"Yes. Do you do that? Does it help you or them?"

"Sometimes I do," she replied. "The patients and families are going through so much. I feel like I can be their conduit to quality care and information, and I try hard to make their ordeal easier where I can. I try not to make it about me. I don't ever go too into the details of what happened." She paused. "But there was this one time. I haven't told many people the story. I don't want them looking at me like I'm crazy, you know?"

"How so?" I asked.

"There was this one kid about a year ago," she said. "He was suffering from brain cancer. It affected his vision, he couldn't focus on anything, his motor control was virtually gone, and he wasn't able to communicate very well. I was the primary for him one day, and I'd take his vitals, check on him, help his family try to feed him, do the things we do. One time I'm in there, alone, and suddenly he says, just as clearly as I'm talking to you now: 'He says he's home and that he's happy watching.' My heart stopped, because I was shocked that this boy could talk in a coherent way. I asked him, 'Who says he's home and watching?' He smiles right at me—he's not shaking a bit—and he says, 'George. He's okay and he's standing next to you, watching.' I ask him who George is. I ask him to tell me what made him say those things. But by then, his focus is gone, and he starts talking incoherently, loses motor control, and goes back to being how he was—just like that."

"What did you do?"

"I freaked out. I talked to his family, asked if he knew a George—you know, the coincidence was too much. How do you explain something like that? They told me there wasn't any George. After I explained what had happened and that it might've been my imagination, I told them about my dad and how he'd died when I was young."

"Did you let them know his name was George?"

"I did. I think about that day a lot, and I'm certain my dad knows how much of a hand he had in my life, and I'm so grateful to have him watching over me."

Standing on a Corner in Winslow, Arizona

I finished day one of my cross-country bike ride at my friend Jonathan's house in Newport Beach, more than twelve hours after the day had begun. I'd put in significantly more than one hundred miles over almost nine hours of biking, had visited with book participants at different locales throughout the Greater Los Angeles area, and had stopped by the Jonsson Comprehensive Cancer Center. As I sat in my friend's hot tub after a late dinner, resting, recovering, and reflecting on the thoughts that had rolled around in my head all day, I knew I had taken on a unique and epic journey.

I wasn't surprised by the meditative benefits of exercising for hours on end, as my mind was always able to find deeper and deeper levels of reflection the longer I ran or biked. What did surprise me was how raw I felt inside once the contemplation began. I could sense—even on that first night, once there was nothing to do but pedal and think, nothing but endless roads with which to work through the mental sludge—that the Cycle of Lives stories would become more real, more consequential, and more revelatory. As I would come to find more and more each day, the irrefutable emotional truths revealed this way took on deeper, earthier flavors. Finding something comprehensible in that rawness, that unrefined truth, became somehow easier as my own physical struggles grew harder.

Day two was another twelve-hour day. I covered 106 miles along mostly quiet seaside bike roads. The highlight was a visit to a huge state-of-the-art proton therapy facility where one of my book participants had received treatment. Dr. Capri, the director of the facility, also happened to be that participant's physician and had offered me much insight and background over many phone interviews. He gave me a private tour and a layman's explanation of how proton radiation therapy works.

At the end of the tour, we stopped at the opening of a hallway adjacent to the large lobby area of the facility, leading back to the five treatment rooms. We stood in front of a polished golden bell mounted on the wall as we rehashed some details about Rick, the book participant whom we'd spoken of during our talks. I stared at the short, thick white rope that was knotted into a small handle hanging from the bell's clapper.

The "survivor's bell," as it's known in cancer circles, is rung by a survivor upon receiving their last treatment—chemotherapy, radiation, proton radiation, and so on. It's intended to signify that cancer is behind them, that they can move forward with their lives. I looked solemnly at the bell.

"Yeah, it's a big deal for those fortunate enough to ring it," Dr. Capri said. "If only we could have every patient ring it for the closure that last treatment brings *and* to announce real optimism for their future."

Back on the bike, I thought about several of the book participants who'd talked about "the bell" and the other objects of significance to their cancer experiences. I wondered if June had had the chance to ring a bell at the end of her treatments. If she had, did she do so with optimism for the future? Or at least some acceptance of the fact that there might not be a long one in store?

Day two ended in San Diego on a similarly heavy note as day one. By the end of my ride, a veritable symphony of contemplation was playing in my mind. I fell asleep to the strains of it, fading away into a deep, hard, exhausted slumber.

Day three was a wicked twelve-hour day through the California mountains and desert. The ride saw me traverse 107 miles—including twelve categorized climbs on my heavy steel touring bike—in 106-degree temperatures. Downhill speeds topped forty-five miles per hour. I'd left the coast and civilization behind and begun a multiday trek through the desolate Southwestern part of the country.

As my body worked to climb and descend the many hills along my route, my mind was filled with thoughts of June. I remembered our childhood, the times I allowed my mom to pick on her and the times I joined in on the bullying—afraid that if I didn't, I'd pay the price and receive negative attention of my own. I thought about the physical fights June and I had, laughing and crying with her, being afraid of our mom together, feeling confused about life as young kids. We'd grown up in a household where our very young mother seemed to hate us, while our very old father—there was a thirty-eight-year age gap between them—seemed to be too old to notice or care. I remembered the times we spent stretches of endless summer days glued to each other's sides, and I remembered the times our lives took paths that kept us distant for years at a time.

On days four and five, as I made my way out of California and into Arizona, I endured twelve-plus hours of biking each day in 110-degree temperatures, difficult climbs, scorching desert headwinds, endless stretches of melting asphalt highways, shadeless terrain, aching muscles, and skin that grew redder from the fire above and rawer from the chafing below.

Several consecutive long days in the intense heat had sapped me of my energy and wreaked havoc on my stomach. Each night left me struggling to rehydrate and take in the calories my body wouldn't let me absorb in the daytime. Each day I awoke stiff and sore, pulling my bike shorts on and prepping myself for the battle ahead, zombielike. I was motivated to move but not quite sure how I was doing it.

True to my discovery on day one, the harsher the physicality, the more penetrating the mental exercises. When I settled into each day's ride, having reviewed my intended route, shaken the cobwebs out from inside my brain, and pedaled out the previous day's muscle soreness, I began the inner dialogue. *Forget the hills and the heat. Think of Patricia's struggles, of Neil's hard times*, I'd tell myself. *With each turn of the pedal, try to focus on Dave's and Joshua's and Karen's pains, not your own legs. No matter how hard it is, June had it so much harder. Just keep pedaling and stop whining.*

By the end of each day, I lay spent and unable to move, crying for sleep yet unable to shut my mind off.

Day six was marked by more heat, more flat tires, and more ridiculous climbs as I made my way through Phoenix, Arizona. Near the end of the day, I was becoming delirious with exhaustion—enough to engulf my senses. I stopped in the middle of the road to change a punctured tube. My fiancée, Erin, was supporting me on my ride, and I'd called her to come back from the hotel some twenty-odd miles ahead to help me, as the darkness, confusion, and fatigue were overwhelming me.

"What the hell are you doing?" she asked when she pulled the truck up next to me.

"What does it look like?" I replied. "I'm changing another flat."

"You *trying* to get yourself killed? Are you serious?"

I looked around, confused. "What do you mean?"

"You're in the middle of the damn street."

I looked around again, with intent. I *was* in the middle of the street. Granted, it was a rather quiet, residential area off the main highway, outside of my intended finishing point in the city of Fountain Hills, Arizona, but I was in the middle of the street. I moved my bike onto the sidewalk and continued working.

"I guess I'm getting a little loopy," I said and shrugged.

That night, she told me all the concerns she'd been holding back: I was pushing too hard; I needed to rest and reassess my schedule. She was disturbed by my lack of judgment and apparent disregard for my safety, and she'd noticed I was becoming more ragged each day, that my control of both mind and body was beginning to erode. I listened, but I knew I could recover enough each day to begin anew. If I continued to push through, I'd get stronger as the days passed. If I just kept moving forward, things would get better. I was relying on years of knowledge I'd gained from endurance events, or perhaps I was just channeling the sentiments of those people whose stories I played over and over in my mind all day. Either way, I wasn't going to ease my intended schedule.

Day seven started like every day previous, except I was a bit more optimistic it would be easier on my body and allow for more restoration of mind and body than the previous days, because although I had more than seven thousand feet of climbing to deal with, I was planning to cover only sixty-some miles in all. I was heading to Payson, Arizona, near the center of the state and near the top of the Tonto National Forest.

The first few climbs were plain merciless on my tattered and wrecked body, shorter route ahead notwithstanding. My early-morning optimism dissipated, and by late morning it became obvious the day was going to be another long one. Between more flat tires, excruciatingly slow climbs, headwinds, and painful recovery breaks—one of which I spent exhausted, lying down on the burning asphalt napping—the day just wouldn't end.

The math of the ride worked out so that the harder I pushed myself physically, the harder my mind worked too. It was also consistent when calculated from a different perspective: The more depleted my body became, the more frayed I became mentally.

Day seven attempted to destroy me and everything I thought I knew about myself and what I was doing. Maybe Erin knew me better than I knew myself. I was fiercely tired, my confidence and motivations had been shredded into incoherent nonsense, and throughout the day, my body had been repeatedly unable to respond to my demands to continue forward.

In my delirium, I tried to grasp on to thoughts that might provide some directional light to follow, some inspiration with which to move forward. I thought of the specific difficulties some of my book participants had gone through, and it pushed me forward. I thought of the time my sister awoke from a twelve-hour surgery smiling, and it eased my pain. I thought of how, only weeks before she died, June still believed she could will herself to overcome her condition and be there to support the people who were going to walk a twenty-four-hour event in her honor weeks later. Galvanized by the memory, I urged my legs to ignore the pain.

I thought of one of my book participants who lived in Florida and loved sunsets, and I asked her to send me a favorite sunset picture to help inspire me to keep moving eastward.

In the later afternoon, I received a timely text from a friend as I lay resting on the side of the road: *Just wanted to let you know Mom passed today. The cancer got the best of her, but she lives on. She always loved hearing stories about what you're doing, and I know she's with you in spirit.* Reading it compelled me to get up and back on the bike.

Regardless of all the inspiration, by nightfall I had to call Erin and my friend Jerry for help. I was severely dehydrated and unable to regulate my body temperature. It was eighty-five degrees out, and I was shivering with cold. My legs were made of heavy cement, and my muscles threatened to seize with each turn of the pedals.

By the end of day seven, my body was pretty near broken, and my mind was smashed into unintelligible little pieces.

With my bike laid in the bed of the truck and me slumped in the back seat, we drove the last five miles to the hotel. Erin had a hot bath, some smoothies, and some comfort food—a burger, fries, some fried zucchini, and chocolate cake—waiting for me.

Once I stopped shivering and was able to ingest some calories, Erin implored me to take a break.

"One day. Just one. Look at you. You can't go on like this," she said. "You have to take a break and recover a bit."

"Taking a break is not possible," I said. "I've got to stay on schedule. I'll be fine in the morning."

"No. You won't be fine in the morning," she argued. "Each day you're looking worse. Each day you end up more tired, more sunburned, more beat up. You're going to hurt yourself out there, and if you don't get run over because you're not paying attention or something, you'll get sick or worse from pushing yourself like this. You're going to snap, and then what?"

I didn't want to discount or patronize her, because I knew that in a very real sense, she was right. But I also knew that even though I was as far in over my head as I'd ever been, I could find the strength to keep going. I would eventually get stronger. I'd get some tailwinds or a day with no flat tires. My stomach would feel better, or my legs would last longer. Things would get easier for me physically, which would help me emotionally.

"Part of the reason I need to keep going is because I have a *choice* to quit," I tried to explain. "Many of my book participants, and my own sister, didn't have a choice to quit what they were going through. I can't quit now, if for no other reason than because I'm fortunate enough to be *able* to quit. I'll recover. I have to get up tomorrow and keep moving."

"I understand," she said. "But you know you *can* take a break, and it won't mean anything against what you're doing."

"I know. You're right. I hear you, but I just feel like I have to not give in. If I do, I might not figure it all out."

"Figure what all out?" she said.

"I don't know. But I know there are big questions in my head, and giving in is not going to help me, that's all. I'm trying to find some answers, and maybe this will help me."

As I clicked the buckles on my bike shoes the following morning, I knew my endeavor was somewhat selfish. I was not just trying to support my Cycle of Lives project, and I wasn't doing this only for the people who'd been affected by cancer. I was also trying to prove something to myself. Maybe I was trying to prove I could beat the ravages of time or accomplish an unthinkable endeavor. Maybe I was demolishing my body and mind hoping to draw out deeper truths. It was conceivable I was simply using the whole thing as a sick and twisted way to bring attention to myself. I didn't know. I *did* know I had recovered just enough overnight to get back on the bike and see if any answers came my way.

About halfway through day eight, after a glorious, hour-and-a-half-long, thirty-mile downhill ride, I rolled into Winslow, Arizona, a small town popularized by an Eagles song. I was on my way toward Holbrook in the eastern part of Central Arizona to have lunch with Erin and Jerry. As I stood literally on a corner in Winslow, Arizona, waiting for them to pull into town, the lyrics from that song played in my mind:

Take it easy . . .

The lyrics ran through my head as the singer sang about not letting things drive you crazy and not trying to understand all the stress and nonsense around you. About just taking it easy.

I imagined the verse was written just for me—so I could feel okay about what I was doing, so I could endure the pain, so I could take it easy on myself, so I could settle into my ride and into the long, powerful train of thoughts that urged me on in search of answers.

Terri, whom I was biking toward, had long lived with her search for answers. They lay, as it turned out, in a series of traumatic events surrounding her monumental battles with cancer, her family and loved ones, and most importantly—herself.

Terri

Relationship to cancer: Survivor, medical professional, advocate

Age: Forty-two

Family status: Single

Location: Albuquerque, New Mexico

First encounter with cancer: Twenty-eight years old

Cancer summary: Diagnosed with Hodgkin's lymphoma. She received a stem cell bone marrow transplant and multiple chemotherapy regimens. She experienced a recurrence one year later and underwent a second stem cell bone marrow transplant and chemotherapy regimen.

Treatment specifics: Hodgkin's lymphoma, stage IV

Community involvement: Terri is a family nurse practitioner. She is active in the wellness community and works with organizations such as Stupid Cancer to bring advocacy and awareness to the community.

Strongest positive emotion during cancer experience: Tenaciousness

Strongest negative emotion during cancer experience: Remorse

How we met: While I was researching this book, my wife, Erin, called me one day from work. "I just saw a post on Facebook from one of the girls I went to high school with," she said, referring to her small Catholic high school in Los Angeles. "She had cancer before, and it's come back. There are at least three women from my class who've had cancer, and another died of it not long ago. So that's *four* out of the ninety-nine total in our class who've had cancer. I don't know if their stories are what you're looking for, or if they'd agree to participate, but you should reach out to them."

Erin hadn't kept in touch with any of the women in more than an ancillary manner, but I reached out to each one and explained the motivation behind my call.

When I called Terri, we hit it off right away. After I introduced myself and explained the reason for my call, she said, "I always thought about how odd it was that four or five out of a hundred of us got cancer before we were forty. If I wrote a book, I think I'd call it, *What the F*** Was in the Holy Water?*"

Terri and I spoke many times after that. She *needed* to talk about the emotions and difficulties brought on by half a lifetime spent fighting with cancer and its after-effects. She often left me speechless in the face of the physical pain and emotional chaos she endured. With Terri, contemplation didn't *solve* issues; contemplating what lay inside only shed light on the endless reflections caused by looking into those mirrors in her soul. It was clear that for Terri, what didn't kill her filled her with endless questions.

Abandonment, Fuzzy Math, and the Meaning of Life

Starting Out Alone

Terri's legs felt heavy and disconnected. The energy required to shuffle along took much more effort than it should have, and she felt short of breath. Her head spun as she made her way down the jet bridge. Her face was flushed, her heart pounded, and her lips pulsed. Terri was certain the people around her could see her anxiety, which only added to the pressure in her head. She felt as if she might just explode right there. She wasn't sure she could make it onto the plane, but she wasn't about to turn around.

Terri wasn't afraid of flying. She loved flying—well, the thought of it, anyway. She'd only flown once as a little kid, and that hardly qualified. It wasn't the getting on a plane that was the issue. She felt overwhelmed by the stark finality of where she was flying to, and away from. At eighteen, she knew that getting on the plane marked the end of her adolescence and the beginning of her journey into adulthood. As she was about to cross over from the jet bridge onto the plane, she looked down and saw a little sliver of California tarmac below. A shiver raised the hairs on the back of her arms and neck as she realized she was about to leave behind everything she knew.

Her parents were against her decision to attend Georgetown, regardless of the scholarships Terri had earned. They believed she should stay in California and not go looking for something out in the world, whatever it might be, that she could get staying close to home. They didn't so much argue with her about her decision to go across the country. Instead, they attacked her lack of understanding about the reality of being out on her own. They gave her warnings intended to persuade her to stay home, but they all fell flat. Her parents hadn't ever given her much support or positive attention, so she had little reason to believe there was anything to gain from staying close to her family. Their judgment fell on deaf ears.

When Terri did try to engage in adult conversation with her parents about going away to Georgetown, her mom just shrugged her off with a platitude, and her dad did little more than remind Terri in an ominous tone that she was at an age to take responsibility for her own decisions, even if those decisions came with consequences she might not be aware of.

On the morning of the day she left, Terri's feelings were more awkward than emotional. Her two uninterested younger sisters were over at their friends' homes, her young brother was obliviously watching television, and her parents seemed intent on avoiding Terri's room. She'd packed two suitcases the night before, so she sat on her bed, waiting for the right moment to begin the goodbye process. On the drive to the airport, there was a lot less said between them than she ever could have imagined might be. Even the hugs her parents had given her at the entrance to the gates seemed more obligatory than loving.

Terri stepped onto the plane. Her heart continued to race, but the pressure in her head was relieved by the knowledge that she wasn't afraid of what lay ahead. Terri could handle things just fine. She strapped in, looked out the window, and began to do some mental math.

During the flight, Terri debated herself on both sides of the leaving-home equation. On one hand, she was scared to move across the country, leaving home and familiar surroundings behind. That seemed a natural response. On the other hand, she wasn't leaving a *real* home: Terri had never been close to her parents. She barely talked to her sisters, and she didn't have much interaction with her brother, who was ten years younger. It was more accurate to say she was moving out of her parents' house than leaving home. She took most of the five-hour flight to search her heart, trying her best to be objective, to uncover some clues that might make her feel less alienated, to determine if *she* had treated her family poorly and not the other way around.

Maybe I was the one who made them treat me like an outsider, Terri thought. *Maybe I was self-absorbed. No, it was them. They just never embraced me the way they should have. They were a cold, emotionless family. But maybe I was the distant one? Did I make myself out to be the black sheep?* Back and forth she went.

These thoughts lurked in the background, direct effects of a melancholic stroll through visions in her head of a disjointed childhood, as she took the shuttle bus to campus. Her head still spinning, Terri checked in with the student affairs office, attended a brief informational meeting, received a schedule for the next few days' orientations, was shown her dorm room, and finally met her roommate. The process seemed too sterile. She'd pictured everything differently, as if somehow there would be excitement in the air, that everybody would be charged up in some way. Perhaps they were, but Terri's excitement felt muted. She was alone, and most of the other students were with parents.

By the time she decided to call her parents and try to take it upon herself to find a way to break through to them, she was almost in tears. She wanted to tell them about her day and her thoughts and the experiences of her first few hours at Georgetown. Terri went to the community phone down the hallway and dialed her parents' number. "Hey, it's me," she said when her sister answered.

"Hang on . . . *Maaahhm,*" she yelled. "It's for you. It's Terri."

Terri wanted to talk to her sister for a moment, but before she could, she heard the phone being set down on the counter. *Not even a "hello"?*

"You okay?" her mom asked.

"I am, Mom. I'm here. Everything's good. I just wanted to talk to you for a minute—"

"Okay, let's talk tomorrow. We're going to dinner now," her mom said flatly.

Terri knew her dad didn't like to go out for dinner, so she asked if she could talk to him.

"We're *all* going to dinner," her mom said.

Terri's tears flowed, but she made sure her voice was steady. She knew they didn't care about her the way she hoped they might. "So, okay . . . tomorrow?" Terri asked.

"That would be better."

A few days passed before they talked, then a few more until they spoke again. The calls were generic, box-checking exchanges, and over the subsequent weeks and months, they happened less and less.

Alone in Chaos

Maybe it was the demanding Georgetown environment, where expectations for high-level academic achievement were set just above stratospheric, or maybe it was the boundless inner drive borne out of her newfound self-reliance, but either way, Terri found that her choice in colleges suited her. She *fit in* at Georgetown. Without much trouble, she learned to manage a demanding academic life and full-time work at a restaurant just off campus. She also found time to develop friendships and take a few first steps into the dating world.

From the start, she spent most holidays in Washington, DC, by herself. Terri's parents weren't big travelers, and they never came to see where Terri lived and went to school. She would have gone home to see them, but her parents never asked if she was going to, so she didn't. Terri didn't really mind—she was building a life on her own just fine. But there were times she dealt with alternating bouts of guilt and resentment. She'd continued to believe that being away from her family might spark something in her or in them that would finally bridge the gap between them, but that spark never materialized. As a result, feeling alone and *being* alone became the norm.

That feature, of feeling both isolated and cut off, changed for Terri when in her senior year she met Phil. Like her, Phil was a bit of a loner; he had no real family to speak of and a small social circle. Also, like Terri, he'd immersed himself in study and work out of a similar, almost desperate need to be self-reliant. There wasn't really anyone either could turn to, so they turned to each other. They dated for a few years while she began working as a nurse and as he went on to study for his postgraduate degree in business. Their lives weren't yet complicated by the demands of too many competing priorities. They were young, they were alone, and once they discovered how much they enjoyed having someone else to rely on, they decided they wanted to build a life together.

Phil proposed marriage to Terri when they were both twenty-six. The identity Terri had envisioned for her future self was a strong, take-charge-of-her-life person who would continue to enhance her education and career, get married, have kids, and cultivate a real family. She accepted Phil's proposal. When Terri shared the news with her parents, no one seemed eager to travel in either direction to celebrate.

By the time Terri took the initiative to focus on planning the wedding, they had been engaged for more than a year. They'd both been working very long hours, he as a research analyst and she as an emergency room nurse. But at close to twenty-eight years old, she didn't want to wait to start a family.

"I'm not feeling so hot," Terri said to Phil after working back-to-back twenty-hour shifts one weekend and feeling especially run-down. "You know what I'm going to do? I'm going to stay in bed all day, and I'm going to research weddings and come up with some ideas for us, and I'm not going to feel bad about doing nothing for a day. We never do nothing, right?"

"No, we don't have much time for nothing," Phil said.

Terri thought she sensed a little nervousness in his body language. "Is that okay?"

"Sure. I think taking a day off doing nothing is a good idea," he said. "Get busy doing nothing so you can get busy planning."

In between long naps, Terri tried to concentrate on what to research, but she was too tired to focus. Throughout that day and the next, her energy level waned until she struggled to even get out of bed. She hadn't eaten because she wasn't hungry, but she was *so* thirsty. She was sweating heavily, totally overtaken by whatever sickness had knocked her on her back.

She made it to work after two days off, but she couldn't seem to shift gears to move faster, and she was having a hard time focusing. In the emergency room, speed and focus were nonnegotiable. She struggled for a couple of weeks, trying to get over whatever she had, but she couldn't get ahead of the deep lethargy. With Phil working so much—and being gone for weekend conferences in New York—she had the freedom to try to figure out what was wrong by herself. What emerged was a nagging, creeping feeling that something more was happening than just being run-down or sick. She wanted to ignore the little voice in her head telling her she should know better. That, being a medical professional, she shouldn't self-diagnose—especially when it came to something that lingers.

One morning, she checked sensitive areas on both sides of her neck and in her armpits that seemed to have appeared overnight. She felt small lumps. There was no more ignoring; she knew she had to go see her doctor. She explained her symptoms over the phone, and they agreed to see her right away. That same day, Terri saw her primary care doctor, who did a complete examination, and a hematologist, who took blood samples, and because her symptoms and examination indicated that lymphoma was a possibility, she was referred to a specialist, who scheduled her for an excisional lymph node biopsy for the very next day. She didn't know how to tell Phil about everything over the phone, so a few days after, when he came home from another trip to New York, she told him what had happened.

Two days later, the results came back, and her world turned inside out. Just like that, Terri went from not feeling well, to suspecting she might be sick, to being told she had Hodgkin's lymphoma.

She and Phil tried to maintain their normal lives over the next two weeks while Terri underwent more tests and procedures to determine what stage she was at before a treatment plan could be determined. There wasn't a waking minute in which she felt anything other than a growing fear that something was hollowing her out inside.

"How bad is it?" her mom asked after Terri gathered the courage to call her parents and let them know what was going on.

"Like I said, they don't know yet. It's not good—they know that. But how bad?" Terri knew from the few results that had come in that her prognosis was probably going to be grave. She didn't know how to show vulnerability to her mom, but she tried. "I'm scared, Mom."

"I'm sure it's not serious. You'll be okay," her mom said.

Terri lashed back. "You don't know that—even the doctors don't know that. It's *cancer*, Mom—like, severe cancer. It might be everywhere. If it is, then *nothing* is going to be okay."

"Well, it might be."

There was no fighting it; her mom was who she was: a distant, unemotional, dismissive person. Terri wanted—she *needed*—more than just Phil's support, but thinking she could lean on her family was a waste of time. A decade before, she felt her family didn't care about her leaving. She felt then that they wouldn't care if she died.

"You're right," Terri said. "I guess it might be okay."

But it was confirmed: stage IV Hodgkin's lymphoma. It was most definitely *not* okay. Not one tiny, wishful sliver of okay. Terri wanted to call her mom and scream, "*I told you so!*" But nothing—not vengeance, not assurance, not comfort—would come of it. Terri went on formal leave. Any type of planning—for work, for a wedding, for living—was pushed aside. There was only one reality to deal with: an expected four months of grueling chemotherapy.

Cancer #1

Terri went through several intense cycles of chemotherapy, each time struggling through every possible physical side effect. She couldn't eat anything, lost all her hair, had sores in her mouth and nose, had unending nausea, vomited up everything she tried to take in, bruised when anything or anybody touched her, slept deep as death for what seemed like days at a time, and barely had energy to move from bed to bathroom to car to chemo chair.

Terri had no idea how to prepare for what she might go through during treatment, psychologically. She knew she felt guilty about other people having to attend to her, and she recognized she felt a fair amount of self-pity, but there wasn't time to feel much more than that, nor the clarity of mind to assess her mental or emotional states. Terri wasn't naturally inclined to submit to being watched over and taken care of. She couldn't always tend to herself, though, and needed to turn to her doctors and nurses, friends from work, Phil, and her closest friend and first college roommate, Marci, for help. She didn't have a choice. She'd gone into chemotherapy thinking she'd be able to balance her life as much as possible around the treatments, but she couldn't. She had to rely on others.

In between cycles, Terri gained back just enough of her wits and energy to call her parents and give them sugar-coated updates. There would have been no benefit in letting them know the details of how hard things were. Her mom would have minimized, perhaps even doubted the truth anyway. During the breaks, Terri could more easily take visitors and act herself. Most importantly, those times gave her and Phil some basis of hope to believe that being cured was a possibility. Survival was the only thing on Terri's mind.

Terri's initial diagnosis happened in late July. August, September, October, and November were stripped away by chemotherapy. In December, Terri went into remission. By the following May, she was feeling and looking pretty normal. She went back to work and began, again, to plan for the future: the wedding, getting her master's degree in nursing, and getting back on track with the minutiae of life. In the months that followed, Terri felt stronger and stronger, and she came to believe that her mom's early proclamation that things would be okay was, in the end, going to be right—a thought that lasted about a New York minute.

In mid-June, the inside-out world of almost a year before could have been described as a walk in the park. Terri was about to take a long, slow journey through a much more wretched place. An every-ninety-days checkup left her devastated. Her cancer had returned, quickly, fiercely, and without mercy.

Cancer #2

Without delay, Terri's oncologist laid out the plan: immediate stem cell harvesting, as the cancer hadn't yet attacked her bone marrow; heavy chemotherapy in an attempt to eradicate the cancer cells that were raging throughout her body; and a subsequent reintroduction of the harvested healthy cells. It was the only chance to save her. She might die, and quickly, if not from the cancer directly, then from the many and severe associated risks. But the doctors let her know that there was some measure of potential success. She had a chance.

As before, everything came unhinged at once. Terri barely had time to talk with Phil, her parents, her friends, or even herself about how to process any of what was going on. She could only react. Cancer wanted to rip her whole life away from her at terminal velocity. When the ship is sinking, heavy thinking is a luxury that gets tossed overboard. Terri was to be immediately admitted to the hospital to prepare for the stem cell harvesting, the high-dose chemotherapy that followed harvesting, and then the stem cell transplant. She expected to be in the hospital for at least several weeks.

In an uncharacteristically benevolent gesture, Terri's mom offered to come to Washington, DC, to be with Terri. Terri knew the idea wasn't feasible. She had Phil and Marci to help her; besides, where would her mom stay? What would her dad do? What's more, Terri didn't know how her body was going to react to treatment this time around, and if it were as bad as before, she wouldn't have the strength to deal with the stresses that would accompany her mom's visit. Not uncharacteristically, her mom didn't put up much resistance when Terri suggested she should stay in California.

On the day she was to go to the hospital, Terri found herself totally alone. Marci had disappeared a few days before. It wasn't unusual for Marci to check out, but the timing wasn't ideal. Phil was delayed on his way back from New York, so Terri took a cab ride to the hospital. She never felt more desolate in all her life as she did in that cab. That is, until her mobile phone rang as she was going through the hospital admissions process.

"Hey, where are you?" Terri asked.

"I'm still in New York," Phil said.

"New York? I thought you'd be here by now. What happened?"

"It's complicated," he said.

"Complicated?"

"Yeah."

"Well, when can you come?"

There was a long silence—too long. Terri's heart sank. She *knew* something was wrong. "Hello? What is it? Did you hear me?" At first, she felt panic, but it quickly gave way to resentment and anger.

What could be so complicated he can't answer me?!

"Well, I don't know what to say," he said.

"Do you know where I am? What's going on right this second? It's not like we've got time for this. Just say what you need to say, Phil. We can deal with whatever it is."

"There's no right time, Ter. It's just, well . . . I can't be there for you. I belong up here."

"Like, right now? What are you trying to say?"

"Someone else needs me right now, today."

"Someone *else*? You're serious? Who in the fuck could need you more than me?"

But she *knew* it must be another woman.

"I'm afraid someone does, and I need to stay here for a few more days," he said. "I've met someone, and, well, she's pregnant, and—"

Their conversation lasted only a few more minutes, not just because Terri was in the middle of being admitted, and not just because what he told her she only needed to hear in headlines, but because her face had turned so white and her mouth had become so dry and her pulse had raced so frantically that the admitting nurse pulled Terri's hand down from her ear, stared deep into her eyes, and mouthed for her to hang up. Terri held the phone in her lap. Phil's faint voice was barely audible out of the tiny speaker from that distance.

"Hang up?" Terri squeaked out to the nurse in a soft, confused breath.

"Yes, dear. You need to turn off the phone now."

Terri looked at the nurse, then back down at the phone, and knew the nurse had understood that something severe happened. She used the word *need* as counsel, not as instruction.

"He's my *fiancé*," Terri said. She handed the phone to the nurse. "Where do I put this?"

"I'll take care of it, dear. We'll put it with your other belongings."

Odd word, belongings, Terri thought. *He belongs in New York with a woman he just found out he got pregnant. And my belongings are being put in a sterile locker in a hospital room. Seriously? Where do I belong? In this hospital? Really?*

Phil disappeared off the face of the earth; he didn't reach out once after that fateful call. He didn't come by the hospital to check on Terri. In the apartment they had shared for almost five years, he didn't leave behind one piece of clothing or personal mementos or any sign that would have pointed to him ever having been in Terri's life. Seven years together wiped clean off the books while Terri was stuck in a cancer ward, going through procedure after procedure, getting endless injections and IV drips, and losing her appetite and her hair, her energy, and every other damn thing on and in her that could be measured.

Hollowed out again in every way possible. Phil was gone. Marci had evaporated into thin air. Terri's family was three thousand oblivious miles away.

But other friends helped raise Terri's spirits; coworkers brought her food. Some came over to clean the apartment and run errands for her. As if by some cosmic reprieve, the side effects of Terri's second round of chemotherapy treatments seemed to be much less severe than the first, even though the dosages were much more intense and concentrated. Maybe her tolerance had increased, or maybe it was her anger at Phil, but something inside of Terri gave her power over her physical constitution and allowed her to overcome what might otherwise have been more debilitating reactions to her treatments.

After more than three weeks in the hospital, Terri needed another three weeks at home to convalesce, follow infection-avoidance protocol, and gain back her overall strength and well-being. There were ups and downs. Terri lost over forty pounds and had such low energy that more than a few times entire days disappeared, any memory of them ripped away by a painful, violent exhaustion.

Somehow, the doctors were successful. She overcame the low odds she was given at the onset. They killed off the cancer cells with harsh rounds of poison and reintroduced hundreds of millions of Terri's own healthy cells into her body. Ultimately, they gave Terri the news that she could expect a near 100 percent recovery. She wasn't going to die yet. There was a long list of potential long-term side effects, and the doctors reiterated that some would and could be severe. A lot of numbers and percentages were thrown around, but anything long-term sounded sweet to Terri.

Dissociation

As she recuperated, Terri began to process her emotions, both from the cancer and from being abandoned by both her fiancé and best friend. Cancer was a vicious, random killer, that much she knew. Somehow, she'd escaped its wrath, but the wounds hadn't scarred over. With Phil and Marci, she could at least try to come up with answers as to their motivation. But she wasn't about to wait around for clarity before getting on with her life. She wasn't going to let cancer or the actions of bad people limit her future. So Terri began to think about what personal and professional steps she wanted to take as she moved forward from what the doctors told her had been, at best, a fifty-fifty chance of survival.

During the weeks that followed her transplant, she applied for, and was accepted into, a program for her to obtain a master's degree in nursing; she joined a support group for people who had recurrent stage IV non-Hodgkin's lymphoma; and she wrote out her ten-year goals:

1. Get my doctorate

2. Married with two kids

3. Cancer-free

A lot had happened in Terri's life during the year following her transplant. Most things were the result of her conscious efforts, such as staying active and involved in her cancer support group, working longer shifts at the hospital, studying for her master's, and doing what she could to take charge of her physical rehabilitation. But there was one event that came very much by surprise: She met someone.

Meeting Bob was an accident. Terri went out for a drink with some coworkers—the taste of alcohol, much like the remnants of Phil, was still acidic months after her treatment had ended, but the acidity was fading. One of her coworkers brought a friend. Terri didn't know if her coworker had told Bob about what she'd been through, and she became nervous about that when she felt an immediate spark between her and Bob.

Just like it was with the cancer, this is a fifty-fifty chance, right? Terri asked herself. *My friend has either told him about the cancer or she hasn't. It's a fifty-fifty chance. That was a spark between us or it wasn't—also a fifty-fifty chance.*

As the talk in the bar continued, Terri continued the conversation with herself. She decided right then that things either happen or they don't.

Everything's 50 percent. What the hell does 90 percent sure or 20 percent sure or sixty-forty odds of something happening mean, anyway? You're either going to get rid of the cancer or not. It's either going to come back or not. Somebody's either going to like me or he won't. I'm going to die or I'm not. My family is either going to come around one day or they're not. Everything is fifty-fifty.

And just like that, Terri adopted a liberating mantra, a comfortably pragmatic mindset.

As it turned out, there *was* a spark between her and Bob. They exchanged numbers, went on a few dates, and after getting to know each other, started dating exclusively. Within months of meeting, they spent much of their free time together. Considering all Terri had been through, their relationship developed relatively stress-free. Terri had settled into her fifty-fifty mindset. She was free to be herself without hedging, guessing, or fretting over the chances of what might or might not happen.

That didn't mean her mind and heart were unburdened. She'd been dragged to death's door and fought her way back alone, and that leaves marks. Terri grappled with existential questions. She had fears about the future and of what lasting long-term medical conditions her treatments might cause. She balanced her need to interact with people who had gone through what she'd gone through with the pain and guilt of watching them die while she was somehow given the gift of survival.

The road to recovery for Terri was often a rocky one. Was a twinge of pain something left over from before, or was it a sign that something new was happening? Did extreme exhaustion indicate her body was repairing itself, or was it a warning? Terri couldn't escape a hypersensitive awareness of her body, and she never enjoyed a span of time completely without fear. Sure, things happened or they didn't, but even the simple act of flipping a coin can torment the strongest of people when done hundreds of times a day, especially when one side of the coin portends living and the other side dying.

Although she was able to climb out of some of the darker dips in the road following the struggles of an autologous stem cell transplant, about a year after things had begun to look and feel normal in Terri's life, her cancer reappeared—only this time, if possible to believe, it was far worse.

Cancer rummages through a life like a tornado can rummage through an unsuspecting town. It has no conscience, shows no mercy, leaves nothing undisturbed. Cancer had taken everything but Terri's life. But this time, like a vengeful spirit, it seemed intent on fulfilling that final objective. *So much for ten-year lists.*

Cancer #3

Her oncologist explained that the cancer had recurred yet again and that it had exploded throughout her body. A bone marrow biopsy had come back positive. He immediately went to the math.

"We have to be realistic, Terri. I don't know if we can find a match for you. People with Middle Eastern heritage, unfortunately, have a low chance of finding a match with a sibling donor. Even if we did find a match, we might not be able to do another stem cell transplant by then. And if we do, odds are very low that we can beat this. I'm afraid we're talking ten percent or less, if we even make it that far. We need to deal with that reality, which brings a lot of other needs to the table—care, planning for end-of-life issues, things like that."

Terri didn't envy the brutal life of an oncologist, but she certainly didn't feel sorrier for him than for herself at that moment. *Well, Doc*, she thought to herself as he held her hand. *I'll take that as fifty-fifty odds. I'm going to die or not. Those are the real odds.*

Terri explained the situation to her family, and all three siblings agreed to find out if they were a potential match. Her sisters were ruled out, which wasn't bad, because Terri hadn't been sure if either would've gone through with it if they were a match. At first pass her brother wasn't a match, but there was enough of a question that they performed alternative tests. As fate and mathematics would have it, there was a fifty-fifty chance he was a viable donor. It was the only hope left for Terri.

The pretransplant procedures were performed in Washington, DC, but the transplant itself would happen in Seattle. Bob agreed he'd take two weeks off to go to Seattle and care for her posttransplant. For the next three to four weeks, Terri's mother had agreed to fly to Seattle and stay with her. By that time, Terri's parents had no choice but to face the graveness of her illness. Banalities like "everything will be okay" just weren't going to cut it anymore. Terri needed her family, and thankfully, her mom and brother came through for her.

Terri packed what little she needed—one doesn't need much for a four-to six-week hospital stay—and Bob dropped her off at the airport so she could fly to Seattle and begin the chemotherapy and transplant process. Terri's brother, who was in medical school in Nevada, had gone up to Seattle during his spring break several weeks before so his stem cells could be harvested and frozen.

Terri remembered how emotional the flight to DC had been when she left for college a dozen years before. As she sat on the plane shaking in fear, donning a surgical mask for protection from infection, she couldn't help but notice the contrast in circumstances between the two journeys. One had taken her to a place where she'd enjoy a lifetime's worth of possibilities; the other was taking her to a place where she'd face the very distinct possibility of death.

A week into the chemotherapy, less than a week before Bob was scheduled to arrive and not quite three weeks before her mom was scheduled to join her, Terri called Bob to give him her daily update call. A few minutes into the call, he dropped a bomb.

"I know you need me, Terri," he said. "I'm just not strong enough for this. I'm sorry, but I thought I could handle it. I can't. I don't know what to say other than I'm so sorry."

You bastards never know what to say, do you? I do . . . how about "go fuck yourself"?

"You're serious? You're not coming?" Terri asked.

"I wish I had two percent of the strength you do. I don't though. You deserve more, some type of explanation or something. I don't know. I just don't have it in me to maybe watch you, well . . . have it be so hard."

"You mean *die*? That could happen. It probably will. Or maybe it won't. But whatever. You don't owe me anything, Bob."

And just like that, Terri was alone on her life raft again.

• • •

Terri endured unimaginable physical, emotional, and mental difficulties during her second transplant procedure. Fortunately, her body didn't reject the donor cells. She didn't get graft-versus-host disease, a condition where the donor cells attack the host cells. She didn't get any infections while her white blood cell count was at zero or as her body took the donor cells and began the process of producing her own; the intense hormone therapy and the chemotherapy didn't result in her contracting veno-occlusive disease, a not-so-uncommon condition resulting in major liver problems and death. She endured it all.

The doctors had given her a less than 10 percent chance for survival. Terri chose to take a less fuzzy-math approach: fifty-fifty.

Terri's Epilogue

When I first met Terri, she was celebrating ten years cancer-free. She told me many stories about her cancer journey: the times she almost died, how she'd been abandoned by the people she wanted to rely on most, how every single person in her support group who went through what she did died except for her. She told me about one particular night when she found herself staring down from a multistory parking lot, contemplating whether she should be the one to determine when her life would end. If not for a timely call from a friend and mentor, she might've flipped a coin to answer the question for her.

Terri had been through the wringer, not just physically but psychologically, emotionally, and every other way. She's had to accept that she won't ever have kids. She might not find a lasting partner. She's been alone too often and for too long. She's struggled with the guilt of knowing she survived when so many others didn't, without a clue as to why. She's struggled with health issues. She lives with a constant fear of the future and can't seem to untether herself from the psychological, emotional, and physical grip of cancer.

"How have you dealt with so much?" I asked her one day.

"I know the sun's coming up tomorrow, with or without me," she said. "But every day I'm still here to see it, and there's a reason for that. I just haven't found out *why* yet. I guess the key for me is that I hope one day to find some answers to that question.

"It's like cancer rips you out of your life," she continued. "It puts you on a rickety raft in the middle of the ocean and sets you afloat. It steals you away from time, or steals time away from you, however you want to look at it. So, you're on the raft, with no protection from the waves or the burning sun. You have no food, nobody to help you, and no idea which way to paddle, because you don't even know how you got there. For me, I just believed that if I didn't die, I'd just keep paddling. At some point, maybe I'll find out where the current will take me, or maybe I won't. Hey, it's a fifty-fifty chance, right? Either way, as long as I can, I'm staying on the raft."

Nobody Talks

When planning my ride, I had to decide whether to take a southern route out of California into Arizona and through southern New Mexico and then Texas or if I was going to take a more northern route through Las Vegas, Nevada. Terri, whom I'd never met in person, lived in Albuquerque, while another book participant, Dominic, lived in Las Vegas. I determined it would be too much to visit both. I decided to take the southern route and avoid Nevada because I didn't *have* to visit Dominic on the ride, as I'd met him in person several times while visiting Las Vegas. In the end, it was the right call. With the necessarily aggressive daily route planning I was doing, I doubt I could have made it through the brutal Mojave Desert and the insane mountain ranges I would have encountered had I gone through Las Vegas. I also might've missed what turned out to be a seminal Sunday brunch with my friend Jerry and his family the night after I met Terri in Albuquerque.

So, days nine and ten saw me stick to my intended route and schedule, departing eastern Arizona to make my way through the Petrified Forest and onto Interstate 40, which I took into Gallup, New Mexico. I then ground through the passes between the Navajo and Zuni reservations and climbed the expansive and beautiful Laguna Pueblo area as I made my way to Albuquerque. As with almost every mile before, the two-hundred-plus miles between Holbrook, Arizona, and Albuquerque, New Mexico, were fraught with challenges: long hills that seemed only to go up, headwinds that came straight at me no matter the direction, temperatures high enough to melt the asphalt, nutrition issues, hydration issues, and hectic highways packed with speeding vehicles seemingly intent on scaring the shit out of me as they raced a few precious feet away from me at breakneck speeds. My impending rest day couldn't have come at a more crucial time in the ride. I was exhausted in every sense of the word.

At the end of day ten, after a huge steakhouse dinner with Terri followed by long, emotional hugs, Erin and I headed back to the hotel where we were staying. My phone rang. It was Jerry, who'd traveled with us all the way from Phoenix to Albuquerque, where he had loads of family.

"Brother," he said, "I got an idea."

"Uh oh," I replied.

"No, seriously. I know you're taking a day off tomorrow, and I'd like you and Erin to go to brunch with my family. My dad, my sister and her husband, and a few other family members want to buy you guys a meal."

Jerry had told me about his sister, a stage III breast cancer survivor who had a bilateral mastectomy, and his father, who was a fifteen-year stage II lymphoma survivor. I agreed.

After we sat down, Jerry had me tell everyone what I was doing and why. Jerry's father, a quiet man in his late seventies who was sitting at the head of the table to my left, tapped my shoulder and waved me in.

"Jerry talked to me about you," he said softly. "I want to tell you, what you're doing, this getting people to talk about their cancer, it's a good thing. I think people are going to learn a lot when they hear the stories of what we go through in here, and here." He pointed to his chest, then his temple.

Later in the meal, Jerry's sister, who was sitting to my right and across the table, leaned in and motioned for me to do the same. "Did Jerry tell you what I went through?" she asked.

"Only highlights, I'm sure. He told me you had a pretty tough battle with cancer about five years ago, and after, you left your career to become a lobbyist for patient rights."

"Yeah, cancer did a tsunami on my life—turned it totally inside out," she said. "When Jerry told me what you're doing, I was so excited. People talk about cancer, but they don't share their feelings about it with each other, do they? I'm sure your book will help so many people."

"That's true, people don't share their feelings," I replied. "So if these stories help people deal with what they're going through or help them learn how to support the people they know who are going through trauma, it'll make a huge difference in everybody's life. That's the whole goal, anyway."

When we finished eating and were getting ready to say our goodbyes, I asked for everyone's attention. "Erin and I appreciate you all taking time for us. Thank you," I said to the group. "It's so refreshing to see a family that's so close. It's rare that you have a man who goes through cancer while staying old-school tough and providing for his family and just plain *dealing*, and also a daughter who went through such a traumatic and life-altering experience, and through it all, to talk and share the way you guys did so you could fully understand each other."

I glanced over at Jerry's dad. He lowered his eyes. I looked over at Jerry's sister, and she did the same.

"Wait. You guys did talk, right?" Neither looked up. Both were silent.

"But you both just got done telling me how important it is! How people need to read a book about people like you so it helps them communicate about their feelings, to better deal with the emotions of cancer. You two didn't *talk* about what you went through?"

Jerry's dad looked up at me. "No, sir. I didn't want to burden my children. I grew up, well, in a time when you don't burden your family like that."

Jerry's sister looked over at her dad, tears streaming down her face. "I kind of knew what he went through. But when I got cancer, I didn't want him to worry, you know, after what he must have went through."

"But you're so close," I said.

"We are." She acknowledged the nodding heads around the table. "We're all close. We just haven't talked about *that* so much."

Almost every person I spoke to for *Cycle of Lives* told me about their difficulties in dealing with the emotions of cancer and about communicating with others about it or any trauma, for that matter. Jerry's family was another perfect example of why I needed to write this book.

Dominic

Relationship to cancer: Patient, survivor

Age: Forty-seven

Family status: Married with three children, one with severe physical and mental disabilities, two stepchildren

Location: Las Vegas, Nevada

First encounter with cancer: Nineteen years old

Cancer summary: Diagnosed with advanced Hodgkin's lymphoma for the first time when he was nineteen years old. He had a relapse at thirty and underwent a stem cell transplant. Diagnosed with mesothelioma during our talks and underwent an immediate and aggressive chemotherapy treatment. In total, he has had hundreds of radiation and chemotherapy treatments.

Treatment specifics: Hodgkin's lymphoma, stage IVB; relapse of Hodgkin's lymphoma, stage IVB; advanced mesothelioma, stage III

Strongest positive emotion during cancer experience: Relief

Strongest negative emotion during cancer experience: Desolation

How we met: A few years ago, a friend and I were in Las Vegas to attend a three-day music festival. At the end of the initial night, we left the venue in the wee hours of the morning and found ourselves wandering among a sea of zombielike festival-goers in search of transportation back to civilization. Out of nowhere, a white van appeared, and the window rolled down.

"You guys need a ride?" a man asked, his eyes darting around nervously.

"Hell yeah, we do," I said.

"Hurry up and get in," he said. "Twenty bucks each to hotels on the Strip. I'll get you there fast and safe."

Fast and safe *and* cheap didn't seem possible. First, the crowd of people and cars was huge. We expected it would take at least an hour or two to get back, as it had taken almost three hours to get to the venue earlier in the night. Second, "safe" wasn't the first impression I got about the driver. He was jumpy, skittish, and shifty. Third, we knew calling a taxi would cost upwards of a hundred dollars, so how was this guy doing it for twenty bucks? But we were exhausted, the sun was about to rise, and we felt certain we could handle ourselves if something went down. We jumped in the van, and the driver sped off.

"I'm not exactly supposed to be picking people up," he said. "But nobody's sweatin' me yet. It's no big thing, really. I don't think they will. This is my fifth trip back and forth. Been driving in this town since I was fourteen. Nobody tells me what I can and can't do—not when I'm behind the wheel. I'll get a couple more trips in tonight, for sure. Hey, where do you guys want to go?"

He continued to talk, but I didn't pay full attention to his words. I was too distracted by his driving. He was all over the place, weaving between barricades, going the wrong way down one-way lanes, passing "Do Not Enter" signs without hesitation—even navigating the open desert next to the highway to pass by the bottlenecked vehicles.

"Name's Dominic. Call me Dom," he said and put his right arm behind the front seat to extend a homemade business card. "Go ahead. Take this, and I'll hook you up tomorrow, too. You got any friends? Twenty bucks a head. You hear that in the back? That noise? That's a full cooler of drinks. Beers, vodka, Red Bulls, Fireball, tequila, you name it. You guys want anything?"

Even at five in the morning, Dominic was a ball of energy. It was easy to surmise that he was part hustler, part concierge. He appeared to be in his element driving like a crazy man—albeit a totally in-control crazy man—and I felt oddly safe in the back of his van. He had an "I got this" air about him that made it easy to relax. I sat back and enjoyed the ride, the nonstop flow of words, the endless lines of cars on the road, and the clouds of dust kicking up behind us.

The next day, my friend and I called Dom for a ride back to the festival. We were refreshed from a hard sleep, a hot ten-mile run, and a few gallons of icy cold water. As we sat in the back of Dom's van, we began to talk about endurance athletics, which led to the topic of the Cycle of Lives project.

"So, you're going to bike across the country? For cancer?" Dom asked, unapologetic about joining the conversation. "You're writing a book about cancer?"

"Yeah," I said. "It's about different people with pretty incredible cancer-related life stories. We're talking about their emotional journeys, not the nitty-gritty cancer stuff. It's more about the psychological side of things."

"Well, if you're writing a book about cancer, I've got a story for you," Dominic said, his eyes meeting mine in the rearview mirror. "And it's a real doozy."

As he rattled off the headlines of his cancer experiences, Dominic zipped between cars and raced perilously along the severely sloping shoulder. By the time we reached our intended drop-off spot, my stomach was swimming with nausea from the ride, and my head was spinning with intrigue from Dominic's story. Both faded as Chad and I made our way into the festival. What remained was a strong sense that I'd found someone else who was perfect for this project.

Waiting to Live

E ven though the heavy scent of fall was in the air, it was still unbelievably hot—like 110 degrees hot. He'd lived in Vegas all of his nineteen years, and the dry desert heat didn't usually bother him, or even cause him to sweat, but that day he stopped running down the court mid-play and walked over to a bench under a tree. Sweat dripped from every pore on his body. It was just a little pickup game. He was barely working. The sweat didn't make sense. He felt lightheaded, and his breathing was heavy. His neck started feeling too weak to hold his head up, and his eyelids were irresistibly heavy. His head fell forward, as if he might pass out. He tried to shake it off, but a darkness was overtaking him, closing in from all around. He could feel himself start to slump off the bench, but he couldn't do anything about it. He was too weak; his sensibilities had vanished. The last thing he remembered was the feeling of his cheek hitting the asphalt.

He didn't remember how he got home and into his bed, but that's where Dominic woke up. His head was pounding, his neck too sore to move. He was thirsty, but his throat felt too swollen and raw to get some water. Besides, he was too tired to get up. He couldn't move even if he wanted to.

What the hell kind of flu is this, anyway? Dominic thought to himself.

He managed the strength to reach up and touch the throbbing area on his cheek. A bandage of some sort covered it. It felt wet underneath.

My cheek was hurt? That's right, I fell. Right on the ground, face-first. But what happened after? How did I get home? I'll figure it out after I sleep some more.

Dominic wasn't just tired; he was *tired*—as though he hadn't slept in a week tired. Sleep came again, and it came easy.

When he woke, it was night. He tried to clear his head, but the only thought that penetrated the haze was that he needed to use the bathroom, and he didn't know how he was going to lift himself out of the bed. He closed his eyes to think. It was either get up or pee right there. Those were the only two choices.

It took all he had, but Dominic managed to get his legs over the edge of the bed and push himself up to a seated position. The urgency of needing to relieve himself hit Dominic in a wave, but he moved in slow motion. The door to the hallway seemed a million miles away, but he needed to cover the distance fast or else he wasn't going to be able to hold on inside.

Somehow, he made it to the door and stumbled down the hall into the bathroom. As he pulled his shorts down, he thought about sitting down, but then he didn't know if he'd be able to get up again. He stood and waited, the pain inside making him swim with nausea. Relief would be so easy now that he stood over the toilet.

He waited, the pressure building, but he couldn't get his bladder to release. He closed his eyes and tried to picture the feeling of letting go, but some kind of clamp deep inside prevented it. The pain sharpened even more, and it felt as if he was going to explode inside, but the clamp wouldn't let go. He felt as if he would scream from the buildup of pressure, but as the scream made its way to his throat, a flash of white light exploded inside him, from his brain down to the middle of his back. He let out a guttural sound of relief. The stream came red hot and fast out of him, and once he let go, the rest of his insides followed suit. He became lightheaded, a thick sweat suddenly blanketing his skin, and he felt as though his intestines were going to fall out of him. He'd been heavily asleep just two minutes before, and now he felt as if he wanted to die on the spot, hollowed out and shriveled like a deflated human-balloon in front of the toilet. He fell to his knees, the stream hitting the front of the bowl, and all went dark.

The next time Dominic woke up, he was in the hospital with an IV in his arm. His dad sat in a chair next to the bed he was in.

"How are you feeling?" his dad asked.

"Okay, I guess," Dominic answered.

"They did some tests—X-rays, scans, blood tests. You've been pretty out of it for a while. They've been keeping you that way," his dad said.

They stared at each other for a bit, and then his dad looked away. His dad loved to talk, to give advice, and to tell stories, but when he didn't want to talk, there was no guessing at his thoughts. He simply shut down. Dominic remembered feeling a creeping sense of worry, and not long after, a team of three doctors and a pair of nurses walked into the room. The air they carried made Dominic's stomach drop and the blood drain from his head.

Three doctors? Seriously?

The doctor who seemed to be in charge spoke first. "I'm Dr. Livinsky. I'm a hematologist. A blood doctor," he said, looking at Dominic. "Dr. Richards is the staff oncologist. Dr. Parito is our chief radiologist."

"Why so many doctors?" Dominic asked, looking at his dad.

"Did you figure out what's wrong with him?" his dad asked.

"Things are not good," the doctor said and paused, allowing the ominous thought a moment to reverberate.

"Not good *how*?" his dad asked.

"We've explored many possibilities in the last couple of days. There's no other way to say it given the urgency of what we need to do. We need to be straight with you both," Dr. Livinsky said. He nodded at Dr. Richards, who continued from there.

"Your son has a very advanced case of cancer," Dr. Richards said. "How advanced, we don't know yet. The CT scan showed that the cancer is in his neck, but there are problems in his chest, lymph nodes, and liver." He looked at Dominic. "The core needle biopsy results aren't in, and we don't know what type of lymphoma you have. Because the cancer's spread in such a quick and aggressive manner, we can't really wait out the results. Your body has no way to fight against it, and it's progressed to a very serious stage."

"I'm just a little sick. What are you saying?" Dominic asked.

"Again, it's quite severe," the doctor repeated patiently. "These things sometimes take a long time to progress to this level. It's not unusual to feel fine until the moment you don't."

"What do you mean?" Dominic's dad asked.

"As you might know, we classify the advancement of cancer by stages one through four, with four being the most formidable," the oncologist said. "We need to do more tests, but we believe your son's cancer has advanced well into stage four. It has metastasized throughout his body. In other words, even with an immediate and aggressive treatment regimen of both radiation and chemotherapy, he most likely cannot survive the cancer. Without treatment, he has no chance to survive it. We still need to determine what we're dealing with, but that won't take much longer."

The color went out of Dominic's dad's face, and he slumped into the back of the chair, as if someone pulled a plug and let some of the air out of him. Dominic had never seen his dad look pale and weak, but at that moment he looked *frail*. Dominic pulled his gaze away from his dad. He couldn't let his dad see him staring at his weakness.

Dominic's head began to spin. He tried to keep his focus on the doctors—their mouths moved, but he couldn't hear them. The spinning in his head drowned out all sound. His stomach became tight and sour, and an acidic flow began to rush up from his gut. It climbed. His mouth started to water. Desperation flooded him. A feeling of nausea overtook his whole body. Before he could find a more appropriate place to do it, the rush in his chest exploded, and Dominic vomited all over the blanket covering him. One of the nurses stepped around the doctors and began to clean Dominic's face; another pulled the soiled blanket off him and replaced it with a fresh one.

"Again, we'll need to begin at once," the blood doctor said, unfazed. "Dr. Richards will discuss what we have in mind for treatment."

"Just cut it out," Dominic said, still trying to catch his breath from vomiting.

"If that were an option, we'd use it," Dr. Richards said. "Your cancer is in the lymphatic system. Treatment is limited, and surgery isn't an option with this type of cancer. Like I said, we'll need to find out more in the coming days, but we should talk about what's in store."

Less than three days had passed since Dominic had simply felt weak playing basketball, but as he watched Dr. Richards exit his hospital room, he knew odds were high he might die before he turned twenty. It was impossible to make sense of.

Waiting to Die

The days that followed were quiet, hazy, and entirely surreal. Dominic was in a kind of heavy waking sleep and felt he was moving through time as if it were quicksand. He struggled to stay awake from minute to minute, trying to maintain awareness of anything beyond his pillow and the phone as he waited for the doctors to call and tell him more. Then the call came.

A couple of days later, Dominic and his dad went to Dr. Richards's office. They learned that Dominic was going to be given large doses of a combination of drugs. They'd scan his body along the way to see where the cancer localized. After the chemotherapy, they would use radiation to kill the tumors. He'd lose his hair and his appetite and be susceptible to infection. His body would essentially be ravaged from all the poison.

"Fuck my hair. How much of a chance to live, Doc? Give it to me straight," Dominic wanted to say.

The doctor told him that if he was lucky, no tumors would turn up anywhere other than his liver and in the lymph nodes in his neck, where tumors were already growing. That way they could minimize and localize the radiation therapy. If tumors cropped up elsewhere, the scans would detect them, and radiation would work to kill them off. If he were strong enough after the chemotherapy and the radiation, his body might not be too destroyed to attempt to recover.

"The unfortunate reality is that a large percentage of patients in your condition don't stand much of a chance to survive treatment that aggressive," the doctor said. "But people do recover. I can't promise you much of a chance, I'm afraid. Onset and progression this rapid is rare, but we'll do everything possible. I *can* promise you that."

Those few days waiting to hear may have dragged on, but once the chemotherapy treatment started—the day after learning he might die soon—entire weeks passed, and Dominic hardly noticed. He was in a constant state of semi-consciousness—a half-alive, half-dead trance punctuated by vomiting, lying on the bathroom floor, being carried from the car to his bed by his dad, and being too tired to get out of bed to pee.

For brief periods, though, stretches that lasted five or fifty minutes—never more, sometimes less—Dominic was aware enough to assess things. When he had those moments of awareness, he'd look in the mirror. He barely recognized himself, and he stared at his reflection as though confronted with an enemy. His skin was a pale, sickly green, and his body was gaunt and skinny. His face was red and puffy. His eyes were yellow and clouded. He was never hungry, and any food he tried to eat only stayed down for minutes. Every once in a while, he could stomach a sip or two of ginger ale, but if he were optimistic and tried a third or fourth, his gut would wrench it right up. He didn't have conversations; instead, he answered questions with a "s'okay" or a "mmnogood" or some such thing. He wanted to talk, but he didn't have the strength or the clarity of mind to make any sense.

When he'd slumped off the park bench on that fateful September day, Dominic weighed about 170 pounds. Four months later, the scale read 120. During that time, and throughout the tormenting chemotherapy, his hair fell out, his teeth became weak and sensitive, his fingernails and toenails turned a cloudy yellow, and he had almost no awareness left. He was an apparition of his former self, not dead but not quite alive. When one day, a doctor asked if he and his dad had made "preparations," Dominic looked at his dad and asked, "S'okay to die?" His dad nodded, and Dominic drifted away.

Life After Dying

But Dominic did not die. He didn't so much put up a fight as he simply never let go of his tenuous hold on life. Over the next six months, his body withstood several cycles of chemotherapy, followed by multiple doses of radiation and a hundred other various treatments. Dr. Richards had told him he had a 20 percent chance of living, but it was the 80 percent chance of dying that got all the attention. It's hard to list everything that *could* have killed him, from the horrible reaction to the first treatment of an experimental drug to the staph infection from an infected port. Everything about his experience with the myriad procedures and treatments (drugs and antibiotics, along with their infections and other reactions) was punctuated by serious talks and warnings of doom from his various caregivers. But nothing killed him.

Eventually, the treatments ended, and when they did, traces of the old Dominic returned: His hair started to grow back, his appetite slowly returned, and healthier blood flowed through his body, muting the rainbow of colors in his complexion that had made him look so sick. He even began to stay conscious of the continuum of days. He stepped back over the line and was very much alive again—at least physically.

• • •

There are many immediate and lasting physical side effects of enduring a battle with stage IVB Hodgkin's lymphoma, and in the months and years that followed, Dominic avoided most of them. As for emotional side effects, there was only one, and it quietly gnawed away at him every single day. It scratched his brain, it scarred his heart, and it drained all the hope and optimism a nineteen-years-young man could ever contain inside of him. He never verbalized it because he couldn't recognize it. The act of accepting his death had forever changed something inside him. *S'okay to die?* became a part of his DNA. Living wasn't even supposed to be an option. After all, his doctors told him he'd die. His dad had given him the okay to die. He had done everything but *actually* die, and that tiny formality came to rule his life.

In his twenties, the decade that could have seen him mature and begin to make his place in the world, meet a partner, maybe build a family, Dominic instead dove headfirst into a dark, swirling world. It was one that brought him ever closer to realizing what he conceived of as his destiny to die young. Except by the time he turned thirty, Dominic wasn't dead, and he wasn't young.

• • •

Las Vegas in the early 1990s was part burgeoning Las Vegas Strip, part urban expansion, and part filth, crime, and seediness. Those immersed in the Strip life saw dozens of hotel and casino transformations take place. Out went the old Sinatra-era resorts, and in came the corporate-era mega-hotels. Americans were becoming wealthier, along with many overseas, and entrepreneurial developers wanted to attract them—and their endless disposable cash—to a glitzier, more opulent Las Vegas experience. As a result, a growing local population began to stabilize, demanding homes, schools, grocery stores, and soccer fields for their young families, instead of the apartments, dingy strip malls, 7-Elevens, and local bars that supported the previous, more transient casino workforce.

Dominic wasn't a part of either of those groups. Those people belonged to the *living*. Instead, he existed in the criminal, drug-ridden, violent underbelly of Vegas, where marijuana, crack cocaine, methamphetamines, and other substances flowed freely. It was a place where people couldn't afford to get on the right *or* wrong side of the tracks. They lived in between the tracks, where a reckless and dangerous train of destruction constantly rolled.

Dominic used drugs and crime to numb himself on his journey toward certain death. At times he dabbled, at times he was addicted, but he became familiar with cocaine, meth, heroin, alcohol, and anything else he could use to get high, make money, or both. It was pain pills, though, that brought him the most trouble. The use of two powerful painkillers had helped him get through his bout with cancer, but that use led to addiction, and his addictions to hydrocodone and oxycodone ultimately landed him in prison for the robbery and theft he committed to maintain supplies.

Doing time in the state penitentiary wasn't easy, but prison wasn't a difficult place for Dominic, either. "Prison wasn't nothin' but a thing, really," he said.

He wasn't a hardened criminal—far from it. He was just a lost soul, but lost souls often wind up on the streets, in mental institutions, or in prisons. Prison was better than the alternatives. Being locked up helped break Dominic of his drug addictions—he wasn't willing to do the things he would have needed to do to score painkillers inside, so he went without. A couple of years flew by in a snap. There were no memories to keep, no benchmarks to measure, no progressions to track—beyond the formality of a couple birthdays spent in prison. In or out of prison, Dominic awoke each day in the fog of death, with nothing to live for, and he lay in bed each night void of any contemplation or hope.

After prison, Dominic got a series of odd jobs. He worked in construction, as a doorman, as a driver, as a host at his dad's strip club—anything that would keep him off the streets but was temporary enough to allow him to drift away. If anything began to settle in, he moved on. This was true in every aspect of his life. He kept his brothers and sisters at arm's length. They couldn't understand what he'd gone through. He kept his mom at a distance, too. She was divorced and struggling to make sense of her ruined family life. She'd had nine children, all of whom were scattered and distant. Dominic even kept his dad at a remove. He'd been such a burden to his dad when he was sick that Dominic was surely a disappointment to him. For more than ten years, Dominic managed to avoid anything and everything that would provide him any identity or sense of belonging.

During those lost years, one of the few commitments he kept was to see Dr. Richards for blood tests every year or so. Dominic didn't put much thought into being tested. He was either going to remain cancer-free or not. He couldn't control it, so he didn't worry about it. Dominic never attempted to look too far into the future, so if the cancer came back, there wouldn't be anything to derail. He didn't get tested because it was the right thing to do, because he could catch a relapse early, or because he had anything to live for. He went because he told his dad that he would. He owed his dad at least that much.

A few months after his thirtieth birthday, Dr. Richards's office called. "We need you to come back today if you can. The doctor is concerned about the results from your blood work, and he needs to talk with you—today, if possible."

Here it comes again. Figures, Dominic thought.

"This Time, You're Going to Die"

"It's not altogether uncommon for the lymphoma to reappear," Dr. Richards said. "But we found no signs just fourteen months ago, and today, well, it's reappeared in a very aggressive fashion."

"What's that mean, exactly?" Dominic asked. His brain flashed back to ten years prior when his dad had asked Dr. Richards the same question.

"I wish I could tell you otherwise, but we don't have many options. Without treatment you'll die—and soon, I'm afraid. The cancer isn't in your chest area again, so we can do both chemotherapy *and* radiation, but the protocol for this type of relapse is rather aggressive and very difficult. We'll need to harvest and freeze your stem cells. A high-dosage regimen of drugs will remove the existing cancer cells from your blood. Then we'll likely aim for a complete bone marrow ablation—destroying your body's ability to produce any new blood cells—with a different chemo regimen and maybe radiation. Once we're at the point where your body can't produce any new cells, we'll reintroduce the frozen stem cells in the hopes they'll help your body to resume production of normal, cancer-free blood cells."

"Doesn't sound like much fun, really," Dominic said.

"Well, it's risky, yes. The cancer's even more advanced this time, but I have to be straight with you—medicine has come a long way in the last ten years, but there may be only months left. We'll do what we can, but the road ahead is going to be tough. Your body will be left without an immune system for a time, and there's a major risk of infection. We could see severe liver injury and mucositis. We'll go over the risks, but we can't promise anything."

"And after?"

"I can't say how things will go. There are a number of factors that could come up, so we'll have to see. I can't make any promises, though of course we'll try everything. Ultimately, a lot will depend on how your body handles everything."

What about my mind, Doc? How does my mind handle everything?

Dr. Richards told Dominic to go home and let it sink in but that soon they would need to complete a whole series of tests and preparations for his treatment. He would have to be prepared to be in the hospital for the entirety of testing and treatment.

Yeah, the whole time until the cancer is gone, or I am.

Everything else needed to be put on hold, Dr. Richards stressed. Fighting the cancer would take everything he had.

On hold? That's a good one. Let me break the news to you, Doc: There's nothing to put on hold.

And just like that, just like before, one day Dominic was fine and the next he'd learned he was going to die.

Dominic stayed up most of that night. He sat out front of his apartment, staring into the distance and thinking of nothing beyond how his dad would take the news. Dominic didn't panic. He didn't feel overwhelmed for himself. He felt numb, like the numbness of being sentenced to jail or having a gun shoved in his face when a drug deal went bad, not caring if the other guy pulled the trigger.

I got a few months to live? It's no big thing, really.

He smoked more than an entire pack of cigarettes as he weighed being straight with his dad versus keeping the news to himself. When he'd finished the last cigarette he could recycle out of the crammed-full ashtray for a couple more puffs, he decided that if he was going to try to fight the cancer, he had to figure out a way to keep the truth about how serious it was from his dad. Dominic knew what his last bout with cancer had done to his dad, and he didn't want to burden his father again with the thought that he was going to lose a son. Dominic thought maybe he should just die without saying anything about it until he had to. But if he was going to fight, his dad deserved to see that Dominic at least *wanted* to live. He fell asleep on the couch before he decided if he could fake that part—the desire to live. After all, Dominic never really *wanted* to live; he just lived.

When he awoke, a couple hours had passed. The sun was still rising over the hills far east of town. He had a choice to make: go get a pack of cigarettes, come home and hide from reality until it killed him, or go to his dad's house, tell him about the cancer, and get ready for the tests.

Dominic drove to his dad's. It took all the strength he had to get out of the car. As he told his dad what Dr. Richards had said, Dominic felt numb. His mind and heart were frozen with shock and dread. No tears came, no blood colored his cheeks, his voice didn't crack. He spoke softly, without emotion.

"We'll just have to see what they say, son," his dad said. "We'll just have to see."

Two days later, after spending almost twelve hours undergoing tests and preparations, Dominic was admitted to the hospital. The commotion, helplessness, disconcerting smells, and unnerving chaos of having doctors and nurses working to save him from a hidden enemy began again.

The following day, as he lay in another hospital bed, doctors told Dominic what to expect. And once again, as was the case a decade prior, Dominic had to watch his dad hear that his son was going to die.

• • •

The initial round of second-line chemotherapy was lighter than treatment yet to come, because they also injected growth hormone drugs into Dominic each day to increase his stem cell count. After about a week and a half, the growth hormone treatment stopped, the stem cells were harvested, and the high-dosage chemotherapy treatments began.

The hardest thing for Dominic in the first two weeks was quitting smoking. Over the years, Dominic had occasionally felt a twinge of guilt about smoking, but only ever a twinge. He'd seen the reality with his eyes: People in cancer wards went outside to smoke. Hell, some of the doctors and nurses smoked, and none of them had likely ever gone through the things Dominic had. Cancer or not, smoking was the one vice he'd held onto. Giving it up felt like giving up a confidante, something he could always turn to for support and comfort. With that comfort gone, Dominic experienced a new level of desperation about his situation. Not being able to smoke was almost enough of a reason for Dominic to pull the plug on the whole thing.

Coming in a close second to the struggle of quitting cigarettes was the embarrassment and demoralization of not being entitled to a minute's privacy. Aggressive treatment for stage IV recurrent Hodgkin's lymphoma came with a slew of side effects, and between receiving enemas for his constipation, filling buckets full of yellow bile to be replaced by empty ones to fill again, the occasional bout of incontinence, and not being able to stay awake even when he was being given a sponge bath or injected with needles, Dominic could do nothing but accept feeling on display and having his body be physically manipulated all the time. *All the time.* And it was both uncomfortable and humiliating.

Being exposed to the world for how frail he was and how pathetic he felt inspired a whole palate of emotions Dominic hadn't known he had and that he was unprepared to handle. As a result, two things happened: He often cried tears of helplessness that seemed to have a will of their own, and he almost stopped talking entirely. He just never knew what to say or even how to formulate words. Instead, he nodded or shook his head. Anger, frustration, sadness, self-pity, shame, and desperation coursed through his poisoned blood, and he fell mute, a silent victim of his own internal emotional collapse.

As weeks passed and his treatment progressed, Dominic became too weak to talk, even if he could have figured out how to express himself. Blinking made him hurt with exhaustion. He vaguely remembered people—his mom, a brother or sister, one of his friends—stopping by to visit, but he didn't speak to them. He just listened, disconnected, as they talked to his dad, who seemed to always be there. Dominic knew he was dying. In fact, dying was the only thing he knew for sure. Throwing up, going to the bathroom, taking shots, receiving radiation—they were all harsh, blurry flashes of memory. Even the comfort of the permanent sleep he thought would ease it all away was lost in the painful realizations of waking up over and over. For years, Dominic had felt that at some point his death would come easily, but lying in the hospital, ten weeks into treatment, he became aware it wouldn't be peaceful.

But one day, a voice came through the fog. Suddenly, he had something his brain was able to focus on, that helped words arrange themselves in a way that made sense.

"S'okay," Dominic heard a female voice softly say. "I'm just checking a few things out. No needles from me now. Promise."

Dominic tried to open his eyes to make sense of the voice, but the light in the room was too much. He attempted to make sense of his surroundings by doing a mental inventory: He was lying down. He couldn't tell if he had the strength to move, but he could at least feel a tingling sensation in his fingers and toes. He could feel a tube coming from his chest and another coming from his arm. He couldn't swallow, but his stomach felt full and bloated. He could feel soft air coming into each nostril, which meant he was being given oxygen. There was that hospital smell he hated. No amount of damage to his senses could blunt that awful smell.

"I'm not dead yet?" he asked. The words had come out, though he didn't remember trying to speak. As he felt warm tears run down his temples, Dominic didn't know if he was crying out of joy or sadness.

"No. You're certainly not dead," the soft voice said. She was a nurse, and over the next few weeks, she talked with him, cared for him, helped him think about something other than death. She also brought him his first real experience of love. His relationship with that soft-voiced nurse ended up being as short-lived as the fuzzy memories of his ordeal, but it wasn't any less real. It ended when Dominic failed to return the letters she wrote to him when he was discharged from the hospital to continue recovering at home. Wanting love and being open to it were still two vastly different things for Dominic.

A Third Chance at Life

Dominic slowly regained pieces of himself. Death went away, and the fog burned off. Soon after, he was able to hang on to thoughts for brief periods of time, and then to speak coherently. He even attempted to contemplate some of the emotional residue left by this latest bout with cancer. He didn't understand much of it: the desperation, fear, despair, hope, gratitude, and disgust. He had no roadmap to help him navigate his emotions, let alone process them. At least he could recognize there was more than just dying to think about.

In time, Dominic gained enough strength to rebuild his life. He went back to working whatever jobs a bankrupt, low-energy, two-time-cancer-surviving ex-con with no college degree could find. He also met someone he could relate to. She was a former drug addict and convict who, like Dominic, spent more days wondering why she was alive than building a life. Within a couple of years, they were married and divorced. In between, they had two kids, and she spent every dollar they could find on drugs, bail, or lawyers, helping Dominic down the road toward a ruined destiny.

Life continued for Dominic as a single dad, but his struggles intensified. Sometimes his ex-wife was in jail, and sometimes, Dominic had to turn her away when she came by the house high on drugs and looking for money. At least she was largely absent. Dominic's health was stable, and his first child, a girl, was healthy too. His second child, a son, was severely disabled both mentally and physically, likely as a result of his ex's drug use during pregnancy.

Dominic's dad helped, as did the occasional family member, but somehow Dominic managed to keep things together mostly on his own. Maybe it was his stubbornness, maybe it was the guilt he felt for bringing two kids into his dark, gloomy world, but Dominic stayed clean. He tried to keep his past where it belonged. Somehow, he managed to keep food in the fridge, help his daughter with her homework, clean his boy's sheets, carry him to his wheelchair, and make it to doctor's appointments.

One night, there was a banging on the door. He barely recognized his ex-wife. She was strung out, desperate. She looked twenty years older than when they divorced just five years previous.

"I got nothing for you," Dominic said, closing the door on her.

"Wait, please." There was something vulnerable, something human in her look.

"What?" Dominic asked.

"Come to the car. I need your help."

Dominic looked over her shoulder. Something didn't feel right.

"It's okay," she said. "I'm alone—except for the baby."

Dominic agreed to take the baby. Without him, the little one would have no father, family, or chance at a life. He demanded only one condition: that his ex never come looking to take the child back.

"We're fine without you," he said. "We don't need you." He looked down at the baby girl in his arms. "She's not ever going to need you either."

• • •

When his eldest daughter was twelve, his son was ten, and his youngest daughter (whom he formally adopted) was six, Dominic's former nurse found him on Facebook. Marlene was divorced and had two kids of her own. Although she'd lost some of the sweetness he remembered, she offered Dominic things he hadn't felt since those days in the hospital many years before: hope and comfort. She gave him a sense that it was all right to just *be*. He may not have thought much about his future, but when he was with her, he could at least live in the present. She was a good person: stable, reliable, *living* her life. It made Dominic think about the future in a way he'd never done. He came to believe he might have things to live for, to plan for, to build toward.

Dominic's Epilogue

In the very first conversation I had with Dominic a couple weeks after we met, we talked about the details of his cancer experiences, his obsession with death, and how Marlene had given him some perspective on life. We discussed how he was still afraid he might die before his dad did, how proud he was of his daughters, and how afraid he was of what would happen to his disabled son if the cancer came back to claim him. Dominic never stopped smoking, even though he'd been diagnosed with degenerative heart disease as a result of all the treatments he'd endured. We talked about regret. Dominic wished he had kept journals, taken more pictures, and done some type of planning to manage his reality. Mostly, though, we talked about how it had taken Dominic forty-seven years to realize that he shouldn't be dead and to believe that he would live to see the future.

Over the next eighteen months, I talked to Dominic many times. I was touched by the depth of his epiphanies. I came to admire his honesty and the way he plainly admitted to having wasted so many years. It was always followed with the kind of optimism and hope that never failed to surprise me coming from someone who'd endured as much as he had.

A few weeks after one of our last big talks, Dominic asked if I would meet him for breakfast the next time I was in town. Less than two weeks later, we got together. He'd lost about thirty pounds in the few months since I'd seen him. He couldn't eat much, he said. Most of his teeth were missing—he needed a lot of dental work—and he was rushing to get it done before his new course of treatment started.

"Mesothelioma," he told me. "They don't know yet how severe, but I've done a lot of reading, and it's definitely a death sentence. I applied to be part of a trial in Chicago. Most likely they won't take me because of my two other cancers. I don't know."

The waiter came to take our order, oblivious to the gravity of the conversation he'd interrupted.

"I'll take a large stack, four pieces of bacon, a side of hash browns, and water," Dominic told the waiter. He turned to me. "I won't be able to eat more than a couple of bites, but I really want some pancakes and bacon. Marlene would kill me, but I just want a taste."

The tumors were primarily in his stomach, and eating was becoming difficult.

"I haven't told my dad yet," he admitted. "I've been avoiding him. I'll have to tell him soon. I don't know—" he said, stopping short to fight back tears. "I don't know what will happen to my son when I die. My girls will be okay, but he's . . . he'll have to be put in an institution. My dad can't take care of him, and Marlene has her own kids to worry about."

"Is there any way to beat this?" I asked. "You've beaten the odds twice, right?"

"Not this time," he said. "They haven't come out and said so, but I've read enough. There's no way I'll survive very long—three, maybe six months, but definitely no more than a year."

"What are you going to do?" I asked.

"I think I need to tell my daughters the truth, about everything," he replied. "I've protected them from so much. My son, he wouldn't understand these kinds of things. I'm going to try and take them away for a few days before the treatments start. I want to go buy journals so I can write some stuff down."

Our food arrived, and Dominic looked at his plate with both gratitude and longing.

"I want to think it's not really a big thing this time, you know? But the third time is usually a charm."

Five months later I attended his memorial.

In one of the last conversations I had with Dominic, several weeks before he died, we talked about his legacy.

"I know I didn't do much in life," Dominic said. "But, you know, I've got amazing kids, Marlene and I had some good years, and I finally did something big with my life. This mesothelioma, it's gonna give my kids and Marlene a lifetime's worth of comfort."

He was party to a large lawsuit and was shortly to receive a substantial settlement.

"Funny," he said. "Could have come from the hospital, could have come from the prison. How many people can say that? Either way, at least my death is gonna count for something."

He also talked about how grateful he was that he finally gathered the courage to open up to his kids and tell them about his life.

There were easily a hundred people gathered to pay their respects at Dominic's service. Many told stories of how Dominic was so selfless and such a good parent, how he did so much to care for his disabled son, how he worked so hard to provide for his family, how he had finally opened up and learned how to love and be loved.

Seeing all those people talk about how much of a positive impact Dominic had on them, I thought about how great it was that he finally decided to live.

Help from Above

Although the route for day twelve was more than a hundred miles, including a lot of climbs along the highway toward Santa Rosa, New Mexico, it was the first day that brought me a tailwind. It was a glorious, strong, leg-comforting, all-day-long tailwind that almost brought tears to my eyes I was so grateful. The difference between cranking the pedals for ten-plus hours into any type of head or side wind versus smoothly turning them for half that time is like the difference between eating habanero peppers and chocolate. One's gonna hurt you inside a whole lot more than the other.

A rest day followed by a tailwind? Someone must be looking out for me, I thought.

I also enjoyed the mental break I got from the exquisite quiet of being pushed along from behind. My mind wandered to a conversation I had with Debra, one of several book participants whose faith played a major role in their lives. I also thought of my sister June, who'd called me one day to explain a newfound spiritual awakening she'd had near the end of her life.

• • •

It was several months before June died, and every time we spoke, I worried that dire news and dark emotion would be at the forefront of our conversation. Yet that day, it was anything but.

"You got a few minutes?" she asked.

"Of course. How's it going?" I always felt awkward asking that particular question as soon as I did. After all, she was dying. But if it was the wrong question to ask, June never said so.

"I'm all right, I guess," she replied. "Listen, there's something I want to tell you, but you need to promise not to laugh. Okay?"

"Uh, no promises."

"Well, pretend you're taking me seriously, then," she said.

"I'll try."

"You know I'm not supposed to drive, right? Well, I went to pick Katie up at school today," she said. "I don't know why, really. It's just something I won't be able to do again soon. But when we pulled into the driveway, I looked at the mileage on my car, and it read 11,111."

There was a long pause as I struggled to find some significance in that.

"11,111," she repeated. "I know it's weird, but then it hit me. I've been seeing ones all over the place. Like, I roll over and it says 1:11 on the clock. I go to pay for something, and it costs exactly eleven dollars. I think of something important and then happen to look at my watch, and the time is 11:11."

"I'm looking right now," I said. "The clock says 1:27, you nut."

"I'm not saying the whole world is ones," she retorted. "I'm just saying it happens *all the time*."

"And?"

"Remember what a numbers guy dad was?" she asked.

How could I not? Most of my childhood memories were hazy, blurred by both trauma and time, but I remember how math and numbers played a big part in his life. The plaque he kept on his desk read: "Dr. David Richman, Poet, Mathematician, and Part-time Genius."

"I remember," I told her.

"Well, when he died, it was one o'clock," she said, choking up.

Our dad died while he was on the phone with June. He was midsentence and stopped talking. She heard his phone drop and *knew*. Although she said the painful memory of hearing him die never left her, she was grateful his last moments were spent talking with her. Twenty-two years later, the memory of that moment was tearing her up, and me along with her.

"Was it?" I asked.

"It was 1:11 in the afternoon, to be exact," she said. "And the time was no big deal then, but it must have stuck with me, because now that I'm seeing all these ones, it makes me think—" She paused.

"It makes you think what?" I asked.

"Well, I know we never believed in a lot of religious-type stuff, but I've come to believe that maybe he's my guardian angel. Like every time I see the ones, it means he's telling me everything's going to be all right. That he'll be there when *I* die. Do you think that's stupid?"

"No," I said. "I don't think so at all."

• • •

After June died, and ever since, it's uncanny how many times I've seen the ones she spoke of. I understood what June meant better and better each time one of my kids' school rooms was numbered Room 111, any of the dozens of times we pulled into the driveway after a long drive at precisely 1:11 or 11:11, all the times my activity tracker happened to read 11.1 miles at just the moment I thought of June, or when the digital thermometer on the dashboard showed 111 degrees just as my kids and I were recounting a June story. Learning to see the ones has allowed us to find comfort in the thought that June is with her guardian angel, that perhaps now they're *both* looking out for *us*.

I'm not certain my faith goes much deeper than wanting to believe, whether backed by coincidence or by a higher power, that some type of absolute peace can come to those who need it, but if it's only that—then that's a start.

As I rolled into the small town of Santa Rosa after an easy seven-hour day, I thought about Debra. In the middle of one of our talks, she hesitated to tell me what seemed—even to her—to be the rather far-fetched, unbelievable story behind her deep faith.

"I don't know if I should continue," she said.

"Of course you should," I urged.

"Well, you might find it hard to believe, not having much faith yourself."

During our first talk, she had asked me about my faith, to which I responded that I was unsure and hadn't yet sought those answers for myself. I decided to tell her about June and the ones. That was all she needed to move forward and share with me the story of a deal she made with the Devil.

After showering at the hotel in Santa Rosa that afternoon, Erin and I drove a few miles to the Blue Hole, a local sinkhole that had been turned into a combination monument, swimming hole, and park. The only other person there at the time was an older man. We struck up a conversation and told him about the Cycle of Lives project. In turn, he told us he was on a quest from Oklahoma to San Diego to put a coin on his estranged brother's headstone. He'd used the coin for over three decades in his chosen profession as a magician-pastor. Now he was ready to give the coin to his brother, a gesture he felt might mend the wounds that had existed between the two when his brother was still alive. At the end of his story, he asked if he could say a prayer for us.

Erin and I glanced at each other, hoping the man didn't see our silent exchange of uncertainty. A prayer? Normally, that would make me feel uncomfortable. It's not that I'm averse to the expression of faith; I just don't have the whole faith thing worked out for myself. But the guy was so kind, and I'd spent multiple hours thinking about the idea of a higher power at that point, so it seemed like a timely idea.

"Sure thing. That would be nice of you," I answered.

Besides, how often would I meet a magician-pastor driving a special coin across the country? He took our hands and made a request to his higher power for my safety.

I ran across many, many people—at least one every day once I was east of Arizona—who either offered, or asked if they could offer, a prayer for me. I'm not saying people west of Arizona don't have faith, but the further east I went, the more open people seemed to be about expressing themselves. I never got comfortable with the practice of holding hands with a stranger while they prayed to their higher power—usually a plea for protection and safety for me on my ride—but the more it happened, the less awkward it became.

Before I fell asleep, I sent Debra a note about the magician-pastor. When I closed my computer and looked at the clock, it was 11:11. I slept deeply that night.

Debra

Relationship to cancer: Survivor, secondary caregiver, and advocate

Age: Fifty-one

Family status: Married for twenty-two years with two children and one grandson

Location: Temecula, California

First encounter with cancer: Thirty-four years old

Cancer summary: Debra was diagnosed with breast cancer and pursued both homeopathic remedies and aggressive conventional treatment. Debra has been in full remission for almost fifteen years. She is very active in the cancer, wellness, and support communities.

Treatment specifics: Inflammatory breast cancer, stage IIIB. Debra underwent a mastectomy, eight rounds of chemotherapy, and radiation therapy.

Community involvement: Volunteer for almost fifteen years at Michelle's Place, a peer-to-peer cancer support group.

Strongest positive emotion during cancer experience: Blessedness

Strongest negative emotion during cancer experience: Sorrow

How we met: I was introduced to Debra through a mutual friend who was excited to introduce me to someone with an amazing cancer story that ended in an unbelievable twist. The friend wouldn't tell me the story but assured me it would be worth including in Cycle of Lives. It took a year to get Debra to open up enough to share the story, and it was well worth the wait.

Replenishing a Soul

....

"How's it looking?" Debra asked her husband. She was shaking off the numbness of the anesthesia, and it was her first and only thought.

"Not good," Kirk said.

Her heart froze, unable to pump the blood that instantly slowed to a crawl.

God, no. Please don't give me bad news, she thought.

"How bad?"

She didn't know if the question had come from her or from her husband—she only *knew* it had been asked, rather than having *heard* the question. The doctor stood at the foot of her bed, and Debra stared at him through what seemed a tunnel as skinny as a coffee straw; through it, she could see nothing but the shape of his lips.

"Very," he mouthed.

She was unable to process anything more than the unmanageable weight of that single word: *very*. It was breast cancer and it wasn't just bad; it was very bad. She closed her eyes as the surgeon spoke about the things that would likely be prescribed by her oncologist: surgery, chemotherapy, radiation therapy.

My oncologist? she thought. *I don't have an oncologist.*

A few days before, she and Kirk were getting ready to do a Sunday 5K run, and he noticed a red mark on the side of her breast. Instinctively nervous about it, she saw her gynecologist the next day, who, after less than a two-minute examination, told her not to worry—it was probably nothing. She wasn't satisfied and called her primary doctor. After examining her more pointedly, he suggested she have an immediate surgical biopsy, and the next night, she was lying in a hospital bed trying to understand what the surgeon was saying—the cancer grade was high, the cancer was aggressive, and she needed to deal with it at once.

How does that happen? One day you're fine, the picture of health, and the next, things are "very bad"? That's not right. Something had to have caused the cancer, right?

As Kirk drove her home, Debra replayed a quick movie of her life in search of clues but came up empty. *I'm healthy. I mean, like, really healthy.* She'd never smoked and wasn't a regular drinker. She completed triathlons, 5Ks, and even a few marathons. Staying active was her passion—hiking, camping, skiing, bike riding. She never got sick . . . *ever.*

Stress? Is that what caused a tumor? She'd had a normal childhood, no real trauma. She and Kirk both enjoyed their careers, and they made enough money to support a full life. Her two sons were fine. She didn't want for anything. Stress was not the culprit. *Genetics?* Nobody in her family had had cancer—she was the first. So, no, not genetics. *But then, where did it come from?*

She thought of one thing—maybe. Was she being punished for something? Subjected to God's wrath for some reason? She dismissed the thought as soon as it came into her brain.

When Kirk pulled into the driveway, Debra looked at their house, nervous to go inside and face the boys. The question kept running through her mind: *Why me? Why me?* As loud as the question reverberated in her head, she was going to have to *give* answers, not focus on finding them.

"What do we say?" she asked Kirk.

"Nothing," Kirk said. "I mean, we don't want to scare them without knowing anything."

"We can't just say nothing. My mom's in there. She'll know if I'm lying."

"Let's say what the surgeon said—you need more tests. That's not lying."

So that's what she said to the boys. Jake was only eight and wouldn't have had the capacity to understand more, unless they had engaged in melodrama. Daniel, fifteen, couldn't hide his worry but seemed to accept the agreed-upon declaration.

Hours later, Debra and Kirk sat on the couch with her mother. "When do they get the results of the biopsy?" her mom asked in a hushed voice. "When do we know if you're okay?"

"We already do. I'm not, Mom," she said in an even softer voice. "They tested the tissue sample right there. It's definitely cancer. They don't know a lot, except that it's serious." She looked at her husband to help bail her out of saying anything more.

"We're going to find an oncologist right away and find out what we need to do," Kirk said. "We'll figure it out. And pray a whole lot tonight."

Prayer was central to their lives. Debra was raised in eastern Pennsylvania, in a small community where religion was a seminal part of most families' lives but not hers. As a child, she was curious about faith, but her parents didn't foster that interest. As a teenager, she explored various religious groups on her own. As a young adult, she found that Catholicism suited her. She found a local church and went through the initiation process. Together with Kirk, she lived her life not just *familiar* with her beliefs but *comfortable* with them. She didn't believe in God and feel his love and his light because she *had* to; she felt those things because she *knew* God loved her. She *knew* he was in her heart—she *knew* to his followers he was a compassionate God, not spiteful or vengeful.

She lay in bed that night, half-asleep, half-awake, not able to keep her mind from swirling around the one question she was trying to avoid, the one that had pricked at her earlier: *Is God punishing me for something?* It pierced her heart as soon as she let it materialize; nothing good could come from asking such a question.

Of course he isn't punishing me. That's a prideful, angry question, and you should be ashamed of yourself for even thinking it.

It was a terrible thought for Debra to have. Her belief in God and her faith were sacred. *Maybe there's a reason*, she thought, *and maybe God doesn't want me to know it right now.* She fell asleep that night resolved to feel awash in her faith, as she always had. The question of *why her* would be answered another way—if it could even be answered at all.

God will show me . . .

Finding Her Path

The first oncologist Debra saw about treatment options simply flipped through the papers on the clipboard—they weren't even the test results—and didn't ask a single question before telling her what was going to happen. Debra walked out without speaking so much as a word to his staff.

She called her primary doctor's office and asked for names of other oncologists. They hesitated, and by the time they called back with names, Debra had resorted to the yellow pages. In a blur of phone calls, she talked to a dozen people. Although some seemed pleasant enough, they lacked urgency, and they didn't seem to understand what it was she was looking for. She wasn't sure either, but she knew she was looking for something and was confident in her ability to ask questions and get answers.

The second oncologist she saw explained more, but Debra didn't like what she heard. The problem wasn't that she was going to have to have chemotherapy, then have her breast removed, and then receive large doses of radiation exposure—she knew that already—it was more that this doctor talked about odds, unknowns, and a lot of play-it-by-ear plans such as "we need to do this right away and then wait and see how your body responds before making a determination about what to do next."

The first doctor knows just what to do, and this one doesn't know anything for sure?

They were two ridiculous extremes, and Debra hadn't gotten any proof, certainty, or consistent information about her prognosis. In her gut, she just didn't feel these doctors knew what they were talking about. Debra believed in herself, and she always figured things out. She prayed, and she had friends and parents she sometimes turned to, but she wasn't given to questioning herself, because she just didn't act on impulse. Her diligence and her drive to ask questions and find answers was part of her DNA, and a quality that allowed her to control the things in her life—she couldn't be any way else, not even about something as ominous and unfathomable as cancer. And after appointments with several doctors, a couple of days skimming stacks of books and magazines in the library, and a hundred internal conversations with herself and with God, she felt that she was the one who had to make decisions about her cancer treatment.

Proof, a sign, something. You need something.

She prayed for an answer. But as she did, she also thought about how she didn't have to have proof of God. He was real; she knew *that* without question. And it made her think that there may be another way to deal with her cancer. She'd always believed in herself. She'd always figured things out. She could beat it her way: with faith, with belief, and in ways that didn't need proving to be real. That approach brought Debra to a holistic healing center.

"Let's not talk about some of the things we may want to do down the road," the woman said. She'd introduced herself as the family medical practitioner.

The woman held Debra's hands in hers and studied her face. "I can see why you're here."

Debra was stumped. They hadn't even talked about why she was there yet. *Great. Another doctor who doesn't want to talk.*

The woman pressed beneath Debra's eyes and asked her to lie on the table. She pressed on her stomach and felt the sides of her neck. She examined Debra's fingers, her joint movement, her underarms, her hips. Seeming content with her examination, she asked Debra to sit up.

"We shouldn't talk about your emotions right now. Your sodium levels are very low—essentially gone. Your cancer is on the left side of your body. Breast, correct?" the doctor asked.

Now, that has to be a sign. Debra's face flushed. "Yes."

"Let's talk, then, about what you should do."

They spent the next hour discussing Debra's medical history—her parents and what illnesses they had, Debra's lifestyle and eating habits, and available treatments. The doctor also scheduled blood, urine, and stool tests. She asked if Debra could get her copies of her scans and X-rays. Before she left, Debra was loaded up with herbs, supplements, and oils and was scheduled for testing and follow-ups. When she drove home, she was certain she was going down the right path on her health. If she ate healthier and took the right herbs and supplements, the tumor would shrink. She could exercise and meditate and do yoga and pray. It seemed reasonable. It seemed *right*. She believed she could absolutely beat cancer—she could rely on all those things, her own determination, and her own body's ability to heal itself.

• • •

Kirk was not pleased.

"I'm not doing it. I'm sorry, honey. You have to believe in me," Debra said, tears of frustration, helplessness, and guilt rolling down her cheeks. "I know you don't agree, but I'm begging you to believe in me."

"No," he said without hesitation. "We'll talk to more doctors until we find the right one. We can't beat cancer with witchcraft. The real doctors don't know all the answers, but they know how to give you the best chance to—"

"To live?" she asked. "I know you think that, but this is what I *believe*. Like our faith, I just believe. That's enough. Don't you see that?"

"Of course, we'll pray," Kirk said. "God will hear us, but we can't turn away from the people who can help you."

They argued off and on for a couple of days, but then Kirk relented.

We'll do it my way, Debra thought. *I have God on my side.*

Debra took dozens of herbs and derivative supplements, rubbed every kind of essential oil and exotic skin cream on her body, and ate a vegetarian diet and drank juices and potions. She did acupuncture and massage and aromatherapy and mineral baths and was involved in a dozen different types of alternative treatments. Over the subsequent several weeks, she got sicker and sicker. Her energy level deteriorated; her ability to focus declined. She started having hot flashes. A pain formed in her breast and became sharper and deeper and *hotter*. Her skin color became paler, dark circles grew under her eyes, and her breathing had grown heavy. Worst of all, she couldn't hide any of it from Kirk.

"Look at yourself in the mirror—like, really look," he said one day. "Do you see what the boys see? Do you want to be stubborn and die? Can't you see? Your way is *not working*. Do what the doctors say. Please, honey. Please . . . for us. Give up on all this other stuff. I don't want you to die."

The Bargain

Debra couldn't fight it anymore. She had to concede. She didn't have the energy to keep pressing forward. She knew it. She had known it for a while, but she was afraid. She went back to the oncologist miserable, not just because she was so sick and not just because of what she imagined she might be in for but also because the people were so unfriendly. They treated her as if she *was* the disease and not as if she *had* a disease. On the first appointment, they told her the plan: a regimen of chemotherapy drugs administered in a series of three-week cycles, followed by a total mastectomy of her left breast, followed by radiation of her chest and potentially her underarm, depending on lymph node involvement. Debra was frightened and nervous and unsure. Her whole foundation had been cracked, and she couldn't rely on herself anymore. She was shaken, deep down inside where she'd never felt things before.

The evening before she received her chemo port, Debra and Kirk went for a walk. They didn't talk much, but she purposely led them toward their church.

"I need to come to peace with what's coming," she said. "Do you mind if I pray alone for a while? I'll meet you at home."

She was certain the doors would be unlocked but was relieved to see that the church was empty. She had to *talk* with God, and she didn't want anybody to hear the conversation. She went to the altar and lit a candle, knowing her prayer would rise up to the heavens. She sat down, anxious to speak, nervous about her intentions. After a few minutes, she leaned forward onto the kneeler and locked her fingers together. She swiveled her head again to make sure she was alone before talking, finding a little courage in the fact that it was just her and God.

"Lord, it was hard to come here tonight," she began. "I know you might feel what's been in my heart the last few days, but also know my love for you has always been strong. I have felt your love and friendship for so long. But I can't help but think you have forsaken me. I feel like you have turned your back on me. I know I shouldn't feel that, and believe me, I've only wanted to be closer to you. But I feel so isolated and distant from Kirk and from my sons—from everything and everybody. I feel ashamed, but I feel *you* have walked away from *me*. I'm desperate and at the end of my rope. Can you understand that?"

She paused for a long time, as if waiting for an answer. When none came, she took a deep breath and sat back down on the pew. She stared at the altar for a while.

"I'm asking you to forgive me for what I'm about to do," she said and then stood and ran out of the church.

Once outside, she leaned against the long door handle and looked at the ground. "Okay. Here I am. Is this what you want? I've walked out. You see? Now you promise. Give me my life—for ten years. Give me that time to get my kids out of the house and finish living and make everything okay for Kirk and them." Tears started to flow. "Give me that time and you can have me. Take me, take my soul, take me forever. Just let me have this time with them. Then I'll do whatever you want. You can have me, you hear? Deal? You can have me forever."

It felt twenty degrees colder outside to Debra as she shook, crying and weak, as if her every last ounce of energy had been drained by making her pact with the Devil. She had to get home. She had to hide from the world and fall asleep and hope she might wake up and everything would have been a bad dream.

But it wasn't. Everything was very real.

We have our deal, you got it? But it's between you and me. Well, God will know. But either way, we have our deal. You better live up to it, she said inside as she lay in bed, crying.

On the second oncology appointment, the following morning, she received a chemo port and underwent further blood tests. The next day, she received her first treatment.

The Devil's Work

The chemo was unthinkably difficult on Debra. After each treatment, she became violently ill for days. The nausea was like nothing she could have imagined. She was both cold inside and hot to the touch. Her sweat was clammy, and it smelled of poison. Her mouth was dry, her throat was sore, and her nose was raw. She was so dehydrated she couldn't close her eyes without putting a wet towel on them.

Her mom took her to chemo treatment when Kirk couldn't, but when she got home, Debra hid alone in her room, away from everyone. Some days were worse than others, but she wouldn't allow the family to help. It would have been impossible not to see how the cancer and treatment were ravaging Debra, but she tried to keep everybody from knowing how bad it really was. Debra wouldn't let them see. She left the lights off and the drapes shut. She wore sweats and a scarf on her head and sunglasses anytime she went out. She crawled into the bathroom, stayed there for hours, and crawled back into bed. Except to come and go for treatments, she rarely came out of the bedroom. All along, she cursed the Devil for giving her the cancer.

It had to have been him. Just so he could trick me into giving away my soul.

As weak as she was, though, she wouldn't give up. No way. She'd turned to the Devil and struck a deal, and she was going to see to it that he lived up to his end of it.

During this time, Kirk tried to have a few conversations with Debra about faith, especially during the tougher spells of her treatment, but Debra told him that she felt abandoned by God and forced to fight for her life on her own. Kirk tried to push the issue with her, but she was either too sick or too closed off to talk about it. There was no way she could ever admit to the *real* reason she wouldn't discuss God. They couldn't come to any agreement on the subject and ultimately avoided talking about it at all.

After three cycles of chemo, the oncologist ordered new scans. Debra sat in the examination room, waiting to hear the news.

Is my soul worth it? she thought. The answer came after an agonizing wait. Her tumor had shrunk.

"We have a long road ahead," the doctor said, "but things are moving in the right direction. The drugs are working, and after a few more cycles, we can move on to the next step."

Oh, something's *working all right, Doc. I hate to break it to you, but it's not the drugs.*

Over the next several months, Debra completed her treatment. In all, she had eight rounds of chemotherapy, had her left breast removed with what the surgeon thought were very safe margins, and received several doses of radiation to her chest—she didn't need it anywhere else, as her lymph nodes had tested negative.

When the cancer was gone and all the treatments were over, Debra underwent reconstructive breast surgery. Within the year, she looked and felt almost normal. On the inside, though, things had changed—she felt softer, more contemplative, more sensitive. Over a year's time, the ups and downs had been so extreme, so far out of the previously narrow range she'd lived in, that she had to accept the reality that she wasn't always in control. When she softened and viewed the world around her from these new perspectives, she saw things differently. Sometimes the views were dark and gloomy, but more often, they were light and hopeful and fresh, as if she had been given a more profound appreciation for life. She felt deeper feelings for Kirk. She reflected on her life and on her qualities as a mom, vowing to do better, to include her boys more, to be more involved in their lives. It was as if overcoming cancer gave her a demarcation point for being given a whole new chance to live.

She had a nagging feeling of dread among all the new and positive epiphanies, though, and when she thought about the deal she'd made with the Devil, a bolt of panic shot through her insides.

I'll never tell another living soul, but you kept up your end of the bargain, didn't you?

A New Life

A year out from the reconstruction, they decided to move to California for Kirk's new job. Debra found a new job as well, and the move gave them more freedom, more stability, and a fresh, new part of the country to explore together.

With her regained health and invigorated demeanor, Debra returned to eating healthy, running, and discovering new places to hike, camp, and boat. Her older son went off to college, and she spent even more time with her youngest, helping him with schoolwork, volunteering for the various sports teams he played on, and living up to her self-promise to be a better, more involved mother. That, in turn, helped her relationship with Kirk, and they became closer than they'd ever been.

In addition, Debra joined a support group for women who were diagnosed with breast cancer, and she became devoted to the process of helping support other women who were going through what she'd survived. In every way possible, life was giving Debra all she could ask for—and she was giving back all that life had given to her.

There was one area of Debra's life that contrasted with the rest, though, and it centered around her faith. Going through cancer had rattled her enough to shake—even destroy—her beliefs. On the one hand, her faith in God became muted, purposely tucked away, not just hidden from her outward expressions but also buried deep enough inside that it didn't interfere with her inner dialogue. On the other hand, she'd bargained away her soul. She'd agreed that if she were cured of cancer and given a chance to watch her sons grow into men, she'd pay the piper. But that thought was so absurd, so contrary to who she was, and so ominous and apocalyptic and private that she couldn't face it. As a result, the years rolled by with Debra having no true awareness of the passing of time in relation to her faith or the arrangement she'd made.

That all changed many years later when a friend asked her if she'd like to attend their church service one Sunday. Debra tried to hide her petrified reaction but knew she couldn't. But it wasn't the thought of *church* that turned Debra white; it was the thought of *time*.

Church? How many years has it been? Debra asked herself.

She scanned a mental calendar. *That was the summer I was thirty-nine—or was I thirty-eight? No, it was thirty-eight.* Debra's breathing became short. She felt faint.

"Oh, I'm so sorry. I didn't mean to intrude," the woman said.

Debra recovered. "No. It's just . . . well, I haven't been to church in a long time."

Like, ten years, Debra thought. *Almost exactly ten years.*

Debra was petrified at the thought, but that night she told Kirk what her friend had explained after she'd initially declined the offer: The church was progressive, the pastor had no centuries-old dogma he was compelled to adhere to, and inclusion and tolerance for diversity were celebrated. She'd said the church was more of a social community than a religious one. Whether to convince him or to convince herself, Debra told Kirk that it was about time they explored their feelings on God again.

Debra hadn't convinced herself it was the right thing to do, or that she could even command herself to go inside once she decided to go, but the following Sunday, Debra and Kirk found themselves driving to the church. They didn't talk on the way there, as Debra was feeling odd, disconnected, short of breath, and even a little claustrophobic. Something was welling up inside of her. She didn't know if it was anticipation or dread.

When they reached the parking lot, Debra's view was closing in, narrowing her appraisal of the activity going on around her, like heavy blood had pooled in her head, drawn there by a flurry of unexposed activity. She felt Kirk's hand, but she couldn't see him. She couldn't see anything that wasn't straight in front of her.

The doors on the church were tall and heavy, reminding her of the doors on the last church she was in. *The last church I walked out of.*

They walked inside, Debra moving to a seat in the middle rows, way off to the right of center. She sat, squeezing Kirk's hand, focusing on the breath that echoed inside of her. With each exhale, she could feel something coming up, something that seemed to be impatient—something that wanted attention. *He wants his due.*

The pastor stepped up to the pulpit. He wore a black polo shirt and khaki pants. He looked out at the crowd and smiled. He had a commanding, comfortable smile, one that lit his blue eyes.

"I was going to talk today about a few different things," he said and paused as if trying to find a way to begin. "But I was in my office earlier, thinking about those topics, and I was overcome with faith. I was suddenly overwhelmed with the need to pray. There was no reason, really, but I sat back anyway and closed my eyes and began a little inner dialogue with God. When I did, my mind began to think of all that we ask him for when we pray. We ask him to watch over us, to keep us safe, to show us how to solve problems, and to give us strength. And sometimes when we pray, we ask for these blessings because of something specific that is going on—perhaps we're sick, and we ask him to help give us the strength to fight through."

The knocking on Debra's brain became even more pronounced. *Sick, like cancer sick.*

"Other times, maybe we are facing a tough decision—do I take one road or the other? We look for him to help guide us."

The frenzy in her head continued, stronger, pulsing her brain, trying to shake things apart.

"And I thought: How often do we ask for help, guidance, or strength for something that is happening at this exact moment in our lives? How often are we focused on where we need to go, and we're looking for help on how to get there? As I sat with my eyes closed, it came to me—sometimes the road ahead was laid long ago in our past. Perhaps the answers to what lies in front of us can be found in the decisions we've made in the past, even years and years ago."

Cracks started to appear inside Debra. She could *feel* things opening up. *You mean, like, almost ten years ago?* Everything inside Debra crumbled away. The bricks of resistance and fear and denial fell aside, leaving her exposed, revealed, powerless.

"I thought about forgiveness, how sometimes we need to forgive ourselves for our mistakes. After all, we ask God to forgive us all the time."

Hot tears started to roll down Debra's face. They found the channels on the sides of her cheeks and flowed against the corners of her mouth. She tasted the salt, and she immediately thought of being drained of sodium, and the cancer that caused her to almost die—the surgeries, the fear, and her faith. She remembered the shame of closing the heavy church doors and striking a bargain with the Devil.

"And I have to believe that we all need to take a minute now and reflect back on the roads we've taken and the paths we've followed, and if we've made mistakes because of the decisions we've made, we need to forgive ourselves. We need to allow ourselves to learn, to understand we should move forward without such heavy hearts. We are all, by the grace of God, imperfect beings."

Through the tears, Debra saw the pastor looking straight at her, as if he could see the pain and anguish and regret and horror that seemed to explode out of her.

Then he said, staring through her with his commanding eyes: "Because I know God is a forgiving God. He forgives us for the mistakes we've made, the wrong choices we've made, the failures we've exhibited in weaker times. Even if, in a moment of weakness, we sold our soul to the Devil, he'd forgive us. If he could forgive that, then shouldn't we forgive ourselves?"

Debra willed her vision to widen. She couldn't turn to look, but she was certain that people—at least Kirk—would be looking at her, seeing her unmasked, wondering why she'd done something so horrible as begging for her life and giving her soul away to the Devil. But nobody was looking at her. Nobody appeared to know her secret.

"Let's all take a moment to do that, shall we?" the pastor asked. "A moment to forgive what we did yesterday, or last month, or even years ago. We are all here to learn, to learn to love God and let him love us. I think we should forgive ourselves as we do."

Debra bowed her head, tears dropping on her and Kirk's hands, and she asked God to forgive her for forsaking him and for bargaining away her life. And she asked him to help her bring him back into her heart.

When the service was over, Debra and Kirk walked through the open doors of the church. Debra looked back. She saw the pastor. He was talking to a group of people, but he caught her glance and nodded slightly at her. She looked back and up at Kirk.

"I think we should come back. You okay with that?" she asked him.

"I think we already have," he said.

Debra's Epilogue
....

Near the end of our talks, Debra was struggling with a tragic event in her life: A childhood friend was dying of cancer. The woman had originally planned to work until she retired a couple of months before needing hospice, so that she could spend some time traveling the world. But the cancer overtook her body much faster than the doctors imagined, and by the time she quit working, she was told she had just weeks left.

Debra has spent almost fifteen years counseling hundreds and hundreds of patients and survivors. Religion doesn't come up often, because in her role as a counselor, Debra feels she needs to give the patients and survivors support in the areas *they* need, not the areas *she* thinks they need. But her childhood friend was agnostic, and Debra felt compelled to urge her to try to accept God. She spoke to her friend about her deep love of God and God's abiding promise, but her friend was not moved.

I spoke to Debra after her friend passed away.

"I couldn't get my friend to accept God into her heart," Debra said. "I tried. We were so close—and I felt so fortunate I could be with her, visit her, and help her prepare to die. That was a true blessing. But it still pains me."

Debra had revealed many realizations about her journey to me but none as touching as her gratitude for being given the opportunity to be with others, to hold their hands through the darkest times. Cancer gave her, she told me, a profound appreciation for life, the beautiful world we live in, and the love of the people around her, as well as a truer and deeper relationship with God.

Days and Days in Texas: Part I

*D*amn *blown-apart steel-belted radials and their little, skinny shards of metal. Tiny pieces of damn havoc,* I thought, changing the fourth flat of the day. I ran my fingertips along the inside of the tire, feeling for a poke from the tiny strand of metal surely no bigger than a fraction of an inch. Sometimes it took several circular passes, but I always found the infinitesimally small culprit. The big things—the wind, the mountains, the traffic, the long distances, the heat—were things I could wrap my head around and figure out how to overcome. But the most miniscule, unforeseen problems—such as a barely noticeable mist of rain on an oily road, an unfortunately placed blister, a sudden rash on the backs of my legs, or the microscopic pieces of metal on the highway that found their way into my tires—worked to chip away at my fortitude. A nick here, a shred there. Fragments that ripped away at my senses, one sliver after the next, threatening to derail my efforts, all day long, every day.

The route for day thirteen took me south from Santa Rosa—and off Interstate 40—along a small two-lane highway, then east along another similar highway at Clovis, New Mexico, and it put me back on the routine of insanely long, drawn-out, difficult days in which I had to deal with several big challenges and endless insignificant ones.

From the start, the wind that day was strong and straight on—no matter which direction I headed, the wind adjusted its angle—and some sixty-odd miles later, I sat on the side of the road, feeling as deflated as the umpteenth popped tube that lay inside of my rear tire. The lonely highway radiated the ninety-five-degree heat, and with the wind, I felt as if I were inside of a convection oven. There was an empty field across the road, and when I stood, having mustered the energy to start working on the wheel, I noticed a herd of cattle off in the distance.

"Any of you want to help?" I yelled at the distant group.

As I worked on my bike, I occasionally glanced over at the field. The cattle, who had been at least a half a mile away when I first spotted them, were making their way toward me. By the time I was finishing up, there were dozens of cattle lined up along the barbed-wire fence, grazing, mooing, and crowding around each other, seemingly intent on checking out whatever was going on across the highway.

"Crazy cows," I said. "What in the world do you guys want?"

Then I started laughing. Not only had I been reduced to talking to cattle, but I thought it equally likely that the cows were confused by me.

"Crazy human, what in the world are you doing in this heat, on the side of the road, in the middle of nowhere?" they asked in my mind.

I had drawn quite a bit of attention on the ride to that point but none as striking as a herd of cattle that came over to see what this crazy human was up to.

Day fourteen didn't involve much laughter, but it did involve hotter heat and windier wind, as if someone cranked the knobs up to high as I crossed out of New Mexico and into Texas. A ten-and-a-half-hour-long, grinding day, multiple flat tires, navigating past bad traffic accidents, and biking through a few thunderstorms all continued to wear me down to the nubs.

As I approached Lubbock, near the end of the first day in the glorious and vast Republic of Texas, I had a harrowing encounter with a vicious-looking pit bull terrier. I was making my way into town, taking smaller highways to avoid traffic. I wasn't wearing earbuds, which allowed me to hear the barking dog, who was ahead of me and across the street, as soon as I was close enough to have drawn its attention. I clenched the handlebars and began to pedal a little faster. The fact that the dog was on the other side of the highway comforted me somewhat, though it seemed the dog became more agitated the closer I approached. Fortunately, the dog's owner was in the driveway, working on his car. As I passed by, I noticed the dog was not tied to a leash. He began to sprint down the side of the road. The man in the driveway pulled his head out from under the hood and looked to see what was going on.

I hope that dog listens to his owner, I thought. I shifted into a higher gear and began to muscle away. The dog was in a frenzy. I pedaled faster and checked on my pursuer. He had crazy attack-dog eyes and an angry-sounding bark—and he was gaining on me.

"Go git 'em!" the man in the driveway called after the dog. "Git that sucker, boy!"

So much for listening to his owner!

Indifferent to any potential traffic, the dog took an angled approach across the highway to make up ground. I pounded my burning legs on the pedals harder. I carried pepper spray for just that type of occurrence, so I reached into the small container attached to the frame, pulled out the mini-dispenser, and bit the cap off. I checked again. He was still gaining on me, his barking intensifying. I readied the spray. My legs were about to give out, and my lungs were on fire from the effort, but just before he got close enough to spray, the dog's momentum petered out and he turned away.

As the dog crossed the road against traffic again, headed back in the direction of his home, I gave the scene behind me one last glance and silently cursed his owner. It took about fifteen minutes for the adrenaline to disperse and my heart to stop bruising my rib cage.

Day fifteen, although filled with a nonstop showcase of roadkill—the sheer volume and diversity of animal was astounding—was absent encounters with cattle, dogs, or any other living fauna. The day was a thirteen-hour, 125-mile, windy broil-fest. By the end of the day, I had to get picked up by Erin about twenty-five miles before my intended finish in Abilene because I was too fried to continue. On the drive to the hotel, I unloaded my frustrations.

"I'm tired of this freaking wind," I started. "I mean, I had three flats by the time I hit Post—three flats in the first forty miles. Making any progress on getting ahead of this thing is impossible. I can't get a break. Could I have one day without a freaking full-on headwind and a million flats and an upset stomach and cars missing running me over by two freaking inches?"

The questions were unanswerable, so Erin gave me a sympathetic smile, and instead, we talked about our strategy for the following days. In the morning, she'd drive me back to where she picked me up so I could get those last twenty-five miles from the day before in, then she'd try to go find new, more durable tires for my bike; give me one last support stop; and drive the more than three hundred miles to Houston, where she'd leave the truck and take a plane back to California. I'd continue on my way to Dallas, then Austin, then Houston over the next several days, and my friend Chad would fly to Houston, pick the car up, and then meet me at wherever I was on my intended route—most likely somewhere east of Houston—to support me for a few days until he had to head back home.

I didn't like that I was demoralized and focused on the difficulties, and I felt guilty about complaining in the first place, but I couldn't help myself. Each day I was overwhelmed with how *hard* everything was. In some twisted sense of reality, I tried to equate my difficulties to the difficulties that some of the book participants and June had gone through. *Imagine what they had to weather each day*, I thought. *Imagine how hard facing the day was for them.* But even with those attempts to put my issues into perspective, it wasn't until Erin came back with dinner that night that I was able to right my mental ship.

"Sorry it took so long," Erin said. "I was talking to this young woman who was helping me. She had a crazy story."

"What's that?" I asked.

"I was telling her about the bike ride, and she started asking questions: Where did you start, and where are you going to finish? How many hours do you bike each day? When's the book coming out? You know, all the usual ones. Then she starts tearing up. 'You all right?' I ask her. She tells me how her best friend just found out her four-year-old has brain cancer. She said she has no idea what to say to her friend or what to do for her. Can you imagine? She said what you're doing is very inspiring, and she hopes your book will help people like her learn how to deal with such difficult situations."

There wasn't a day when I didn't hear stories like that, either about what people were going through or had gone through or about what people they knew were going through or had gone through. But it just kept hitting me that so many people were so open to talking about not knowing how to talk to people, about not knowing what to do or what to say to loved ones. It was so pervasive. What *could* one say to a friend who was just dealt the news that their kid has brain cancer? I didn't know the right answer, but I did know that people wanted to learn how people like them found some of the answers about how to deal with those types of emotional issues around cancer.

I didn't set out with the Cycle of Lives to analyze people or give advice or counsel or guidance about the psychological and emotional issues faced when encountering cancer—I'm not qualified in any way to do that. But I also knew most people weren't going to seek any type of professional help about those things.

I decided I shouldn't think of my daily struggles in terms of how they related to the difficulties the fifteen book participants had, or my own issues over having lost my sister, nor should my journey be considered from the perspective of navigating through days and days of difficulty that spanned these vast distances between a handful of people whose stories might provide some answers. Rather, I decided I should just picture each and every person I encountered all strung together—a cross-country collective of humanity. And they would all likely be looking for answers at some point in their lives. My ride wasn't about my difficulties riding across country, or the fifteen book participants and their struggles, it was about every person's inability to deal with cancer, the prospect of death, and the pain of seeing people go through such difficulty and confusion and anguish as that brought on by one of humankind's most inexplicable and troublous maladies. If I could think about the ride in terms of the few pedals between people and not the hundreds of miles between destinations, it might just become easier.

When I awoke for day sixteen, I felt less burdened, less intimidated about what lay ahead, less desperate to encounter some good luck to help me get from here to there. Instead, I felt I could take it one pedal at a time, passing one person along the continuum after another, staying present in the moment, one moment to the next. Obstacles, struggles, confusion, roadblocks, wind, flats, tired legs, and long days were just things I needed to deal with. And everyone deals with the things they need to deal with while trying to get through each day, in search of answers or not, dealing with supreme adversity or not, and pondering the greater meaning of life or just living.

My refreshed disposition came at the right time. Day sixteen turned out to be the most physically challenging day of the ride up until then by a long shot: sixteen hours of biking, 146 miles, four thousand feet of climbing, ninety-five-degree heat, five flats, and my first day self-supporting. That meant panniers full of all the clothes, supplies, tubes, food, and more I'd need for the next several days and no chance to call anybody for help. I spent most of the day heading east on Interstate 20, loaded down with full front and rear saddle bags, pedaling into a fierce, scorching wind; spinning through the mental Rolodex; pondering book participants; thinking of all the people I'd encountered in the previous year or two; and contemplating the emotions and the ways in which I might try to write about them. I finished the day beyond exhausted, rolling into the parking lot of my hotel in Weatherford, Texas, around midnight, depleted and dehydrated, a deep fatigue roiling my muscles and joints, but my emotions and mental state were holding steady, the result of having committed to my newly discovered perspective.

Day seventeen was a short day—seventy miles to Dallas. In addition to the accumulated fatigue, I'd developed a bad rash on the back of my legs, the result of too much sweat, sun, dirt, and friction, and I was looking forward to a shorter day so I could rest before going to dinner with friends who lived in town. About thirty miles outside of the city, after yet another flat, I was down to one extra tube. It was a Sunday, and I was nervous that if I didn't find a bike shop, I'd be in big trouble.

In any major city, the freeway system can be difficult to navigate upon the first encounter—and navigating is particularly challenging if you're doing so on a bicycle—but the freeway system around Dallas is *chaotic*. As I made my way into the Dallas area, several times I fell victim to the seemingly order-free roadways, and I found myself biking along shoulders that suddenly disappeared, winding up on the wrong side of a merged lane, or plain stuck in too dangerous a position to continue along my intended route. Add to that being on the receiving end of impatient honking and frustrating drivers, and I was pretty frazzled. One car lay on the horn and pulled to the shoulder about a quarter mile ahead of me.

Oh shit, I thought, *this is Texas. He'll probably jump out, guns blazing—or let his dog out to come get me.* I readied myself for confrontation.

A man came out of the car. He was barrel-chested, wore a blood-red bandana on his head, and hid his eyes behind huge dark sunglasses. He began to lumber toward me wearing a tight red shirt and bright red shorts, flashing a crazed grin and wildly waving his arms. I slowed down to assess the situation: He was either warning me of danger, or he was a madman. Either way, I was about to be in big trouble. I came to a stop about twenty yards in front of him.

He pulled his sunglasses up on his head. His face was red, and his big brown eyes crinkled at the edges as he grinned with soft wrinkles. Upon close inspection, dressed up in all red, the guy looked like a skinnier, semi-clean-shaven Santa Claus impersonator. He laughed an animated, hearty laugh.

"I was driving along and went flying by you—on the freeway!" he said. "You do know you're on a busy freeway, right? 'Does this guy have any idea what he's doing?' I ask myself. 'Of course he does. He's geared up for the long-term,' I say to myself. 'I have to see what this guy is up to,' I say."

I noticed that his red shirt was a cycling jersey. It read *Razorbacks* all over. His shorts were cycling shorts, and his socks were cycling socks too.

"Yep, I'm a Razorback. Just finished a forty-miler, as a matter of fact," he said. "I got off, up a way, then I turned around. I stopped to see what this is all about. Where are you biking from?"

"California," I said.

"California? Where are you biking *to*?"

"To Austin, then Houston, halfway down Florida, then across and up to New York."

"How many months?"

"Forty-five days, actually."

"What?" he asked and laughed. He had a deep, natural laugh. "That's gotta be like a four-thousand-mile sprint."

"Closer to five," I said.

"A 5K sprint? On that?" He looked over my bike. "How much that thing weigh?"

"Too much."

"What do you need? Water? Food? Anything?" he asked. He asked me about the trip, the reasons for doing it, details about the biking, the nutrition, and the heat. Then he told me he knew a few people who had fought cancer—even a close friend who was going through cancer right then—and that he would help spread the word to his biking community. I told him about all the flats I was getting on the freeways, and that I had no tubes left, and asked him for a suggestion on a bike store.

"I knew it!" he said. "What are the odds? I'm glad I circled back."

He directed me to a bike shop he knew well that was about a forty-minute's ride away. We shared numbers, and then he gave me a genuine and comfortable high-five handshake, interlocking my fingers in a tight grip and shaking my whole body as he thanked me for what I was doing.

"I'm gonna live off this story for a month," he said. "You tell 'em at the bike shop Keller sent you. You got it?"

"Keller. Got it," I said.

When I got to the bike shop, there must have been a dozen customers and half as many employees there. I asked for help with picking some tubes and told the guy helping me what Keller had said.

"You're the guy on the freeway?"

I nodded.

"Hey, everyone," he announced over my shoulder, "this is the guy Keller just told us about. He's on his way from California to New York, biking for cancer."

I looked around to see if Keller was there. He wasn't, but all the people there had stopped whatever they were doing and began to clap.

"He stopped in for a minute," the guy said. "Put his credit card down. Said he'd pay for whatever you need."

I didn't know when I'd hit another bike store—or how soon I'd need another restock—so I loaded up on tubes, glue, a fresh patch kit, and carbon dioxide cartridges. The cashier refused my credit card, and then the manager came over and let me know that the store wanted to donate the items so no one would be charged.

"Anybody who's racing across the country five thousand miles deserves a little support," the manager said. "We got you."

After thanking everyone, I loaded my bags with the several additional pounds of gear; rerouted the fifteen miles to the hotel on my GPS, making sure to stay on streets and off the crazy Dallas freeways; and rolled off—refreshed, restocked, and reinvigorated by a stranger's kindness.

With no stresses to distract me, my mind wandered. I thought about coincidences, how I ran into someone who could help me with just what I needed, when I needed it. I thought of what Keller said to me on the freeway about sprinting. *Five thousand miles*, I thought. *Thousands of miles, and I ran into that guy at the right time. So many coincidences. "A 5K sprint," he had said. A 5K. Three-point-one-miles. The run on a sprint triathlon is that. Triathlons . . . One of America's most elite triathlete and long-distance runner ever . . . whose coincidences saved his life . . .*

Rick

Relationship to cancer: Survivor

Age: Fifty-nine

Family status: Married for sixteen years with three grown children

Location: Denver, Colorado

First encounter with cancer: Thirty-eight years old

Cancer summary: Testicular cancer at thirty-eight; second diagnosis, prostate cancer at fifty-six

Cancer specifics: Traditional chemotherapy and radiation therapy for testicular cancer. Engaged in proton therapy treatment for prostate cancer. Currently, Rick is cancer-free.

Strongest positive emotion during cancer experience: Gratitude

Strongest negative emotion during cancer experience: Shame

How we met: I met Rick as the result of an unlikely chain of events, which was apropos, considering major aspects of his life, as well as his cancer story, centered around a series of outlandish coincidences.

While looking for book participants, I called around to various cancer centers, canvassing for interesting stories. One center initially turned down the idea of referring anybody, but after I sent the communications director a copy of a long-distance-athletics-slash-business book I wrote as a means of thanking him for talking to me, I received a call back. As it turned out, he was a cyclist and triathlete, and the book was "right up his alley." He suggested I call a prominent radiation oncologist—who happened to have been a notable athlete back in the day—and pitch him my story. That doctor declined. I went back to the communications director, who gave me another shot.

"I've got someone else in mind," he said. "He used to be somewhat of a public figure and let's just say a big athlete, too. I don't know if he'll be interested, but I can find out."

By the next week, I had a call lined up with him. I was excited to talk to Rick, because he wasn't just a public figure; he's a *legend*. An accomplished runner and triathlete with an endless list of records. I explained the book project.

"I'm not sure that would be something I'd be interested in, to be honest," Rick said. "My cancer story is not that exciting, and everybody already knows the rest."

"Well, I doubt they know *everything*," I said. "I read a recent article about you and noticed your radiation oncologist is in my backyard. I've spoken with him—not about *you*, of course, but about the Cycle of Lives project." I tried to keep the conversation going without letting Rick know that his oncologist had declined to speak with me. I wasn't trying to mislead him, just giving him a reason to keep talking.

"Well, everybody knows the juicy stuff, then," he said. "Maybe not about me and him, though. That's a pretty unbelievable story how he saved . . . well, I don't know if he saved my life exactly, but in one sense, he did. He didn't tell you about that?"

A Matter of Timing

The first time Rick was diagnosed with cancer, it came near the bitter end of his illustrious athletic career. He was close to forty years old, unable to compete at an elite level anymore, embattled in a rancorous divorce, and facing financial hardship. It felt as if his life was crumbling, and testicular cancer was just one more nasty problem to solve.

The good news was that Rick's years of competing at an elite level had taught him how to endure pain and tackle hard problems. He was well-prepared to handle the treatment without much fanfare, and he did—though anyone who had known him as a child probably wouldn't have believed Rick would grow up to have that kind of grit.

Born on the outskirts of Los Angeles in the late-1950s, Rick's upbringing was very *Ozzie and Harriet*. His all-American family centered around a somewhat strict, very intelligent, and active mom who'd stopped working so she could raise her three children before returning to her career in school administration. They also had a hardworking, conscientious father who was

only absent from some of the day-to-day home life because he was committed to his practice as a family physician.

Rick's parents weren't perfect, but they were good, stable parents. No
bombshells were ever dropped in their family. They had no dark secrets waiting
to be unearthed or double lives just waiting to be revealed. Life was normal,
quiet, and uneventful.

Rick didn't have many aspirations growing up. He knew early in life he
wasn't as smart and driven as his brother and sister—who were intent on succeeding in school and then pursuing professional careers, like their parents.
Rick was athletic, good-natured, and charming. He relied on those qualities to
skate through to his teenage years. To his parents' displeasure, Rick's focus was
on seeing not how much he could accomplish but how little effort he could
put into the things he wasn't naturally gifted at.

As a freshman in high school, Rick noticed the athletes got all the attention
from all the right sources. He hadn't participated in a ton of organized athletics
before then, but then again, some of the payoffs for doing so didn't exist before
puberty. He was a natural at several sports, swimming, soccer, cycling and settled
on trying to make the baseball team—until the running coach saw him.

"You ever think about running?" he asked Rick.

"I sometimes run with my mom." It was an exaggeration, since no matter
how often she urged him to join her on her daily run, he had only gone a
handful of times.

"I've been watching you run around the field. You're darn fast," the coach said.

"Am I?" Rick asked.

"Yup. With some hard work, you might just be *fast*."

Hard work? he thought. *I don't think so.*

"Don't look so skeptical," the coach said. "Come to one practice and let me
show you what we do."

Rick went to the practice, and he fell in love—not with running, not at
first—but with a dark-haired runner on the girls' team who happened to be
training at the same time. One and a half laps into the workout, Rick had won
the dumbfounded stares of the group of runners, and a generous smile from
the girl. He *was* fast, and he wasn't even running hard. He joined the team.
After all, he had to get to know that girl.

Regardless of Rick's lackadaisical attitude, his coach took a deep and personal interest in his running development. Rick soon found out he excelled at most distances between 1,500 and 10,000 meters, one mile to six miles. He also found out that runners were as popular with the girls as the other athletes were.

When Rick had watched the 1972 Olympics—the exact time that American running had started to become a cultural phenomenon—his mom was hooked. Some of that had obviously rubbed off her and onto him, but when the sport of triathlon emerged at the same time, Rick became a little obsessed. Besides track, he joined the swim team. Over the next couple of years, Rick's confidence and ability grew, and by the time he graduated high school, he was an accomplished swimmer, an almost junior pro-level cyclist, and one of the top distance runners in California.

Rick's track coach got him to understand how gifted he was, and then to understand the physical and mental intricacies of competition. He sparked something in Rick that motivated him to put forth unmatched training efforts and, by doing so, helped him to believe he could realize the full potential of his gift, no matter how fast he aspired to be, nor which sport he ultimately committed to pursuing. He wasn't a top swimming recruit, he wasn't a good enough cyclist to go pro, but he could do both at an elite level—and he could run with the best. Rick had come to the track as an uninterested, lazy underachiever, and by the time he accepted a scholarship to attend the respected running program at one of the top collegiate running programs in the country, he believed there was no stopping himself. Then came the harsh reality of swimming, running, and cycling with the big boys.

At his peak in high school, Rick ran forty miles a week, made most of the swim team's workouts, and rode no less than 100 hard miles a week. The first week in college, the running coach gave him a rude awakening—120 miles, *running*—doing two, sometimes three runs a day, with runs from five miles to fifteen miles. He'd never imagined running so hard in training, but he soon saw how hard elite collegiate runners in the country worked, and his appetite to experience the pain of running extremely long and intensely hard became voracious. He wanted to be the fastest distance runner, no matter what it took. Along with this new hunger and a limitless desire to train came continued and elevated success on the track.

He continued to swim and bike on his own, while managing as light an educational load as he could. Rick even started driving to San Diego some weekends to race (and often win) against the newly emerging triathletes, many of whom were curious collegiate athletes themselves.

Similarly, success came to him in his amorous pursuits as well. After all, life wasn't just about athletics.

On the track, in the pool, and on the roads, Rick worked hard. In the training room, he worked even harder. And when competing, he was fierce. His college coach became equally a mentor to him as was his high school coach, and by his junior year, Rick had won several national titles. Although he was competing with the top long-distance runners in college, at the same time, he was becoming a name in the burgeoning world of long-distance triathlon, running, swimming and biking toe-to-toe with the best emerging multi-disciplined athletes. He even dared to believe that he might become one of the best triathletes in the world. But the Olympics were calling him, and he set his sights on running the half and full marathons for the United States in the 1980 Summer Olympics in Moscow, two years away.

In 1979, Rick was twenty-two and had reached a level where the world's best athletes competed. While running ever faster times in preparation for the Olympics, he started chasing records and decided to stop chasing women. He married his high school sweetheart: the dark-haired girl from that first day on the track.

The Olympic trials were approaching, and Rick was focused. He was peaking. He was *flying*. Everything was primed for a golden run at the Olympics. And then ...

The Russians had invaded Afghanistan, and the United States decided to boycott the Moscow Olympics. It was devastating for Rick. His chance to shine, to run with the the best in the world, to make his family and a run-crazed country proud, disappeared like the flashes on the cameras at the president's fateful news conference announcing America's decision to boycott.

It took a while to recuperate, but Rick did bounce back. Fortunately, he had triathlon, and triathlon was beginning to explode.

Making a living as a competitive triathlete during the golden age of running popularity in America was not easy; it was still a fringe sport. But it was gaining popularity. Rick was doing what he loved, but it had become a grind. For years, he lived out of a suitcase while he traveled the world competing. Financially, he was struggling. The world of triathlon was not like many upper-echelon professional sports. Promoters were sometimes shady, sponsorships came and went, and promised payments often never materialized. Rick had to work hard to make ends meet, and when he wasn't on the road, he was grinding through training and public appearances. The stress was compounded by his giving in to temptations he found while out on the road. He and his wife—parents now to three children—became distant and combative. He loved competition. After tasting success, he still wanted to become the best ever at something, but he was broke and struggling to provide for his family.

Through all the struggles, his addiction to competition was the thing that made him come back after every event, but it was the fans that made him stay in the game for as long as he did. Both running and triathlon brought dedicated fans, and Rick embraced his role as a top runner and middle and long-distance triathlete, winning more events and races than he could remember, and even attempting to qualify for the 1984 and the 1988 Olympics.

But a quiet desperation crept in during the early 1990s as Rick was coming to the realization that his career was ending. Not competing was unthinkable, yet his body could handle only so much. He knew that hocking product, coaching, or who knows what awaited him. He was unprepared for the next step. He liked being something of a vagabond, answering to no one, doing what he pleased, and continuing to see how hard he could continue to press forward.

But although the triathlon lifestyle worked as a backdrop for Rick's athletic pursuits, it also fueled his infidelities, inflamed the turmoil at home, and led to a deep unsettling of his psyche and moral compass. Rick's private life was in shambles, he had no plan for what to do with his life, his marriage was a disaster, and his relationship with his kids was distant and strained. The solace of hiding himself in the public eye—and away from the off-road realities—was slowly disappearing. But he had one more pinnacle to achieve: set an American record in the half-marathon and marathon in the 40 and over age group, *and* win a world championship in long-distance triathlon—a nearly impossible combination of feats to consider.

Seeking Shelter in the Storm

By mid-1993, life at home had become unbearable for Rick. He and his wife were ensnarled in a contentious divorce, training for his last major athletic goals was intensely difficult, anxiety over what his post-competing days would hold was thick, and he was barely able to make it through any twenty-four-hour period without feeling desperate and lost. He was as far away from the happy, mellow, lighthearted Rick as he could imagine.

Rick's world had built up from the wonderfully barren landscape of calmness he'd enjoyed throughout his precollege years into a frenzied pile of stress, bitterness, scandal, aggravation, lost dreams, and a crumbling life. Within the next few months, two things happened to make his situation even more complicated: First, Rick received a diagnosis of testicular cancer. He'd felt a heaviness in his abdomen, and routine testing had uncovered the cause. Testicular cancer when caught early is very treatable, but it's still cancer: terrifying, exigent, and potentially life-altering. Rick's Olympic dreams had been dashed by Carter; his over-forty marathon and triathlon records dreams were dashed by cancer.

Testicular cancer was a problem he had to deal with, but it was curable. So Rick attacked the cancer the way he attacked a difficult race—workmanlike and with no doubt he'd prevail. Besides, he had other crises to attend to. In between and around treatment, Rick continued to find peace in competition, even though he couldn't compete at the elite level of his glory days. In late-1993, while competing in a local marathon, he encountered that second source of complication: another woman.

Rick met Jessica, an elite triathlete and long-distance runner herself, in late-1993, and sparks—more like lightning bolts—flew between them. But, with everything going on at the time, Rick couldn't add another source of turmoil. He needed to pursue *solutions* to his problems. He chalked it up to bad timing and moved on.

A few months after that local event, Rick received a call from a sponsor asking him to fly to an event with another athlete to represent their products. Serendipitously, that athlete turned out to be Jessica. Alone on the road together, the electricity between them was unavoidable. Rick and Jessica began a relationship during the height of his turmoil, and they quickly fell in love. But Rick was still married, and months into the affair, Jessica told Rick she was in too deep.

"I'm moving to Arizona," Jessica said. "I can't be the other woman. Find me after you're done, if you want. If you've decided who you want to be."

Rick's divorce had been in progress before he met Jessica, and he didn't wait too long after his divorce was final to try and win Jessica back. Although some of the madness in his life had subsided, the flurry of discourse didn't: He'd been driven to do things he either couldn't sustain, competing, or couldn't be proud of, infidelity; his professional athletic career was over; his marriage had ended in failure; he fought with difficulty to maintain relationships with his kids; and he pursued every reasonable lead in the product-repping game to eke out a living. Thankfully, there was one shining light for him: Jessica. By then, the cancer was gone, but even with her at his side, Rick still very much wrestled with who he was and who he wanted to be.

During the subsequent few years, as he shifted to a new, post-elite-athlete life, Rick confided in his old college coach, who continued to mentor him through the process of transitioning his life. He helped Rick get into coaching, helped him to become a better person, and led Rick to Christ. As a result, Rick's personal life started to develop new meaning, and he began to rely on more than just swimming, biking, and running as a source of self-evaluation.

Rick became the running coach at a Division II school in Texas, then Colorado, and finally in Southern California, where he coached both the men's and the women's track teams. He spent the next several years learning how to be content with who he was and what he'd accomplished and forgive himself for the mistakes he'd made. His sole focus was on living his life in ways that were meaningful and fulfilling. And over time, he found a place of satisfaction, acceptance, and optimism. He and Jessica pushed forward together, with a deeply committed love and trust, finding their way through years of counseling, individually and as a couple; through learning how to embrace their faith; and through working together to navigate the ups and downs of life.

So when the second cancer diagnosis came—prostate cancer this time—it shook him to his core.

I'm finally in the middle of the perfect run I want, and I don't want it to end.

Choices

"So, what are our options?" Rick asked the doctor.

The urologist explained that the tumor was surrounding a bundle of nerves on either side of the prostate, and those bundles were responsible for sexual function and continence. Radiating the tumor or removing the prostate through a procedure called a prostatectomy would likely leave Rick impotent and incontinent.

"Let me get this straight," Rick said. "I'll have to wear diapers all the time and give myself a shot in my penis each time I want to have sex with my wife?"

I'd rather die, he thought.

There were other treatment regimens available, such as chemotherapy, hormone therapy, and cryotherapy, but the doctor believed surgery or, at the least, radiation therapy was the best choice based on all the circumstances. "Don't take this the wrong way, Doc," Rick said. "But my gut is telling me to find a couple more opinions."

"I'd do the same thing," the doctor responded, "although you will find that treating prostate cancer is not as much of an art as with many other cancers. We've come a long way in narrowing things down to what works."

Rick sought another opinion, and the second doctor's treatment plan paralleled the first. Treatment for his prostate was available, accessible, reliable, and proven, and because he'd caught the cancer early, prognosis was favorable. The side effects were the problem.

"I know you're afraid that your manhood will disappear," Jessica said to him late one night. "But that could never be the case. We'll figure out how to work through those things. God doesn't want those things to get in the way of me having my husband."

"I won't *be* a husband to you if I'm in diapers," Rick argued. "And not making love to you unless I put a pump on me or stick a needle in my balls—it can't be that way."

By the time they decided to go with surgery, they had prayed, argued, discussed, cried, and hashed and rehashed their points, attempting to persuade the other to see their perspectives. But Rick couldn't argue with the ultimate truth that there was more to their relationship than uncomplicated sex and bathroom habits. They scheduled the surgery for a few months later, after the spring running season was over, so Rick wouldn't miss coaching his team through the collegiate competing season.

As that spring unfolded, a series of extraordinary events rocked Jessica's world, and then Rick's. He would never go in for the surgery he feared so much.

Bad Timing

Rick knew that no matter the specific timing, cancer would not have been less distressing, but the timing was *awful*. Not only was he balancing a busy and tense schedule coaching his college running programs, but he was trying to wrap his mind around what lay ahead of him with his cancer. At the same time, Jessica's mom was dying. They visited her as often as they could, and on one of those occasions, her mom felt the need to tell Jessica something she'd been hiding from her for her entire life—and it was a bomb.

"It's about my dad," Jessica told Rick. As she spoke, she was white as a ghost.

"You already know about all that," Rick said, confused. Jessica's dad had come out as gay when he was forty.

Jessica shook her head. "No, it's not that. Mom said, 'Your dad is not your father. Your *real* father is a man named John Danker.'"

Over the next several weeks, during the height of anxiousness about Rick's cancer, Jessica struggled to make sense of what she was told. Rick tried to help calm her while she scrambled to discover some of the details of an extraordinary story; at the same time, he leaned on *her* to help calm *him* about the upcoming treatments. Once armed with enough information to explain what her mom had told her, Jessica wrote a long letter to one of John Danker's children, a woman name Beverly Danker, and finished it with an invitation to reach out with a phone call. About a week later, Jessica's cell phone rang.

"Hello . . . Yes, it is. Beverly?"

"Is it her?" Rick asked in a hushed voice. Rick and Jessica had been married long enough to know each other's subtle facial expressions, and Rick read shock and panic on Jessica.

Jessica poked at the speaker icon a few times before she hit it—her hands were shaking. "Okay," she said into the phone, looking at Rick for comfort. "I'm here."

"Hi there. This is crazy and, well, not so crazy," the woman said. "I know we all only just found this out . . . but Dad . . . he's just the gift that keeps on giving."

She spoke with Beverly more than an hour, and over the next several weeks, as Rick's surgery drew closer and the prospect of those horrible side effects became more real, Jessica uncovered little pieces of a wild and complicated picture, and they came to learn a remarkable set of stories about her long-hidden past.

Seeds of Secrecy

Rick and Jessica would often joke that Rick's parents might've been cast in the mold of *Ozzie and Harriet*. If that were the case, what they found out about her parents might've made them the exact opposite.

Jessica's mother, Elizabeth, a beautiful, light-skinned, blonde woman, grew up in Madison and was trying to find the beginning steps of her path into adulthood after a traumatic childhood: Her father had killed himself when she was eight, and her mother had struggled to raise her on her own. When she was nineteen, Elizabeth applied to work as a secretary at one of Madison's largest car dealerships. John Danker was the larger-than-life owner of that dealership, and even though he was married and had five children at home, he loved to prey on the women in his employ. John targeted Jessica's mother, and as any strong male might have done at that point in her life, lured her into his trap. Weeks after beginning work there, Elizabeth became pregnant.

A nineteen-year-old, single, pregnant girl in Madison in the 1950s didn't have many options. Running away wouldn't have been feasible; an illegal and dangerous abortion was out of the question; and raising a child on her own— seeing what it had done to her own widowed mother—would have been too difficult and disgraceful. But apparently, Elizabeth had one option: Her friend had just told her about a pleasant twenty-two-year-old marketing associate named Robert, who she thought needed to find a wife and start building a family. It was a timely stroke of luck. Elizabeth's friend didn't know Elizabeth was pregnant nor that Robert was living a hidden life: he was gay and had to keep his true identity hidden.

Elizabeth's friend arranged for the two of them to meet on a blind date. Unbeknownst to Elizabeth—and unspoken between the two of them—they *both* had pressing agendas. Robert's was to quell the hushed talk about him not having any girlfriends at his age, and Elizabeth's was to find a husband and fast. Armed with the most unlikely of aligned hidden agendas, each was able to advance toward their goal without resistance. Within a few days of that first date, Elizabeth coaxed Robert into bed. Even if uncomfortable, his first interlude with a woman was successful. He'd found the cover—albeit a severely dysfunctional one—he so desperately sought. Weeks after their assignation, Elizabeth revealed, to her questionable astonishment, that she'd missed her period and was afraid she might be pregnant.

It was a lightning-quick capture for both of them. They hastily married, and about eight months later, Jessica and her twin brother were born. Robert camouflaged his being gay with an instant traditional family, and Elizabeth had found a way out of a very difficult predicament.

When Jessica was six, her mother had another child. Jessica had told Rick how, even when young, it was hard not to notice how that baby looked so much like her parents and how little she and her brother did, but she didn't know enough to think oddly of it, and to her knowledge, nobody had questioned appearances. Her mother had successfully kept her secret hidden. Jessica had told Rick it nagged her a little as she got older, but her life until just then had given her little reason to believe it was anything more than just odd.

When Jessica was in her forties, her dad told her he was gay and that he had been his whole life. Then, once Jessica learned her mom's big secret, which explained some of what she'd suspected growing up, she pieced it all together with the help of a DNA test the dad she'd known her whole life reluctantly agreed to take. The history behind Jessica's true identity became clear: John

Danker and his wife had raised their own kids, ignorant to the reality that he had fathered twins with Jessica's mother. Jessica's dad was able to hide being gay through four decades of marriage because Jessica's mother was hiding a much bigger secret: Jessica's dad was not her brother's father or hers. Jessica's sister was, in fact, her half-sister, and Jessica and her twin had a slew of half siblings whose namesake was Danker.

Signs?

Out of all that unlikely craziness came a conversation that proved monumental in Rick's plan to fight his advancing prostate cancer. After one of her talks with Beverly, Jessica called Rick.

"The topic of your cancer came up," she said. "Beverly asked me if I'd heard of proton radiation therapy—someone her husband knows had just successfully undergone that treatment. She sent me an article on it. Proton radiation is a lesser known—but not new—way to treat cancer. We should look into this before your surgery. There's a few facilities right there in Southern California."

"I don't know, honey. We kinda know what's what at this point. Dr. Morrow never said anything about it."

"I looked some stuff up online, and it's interesting. It can't hurt to see," Jessica said.

"I don't know. What's the point, really?"

"Come on, babe. Coincidences like this don't just happen—I mean, having found out about my family and Beverly's friend, and the center's right in our backyard. Maybe it's a sign."

"I hear you. It would be great if coincidences were more than just that, but we've got to accept what's going to happen and figure out a way to move forward," he said. Rick had learned not to look back with the hopes of changing the outcome. *Things were what they were, and they are what they are. You gotta look ahead.*

But he also had learned that Jessica was going to get her way, especially when her argument sprung from a place of her love for him. "Okay, honey. Make the appointment. We'll go see what it's all about," he relented.

Hope was not running hot through Rick's thoughts as they drove to the proton radiation oncologist's facility. He was resolved to try to learn how to accept what would be his new reality—diapers and a shot every time he wanted to make love to his wife. Hope had no place there.

Once inside the new-looking building, the receptionist greeted them. "Dr. Capri will be with you in a moment," she said.

"His name is Dr. Capri?" Rick asked.

"Yes," the lady answered.

Jessica turned to Rick. "Why'd you ask?"

"No reason. Name's familiar." Rick remembered bumping into a guy—a former budding athlete—named Doug Capri at a big swim meet in Long Beach and at some other local races. He remembered the guy was a doctor and might've been some kind of coach as well.

"Dr. Capri is pretty excited you're here," the receptionist said and smiled.

Nah, can't be the same guy.

When called, Rick and Jessica followed the nurse. Once in the hallway, Rick glimpsed a view of what looked like four or five treatment rooms off to the right, and a shiver ran down his back. On an adjacent wall, he saw a bell, centered and solitary, with a thick, short rope with a knot at the end hanging down from the clapper.

A bell? Rick asked himself. *Odd.*

A nameplate was on the wall outside of the office they were being led into: *Dr. Doug Capri, Chief Radiation Oncologist, Director.*

When they walked in, Dr. Capri jumped around his desk with a huge smile on his face. He was a small-framed man in his young fifties but spry enough to be half that age. Rick guessed about five foot eight, a hundred and forty pounds—a runner's body.

"When I saw the name come through, I knew it!" he said.

"You're *that* Doug Capri?" Rick asked.

"I'm sorry," Dr. Capri said, reaching his hand out. "You must be Jessica. Nice to meet you. Please sit down. Let's talk. You've no idea how much I idolized your husband growing up. He's the reason I was a runner and swimmer—do run and swim—and coached."

"Really?" Jessica asked.

"Without a doubt. Can I tell you a quick story? You don't mind, do you, Rick?"

"I always like a good story about Rick's past," Jessica said, winking at Rick.

"It must have been just before high school. I was a runner, but when I read about Rick going sub-sixty-three for a half . . . God, did I want to be that fast. I mean, *sub-sixty-three*. So, I make it on the track team, and me and my teammates are running a 10K in Orange County, and who is there but your husband? We walk up and bug him about autographs, and he asks, 'So, where do you guys run? What type of events do you do? Do you train in other sports? What's your team like?' He—you—were so unbelievably friendly. We talked about it for three years. And then, building up to the Olympics, you were on fire. . The guys and I were so crushed about the Olympics."

Rick waved him off, and Dr. Capri continued. "So, my story. *I* beat this legend in a race. It was years later, in 1987. So Rick was doing a tune-up race in Ontario. You were starting to win every triathlon. I was the leader's bike escort on the run. Rick comes out of the water, smashes the bike, and then comes out of the run transition like a man on fire. I almost make him run into me, because I'm looking over my shoulder in awe. I pedaled like crazy and then kept my distance. He won the race, of course, but I beat him to the finish. I always brag about beating you in a race."

For the next half hour, Rick and Dr. Capri talked endurance athletics, Olympic trials, and coaching. Finally, Dr. Capri asked Rick about his diagnosis and what the other oncologists had told him. "Both biopsies confirmed that both nerve bundles are affected?"

"Wrapped around them both. Don't you want to get my records?" Rick asked.

"Of course. My first consultation is usually very general in nature, though, as I've found many people don't know much about proton therapy."

Dr. Capri explained the basics of the therapy—highly charged protons kill cancer cells, and they're able to administer the radiation to specific cells via mapping the exact location of the tumor. A very expensive machine called a cyclotron charges the protons, then they're sent to the tumor and attack specific cells, unlike traditional radiation, which continues to irradiate an area around the tumor as the radiation leaves the body.

"An analogy people usually understand is that the procedure is like a 3D printer: The model—the tumor—is 3D-printed, then we hit the tumor with protons, one exacting cell at a time."

"Why didn't my urologist and oncologist talk to us about this?" Rick asked.

"I could talk about that for a long time, but really it comes down to money. It'll go down, but it costs about one hundred million dollars—and a lot of space—to set up a facility, and, without being rude, because it's so expensive, proton therapy is not very prevalent. A great percentage of urologists and oncologists just plain don't know enough about it," Dr. Capri said.

"What's the catch?" Rick asked.

"Besides the cost, none. In fact, just the opposite. I can't promise anything, and I'll have to review your records, do some scans and other tests, but my team and I do the treatments here, on an out-patient basis, and there's no pain. Failure rates are about the same for all treatments, but depending on several factors, we can often avoid—or at the least, minimize—the side effects."

Rick gave Dr. Capri a questioning look.

"Yes," he said. "Little or no chance of incontinence, bowel and other gastrointestinal issues—or reduced sexual function."

Little or no chance of losing my ability to get an erection? No diapers?

On the drive home, Rick and Jessica were silent. Rick was stunned, and he could tell Jessica was as well. They barely spoke a word until they walked up to the house.

"You want to go for a run and talk about it?" Jessica asked.

About a mile into the run, Rick spoke. "I was thinking. So, no chance I meet you and that you'll teach me so much about love and life, right? And no chance I get cancer at just this crazy time in our lives, right? And we do pray for guidance and answers and for a miracle to help us out, right? And there's definitely no chance you have a whole secret family, or that one of them tells you about this procedure we never found out about, right? And just to make it totally improbable, it's that guy who's the doctor. I got that all right, right?"

"Yeah, too coincidental and too impossible to ever happen, honey," Jessica said.

"So there's nothing to talk about, is there?" Rick asked.

"Nope. Let's just run."

Rick's Epilogue

Rick and I spoke many times, and no matter the topics we addressed—the successes and the failures of his athletic career, his ability to continually make bad choices in his past, the beautiful and sometimes terrible dynamics he experienced with his kids, the challenges he and Jessica faced until they finally learned how to love and be loved—I could sense his humility and gratitude at the end of every story. He'd describe his frenzied attempts to control life and the outcomes of his efforts, and then something would happen to show him that he was not in control.

"I'm very much my own guy," he said to me during one of our talks. "You've figured that out by now. I do what I want, how I want. But it's taken me a long time to understand that I'm not in control. Growing up, I didn't give my trust to anybody, except my high school coach and my college coach. They came along at the exact perfect moment for me. Just like Jessica. Just like God. Just like Dr. Capri. I thought I was master and commander of so much in my life—my first marriage, my kids, my career, my health, *everything*—but I wasn't.

"Life is kind of like running the last mile of a competitive marathon. You think you know what's coming . . . *it's what you do*. You've been through so much and done unbelievable amounts of training. You believe in yourself and your ability to push through anything, you're in command, and you've got the balls to put it all out on the line . . . and then the last hundred yards comes. You can see the finish line, you've crossed it before, you know what's coming and how to deal with it, but the pain burns a hole through your chest and shreds your legs through a meat grinder and rips apart your lungs. And you start to question everything. You start to doubt. The pain is unbearable, unimaginable—much worse than you think you can handle—and if you try to control it, you're going to lose. The only way to make it to the finish is to give in to the pain, to let go, to embrace the unknown and allow some higher power, some unknown source, something outside of yourself—because you have nothing left inside—to take you forward, across the line. I'm blessed to have at last learned that kind of relinquishment in my personal life."

If not for a life filled with timely and remarkable coincidences, Rick might not have ever learned how to get through the pain of letting go, putting his fate in the hands of the powers that be—and in people who help push him forward—instead of always having to race to the line under his own power, alone, with nothing but pain in his pounding heart.

Days and Days in Texas: Part II

I heard it at a comedy club, decades before I found myself biking into and down and across Texas. "I grew up in Texas," the comedian said. "Texas is flat, let me tell you. How flat, you ask? Texas is so flat, when you look out over the horizon, you see the back of your head."

Until you've biked a thousand miles all over Texas, you don't know how *not* flat Texas is. On day eighteen, I left Dallas and headed toward Waco, Texas, 101 miles and 2,300 feet of climbing away. By nine o'clock in the morning it was almost ninety degrees and Texas-sticky. Before I even started, the salty sweat began to aggravate the rash on the backs of my legs, which went from the bottom of my bike shorts to halfway down my calves.

The shortest route to Waco had me on back roads, dirt roads, and single-lane highways as I zig-zagged south—and into a menacing southeast wind. I ran out of fluids twice—the first time for almost two hours. But it wasn't a result of poor planning. Rather, I was taking in four pounds of water an hour to keep ahead of my sweat rate, and I was two to three hours between one-stoplight towns at a time.

I had a lot of time to think that day. For eleven hours, I was on desolate, empty roads, passing miles-long fields that separated one rural farm house from the next, which all had the Star of Texas, the Seal of the Republic of Texas, or Texas itself painted prominently on the public side of the barn or on the front of the garage, sculpted on the roof or as a free-standing display, or flying atop of flag poles that stood in tall defiance of the mostly treeless, bucolic landscape. Texas has a diverse terrain—expansive and lush, bone-dry and dusty, rocky, hilly, pancake flat. The surroundings are anything but uniform. But the one unfailing sight, no matter the landscape, is the prominent displays by Texans of their love for Texas—it's unbridled and inescapable, and every turn of the pedals revealed another Texas-sized exhibit of that passion. As my eyes roamed that living mural of glorifications, my mind wandered among the stories of the people involved in the Cycle of Lives. I thought about their passions and the ways in which *they* emblazoned their particular affections.

None of the participants was a one-dimensional illustration, defined only by the emotions that most prominently characterized their cancer ordeals. Each was a multilayered, complex collection of experiences and perspectives. But in the narrow context of the Cycle of Lives, each did have a love-of-Texas-level manifestation or two that symbolized their journey. Jen's was her quest to become a pediatric oncology nurse, Bobby's was to learn how to love and be loved, Dominic's was a lifelong battle against himself, and Debra's a fight to overcome her loss of faith. My own journey—cancer or otherwise—was unclear. Even a decade past losing June, I was still trying to figure out the greater meanings surrounding the challenges, blessings, and hardships that existed inside of my more than five-decades-long maze.

Maybe my life is symbolized by just that: long, contemplative journeys in search of answers, in search of some clarity, lost in the tumult, looking for a way out through all the questions that were blocking my view.

I started out day nineteen with both dread and anticipation—dread for a 102-mile ride from Waco to Austin, Texas, with over three thousand feet of climbing and an anticipated heat index of 110 degrees, and anticipation for the rest day scheduled for day twenty. Thankfully, my friend Kristy in Austin offered to drive up and relieve me of my saddle bags. She met me at about the seventy-five-mile mark. Relief couldn't have come at a better time—sweat was flowing from every pore on my body, and the hills, never a knockout punch but rather a constant barrage of body blows, caused my legs to burn with as much intensity as the cement below me. In addition to the sheer beating I was taking thanks to the elements and terrain, with all the added weight from carrying extra fluids and from having stocked up at the bike shop in Dallas, I was pushing thirtyish pounds more than when Erin set me off alone four hundred miles back. Although I still struggled to the finish point that day, being free of the panniers for the last couple of hours was a glorious respite.

After resting a day in Austin, I took off on day twenty-one, ready to continue my unending trek through Texas. Brenham, Texas, was about ninety miles away, and Kristy offered to drive my saddlebags there so I could have a light ride. Again, it was the help I needed when I needed it, because that repetitive trio of doom—headwind, heat, and hills—was relentless in its consistency, and lighter bike or not, I was at it for more hours than I should have been.

My friend Chad arrived that night, which meant that I could rely on his help for the next few days. I'd enjoyed the challenge and contemplative solitude of self-sufficiency, but there was no denying that without the support, I wouldn't have been able to keep up the schedule as planned. All the help I'd been given was what allowed me to keep moving—and moving with focus and purpose.

Focus was important on day twenty-two—a harrowing, 111-mile ride from Brenham to Baytown, Texas, along dangerous, bumpy, traffic-jammed, shoulderless roads leading into, around, and through the massive construction zone known as Houston—another in an endless string of long, smoldering, dusty, windy Texas days. An accident was a minute's lack of focus away.

As I rolled into Baytown, my excitement for being done with such a meaty part of the country was only overshadowed by my gratitude for all the help I collectively received on my adventure through the Lone Star State.

Help is a funny thing—sometimes you don't know when you'll need it, sometimes you don't know in what form it might come, but if you're in need of it and you don't have access to it, help can be the only thing that matters. Somehow, I'd made it three days and more than three hundred miles without a flat tire; I hadn't had a single one since receiving help from Keller back in Dallas. In retrospect, I hadn't needed to carry all those tubes, but I knew that even if not directly then or in that form, someday, somehow, I'd be much worse off had he not stopped to help me.

I had never been comfortable turning to others in my life, but I was learning that help can be immediate or it can be tucked away and used at another time, but its effects can be forever lasting. And the idea of help often brought me to the story of Maggie.

Maggie

Relationship to cancer: Caregiver

Age: Fifty-eight

Family status: Single

Location: Westchester County, New York

First encounter with cancer: Thirty years old

Cancer summary: Maggie was the primary caregiver for her grandmother and then her other grandmother. Then she became the primary caregiver for her mother, who died of liver cancer. Now, she is the primary caregiver for her elderly father, who has prostate and stomach cancer. She has also been a primary and secondary caregiver for others in her life.

Strongest positive emotion during cancer experience: Acceptance

Strongest negative emotion during cancer experience: Melancholy

How we met: When I worked on Wall Street, one of my jobs was to recruit top talent from the competition. The recruiting process, precommitment, was all sales, but once the recruit committed to join our firm, the real work began. Transitioning a wealth advisory practice from one firm to another is both a complex operation and an emotionally taxing process for the recruit. Success is based solely on the receiving firm's ability to tend to the endless administrative details while helping the recruit navigate ups and downs along the way.

That's where Maggie came in—she ran the division responsible for dealing with all facets great and small related to helping newly recruited advisors successfully transfer millions of dollars of collective revenues per year. Maggie was the perfect person to take responsibility for the well-being of dozens of advisors and their thousands of clients. Caring for others during their most difficult times is what Maggie does and what she has always been about.

I befriended Maggie early in my career. I knew it was critical to my survival to make friends with someone so important to my success and growth. During the twenty-plus years I've known her, she's had a reputation for being the go-to business resource. But it was only through this project that I came to know how much of a caretaker Maggie really is.

A few years after I left the firm where we both worked, Maggie reached out to me. She'd heard about the Cycle of Lives project, and she'd called to learn more. Maggie had always offered financial support for the fundraising events I did, and after hearing about this one, she offered her support again. Only this time, she asked that I accept her donation in support of her mother, who was nearing the end of her battle with liver cancer.

"Of course," I said. "Tell me about what's going on."

While we talked, I learned how Maggie had taken care of one person after another throughout her life. As we continued to talk on a more personal, purposeful level, I came to understand how a lifetime of caregiving, one that I'd have thought burdensome, was to her an oft-repeated privilege.

Caring for Others

The Origins of Care

Maggie loved horses. She was *born* loving horses. One of Maggie's earliest memories was of her grandpa holding her on a small pony that her dad had rented for a party. She couldn't have been old enough to hold on by herself, but she remembered feeling as though she *belonged* on the horse. Even after she fell off the small pony that her grandpa found for her first solo ride a few years later, Maggie wanted nothing but to be on a horse. She had run up to her dad that same night, bruises and all, and begged him to let her buy a horse. "How 'bout I give you a dollar, and you can buy four quarter horses," he'd said, laughing.

Maggie grew up in Ossining, New York, a small town on the Hudson River about an hour's drive from New York City. Her parents met on a blind date, married not long after, and enjoyed more than fifty years of marriage.

Maggie had two sisters and two brothers. She was born second, almost four years after her eldest sister. Each of Maggie's younger siblings was born almost exactly every two years after her. Mom stayed home to raise the kids, and Dad owned a local beverage distribution company and retail store. Both spent their time busied by the primary focus of their lives: Dad worked unending hours at the store, at least six days a week, while Mom tended to the endless stream of kids, grandparents, aunts, uncles, and cousins who constantly filled the house. Many of Maggie's relatives lived nearby, and they came and went as casually as if they all lived together. The house wasn't chaotic, just busy. There were always things to do and chores to attend to and meals to cook.

Maggie's parents had always celebrated one collective birthday for all the kids, as there was not much free time for celebrations—other than Easter and Christmas. The family took two trips each year—the first was to the Catskill Mountains for a few days, where they'd do things like visit the exotic animal farm, hike to Kaaterskill Falls, and have picnics late into the afternoon. The second trip was a yearly visit to Playland Park, an amusement park in Rye, about thirty miles away from Ossining.

What Maggie's family might've lacked in birthday celebrations and extravagant trips, though, they made up for in hearty nightly family dinners; an overflowing and vibrant, warm home; and weekend outings with her mom while her dad worked.

All the children had chores growing up, but Maggie seemed to be the only one who didn't need coaxing to complete them—especially when doing so left time for a drive to the library or a walk around town, or better yet, to a field or a river's trail or a country road. She never complained about cleaning, watching her baby brother and sisters, or helping in the kitchen—especially when her grandma was over baking Hungarian cookies. Maggie learned early that work and chores and taking responsibility were simply part of life—service in response to need was never questioned.

Finding Horses

One Saturday when she was eight, Maggie was in the back seat of her dad's 1957 Chevrolet Bel Air. Her mom hummed to a song on the radio and slowly navigated Barnes Road, a thin, bumpy stretch of dirt off Route 133 that led toward a small park surrounding Echo Lake. Maggie sat between her older sister—who, at twelve, was way too mature to give any attention to her younger siblings—and her younger brother. Her sister opted to ignore everyone and looked out the window and sang along to a song a lady sang about buying cars and having fun in San Jose. Her brother kept vrooming his Tonka Truck down Maggie's right arm and onto the fading tan leather seat between them. Her four-year-old sister stood in the front seat facing the back to show her oldest sister how well she could dance. The baby was with Grandma. Dad, of course, was at the store. It was a typical Saturday in December.

Mom hit a huge hole in the road, and Maggie's baby sister went flying up and bumped her head on the roof of the car. Maggie leaned forward and grabbed her sister's wrist to steady her in case another bump came. Nobody but Maggie seemed to notice. Maggie didn't mind; she thought things like keeping her baby sister from bumping her head were *expected* of her. They pulled up to the lake's shore, and Mom stopped the car and turned the music louder.

Her mom sang loudly along with the radio and laughed. Her older sister opened the door to get out, and Maggie rushed out behind her. The week before, Maggie had stumbled on fresh horse droppings at the same spot by the lake, and she was excited to go looking for more clues that a horse might be near. Maybe she'd even get to see the horse this time.

After promising Mom she'd stay close enough to be seen, Maggie walked along the stream that fed the small lake. She jumped from rock to rock, moving away from the field where her mom had set up a blanket, and made her way up the water's edge. She glanced back once but then, forgetting her pledge, set off in search of the horse. Not two minutes later, a loud whinny came from the woods. Maggie froze; the only sign of movement was a faint fog coming out of her mouth. She waited, hoping to hear that wondrous sound again, and just when she was about to turn around, the sound came again from the same direction.

Maggie felt a ping run through her, the ping an eight-year-old feels, but doesn't recognize, when she is about to do something a parent told her not to do. She brushed the ping off and started walking through the trees toward where the horse might be. About twenty yards in, the trees cleared to an expansive field wrapped by a weathered, split-rail fence. At least another thirty yards past the fence, a tall man, who looked older than her grandpa, stood next to a huge barn. He wore high black boots and a long apron that wrapped over his pants and jacket. He held a rope behind him that disappeared into the open side doors of the barn. The man gently pulled on the rope, but only when she heard another whinny come thundering out of the barn did Maggie understand that the horse was so close.

Maggie climbed on the lower wrung of the fence. She watched the man as he stepped backward, attempting to pull the horse out from the barn. Maggie leaned over the upper railing, excited to see what a horse whose whinny was that loud looked like. The old man appeared to be talking toward the inside of the barn, probably to try to calm the horse, but it didn't hide that he was struggling a little against the rope. After a few more uneven steps back, the man had tussled the horse halfway out.

The horse was majestic. His dark brown hair glistened, reflecting the light gray sky, and as he moved, his muscles flexed, showing definition and strength and power. His nose was higher than the top of the man's head. The horse shook his head and chewed at the bit in his mouth; his mane swept from side to side, brushing against his long neck like waves against the shore. The horse stamped a little as he resisted the man's pull, and he breathed loudly, showing his displeasure. Maggie took in every detail. It was like the fence was ten feet away, not a hundred feet across the field.

"It's okay," Maggie whispered quietly. "It's all right, boy."

Just then, the horse turned toward her, paused, and looked straight at her, as though he'd heard her whisper. As he locked eyes with her, the horse slowed his breathing and relaxed his gait. The rope between the man and the horse drooped, removing the tension between the two. Maggie stared down the horse, and the horse stared down Maggie. Maggie felt as if she could have reached out and touched him—and she was sure the horse wanted her to rub his neck and whisper to him—if only it were just a little closer.

The old man turned to see what had caught the horse's attention, and when he saw Maggie, he tipped his head and smiled at her. The man led the calmed horse to the front of the barn and toward a round pen near the other side. He stopped and waved Maggie over, but there was no way she would.

Maggie knew that house. It was the largest one in that part of town, and everybody knew that a mean lady lived there. Maggie had never met her, or even seen her—and she didn't know anybody who had—but she wasn't going to take any chances. She shook her head and looked down. When she looked back up, she could see that the horse remained untroubled as the man opened the gate, then began to walk him around the inside of the pen.

"There you are," Maggie heard her older sister's voice say behind her. "Mom sent me after you. Didn't you hear me calling you?"

Maggie turned her head, eager to show her excitement, but her sister had already turned her back and started to walk away. "No, I didn't hear you." Maggie said to her sister's back.

"You weren't really thinking of going on that woman's property, were you? She'd probably have eaten you up."

Maggie stepped down from the railing and looked one last time in the horse's direction, then she turned away and ran to catch up with her sister.

In the summer of Maggie's tenth year, her parents sent her to a horse camp—a present they and her grandparents had given to her the previous Christmas. Waiting for the camp was a painful exercise in restraint, yet summer came, at last, and the camp further deepened her love for horses. She learned what it took to clean, feed, and exercise the animals. She learned about the gear, tack, and shoes. She learned what to look for in the mannerisms and actions of the horse, which might indicate the horse's health and emotional state.

The following summer, one of the women who ran the camp offered to sponsor Maggie for a job at a stable owned by the Rockefellers. Although not far from Ossining, it was light-years away in terms of wealth. Even at eleven, Maggie understood that money made all the difference in the world when it came to horses. She was paid to walk, trot, and canter jumping horses. She saved the money she made that summer and even mowed lawns to make more. She was secretly saving for her own horse.

By the time Maggie was thirteen, she'd worked her way up to a trail guide and had saved enough money working at the stable to buy her first horse—if she could partner with her cousin Carol, who loved horses almost as much as she did, and get a little extra help from her dad. Maggie had a horse in mind at the stables where she worked—Dandy—a quarter horse like Dad had joked about when she was little. Dandy was small and gentle, and the girls knew they would be able to care for him. They found a fifty-dollar-per-month stable, and Maggie told her parents she'd do extra chores and odd jobs to pay for her share of the boarding. Her parents agreed.

Dandy was a strong chocolate-brown nine-year-old sprinter. He had effortlessly carried Maggie around the riding pen and on short rides, and both Maggie and Carol clicked with Dandy's moderate, patient personality. Maggie was proud she'd saved her portion of the 350 dollars it took to purchase Dandy. She'd worked so hard and been so patient saving her money, and as she brushed Dandy the first day she owned him, she understood the warm satisfaction of having done what she needed to do to realize her dream of owning her own horse.

Learning to Be Tough

Eight days into owning Dandy, he was injured in a freak accident on a short sprint and came up lame. He had to be put down. Maggie cried for days. She was heartbroken. Owning Dandy was a dream come true, one that ended in a nightmare right after materializing. She didn't know what to do or how to even think of moving on. Days later, the tears had lessened, but Maggie's heartache hadn't. She moved a little slower through the motions of each day: She made her bed, did her usual housework, and helped with her younger brothers and sisters. Her mood was gloomy, and her normally spirited aura disappeared, sucked away by an inconsolable misery.

"Death is a part of life," her mom finally told her. "It's unfortunate the way it came so quick, but death is something you can't often plan for, and it never comes at the right time."

"I don't know what to do," Maggie said. "I worked so hard and waited so long. I wanted him so *bad*."

Dad sat back in his chair, arms folded, squinting in contemplation at Maggie.

"Did you have fun while doing those things?" her mom asked. Maggie looked at her questioningly. "The work and the waiting, that wasn't all bad, was it?"

Maggie shook her head. "But having to put him down was the worst thing ever."

"You do know what to do," her dad said, his expression unchanged. "Just like when you fell off that horse with Pop-Pop when you were little. That's what happens, and it happens all the time. You fall, you get up. You don't go and hide and stop doing what you love."

And she didn't. Working as often as she could—cleaning tack, grooming, feeding, cleaning barns, guiding, and doing any job around horses she could find—Maggie soon earned enough to buy Scout, a Tennessee walking horse. She rode him for about a year.

When Maggie was sixteen, she asked if she could move into her grandma's house. Maggie loved being around her grandma, and she liked helping her grandma, as she was becoming frail and needed more help day-to-day. Although her grandpa had died of lung cancer years earlier, her grandma seemed to age faster after her youngest son died of cancer just weeks after being diagnosed. Another reason she wanted to move in with her grandma was that her house was closer to the barn where Maggie was going to keep her newest horse, Sebago. Sebago was a beautiful, strong thoroughbred, and Maggie wanted to be around him as much as possible.

Prior to moving in to care for her grandma, Maggie had sold Scout and bought Sebago. By then she was driving, which allowed her to pursue better jobs with better clientele and also offered a chance to compete in shows. She'd grown to love jumping, and although it was difficult to successfully compete on the horses she could afford, Maggie didn't care—a saddle, any saddle, was where she wanted to be.

Outside of school, when she wasn't around a barn or a stable or jumping at shows, she was home doing chores for her grandma, driving to her parents' home to help them, or doing things with her brothers and sisters. There wasn't time for anything else but school, family, and horses, and if there were time to choose another pursuit, Maggie would only have opted to do more of the things she was already doing.

Maggie's life during college went along much as it had before: Maggie bought and sold horses, sometimes making money, sometimes not; she cooked for and with her grandma; she took care of the house and helped her parents;

she continued to work around the stables and give riding lessons; and she jumped in shows whenever she could. Her busy life flowed naturally because she loved her family and helping tend to their needs. She loved each of the horses she owned, even the ones she'd had to put down or had died or she'd sold, and she loved knowing what she loved doing—there was no hazy and itching ambition about the future. Maggie found peace and comfort in the saddle, in cleaning out a stable, in taking care of her grandma, and in helping her family, because *those* things were the things she wanted to do.

Maggie was becoming more competitive and making more of a name in the horse community. She continued to buy and sell horses, eyeing ones that might be an investment and scouting for ones that might take her jumping career further. But at some point, she'd have to realize her limitations. Without limitless funds, she would never be an elite showman.

Maggie wasn't sure what she was going to do after college, but she wasn't worried about her direction in life. She wasn't going to leave her grandma's house—she was in her eighties and needed more care—nor was she going to stop jumping in competitions, working around stables, and teaching riding.

A few years after graduating college, a hedge fund manager she'd met through riding asked her if she had ever thought about going to work in the financial business. He told her he thought she'd have the steadiness and drive to thrive in a corporate environment.

Maggie impulsively answered, "No." But she did need to earn more money if she was going to continue to go up against the one-percenters who dominated the sport of jumping. So she talked to her parents and a few of the friends she'd made in college and decided to give it a shot. The hedge fund manager introduced her to some of his friends at a few firms, and Maggie soon found a position that suited her skills and natural tendencies: supporting advisors through the emotional and operational upheaval of transitioning a practice from one firm to another.

Although working at a prominent Wall Street firm impeded her ability to help care for the family as much as she wanted, and it took her away from the stables more than she liked, the earnings did support her—and she continued to compete and invest in more expensive horses.

As the years passed, Maggie's life focused around work, spending time with her family, and caring for her grandma—whom she still lived with while commuting into the city—and her horses.

Measured interruptions came along, and Maggie always prioritized those over herself and her horses because the disruptions centered around her needing to help others. There was the time when her sister died unexpectedly, and Maggie attended to many things around that tragic death that her parents and siblings didn't seem able to deal with. There was the time Maggie took a leave of absence for a stretch of time to help care for a college friend who'd been shot—and shortly thereafter died—as a result of a dispute with one of his tenants. There was the time when she did all she could to help take care of her brother and his kids when his wife went through terminal cancer. The list went on.

The Mean Old Lady

There was even the time she took care of the allegedly very mean lady who lived in the big house she'd seen that day she wandered off as a young girl in search of the horse behind the whinny. Meeting that lady happened one October day when Maggie was feeling the weight of Grandma's deteriorating condition, the fear brought on by her mother's discovery of some potentially major health issues, the lingering heartbreak of losing her college friend so tragically—because it pained her so that he was so afraid of dying—and a myriad of other emotional weights that had managed to overtake her normally calm mind.

Maggie needed to get away. She drove aimlessly, not wanting to head toward the city but not wanting to go back to her grandma's, her mom and dad's, or any place where she knew people were dealing with heavy stuff. When she came to Route 133, she remembered the wintery picnics Mom had planned and the whinny through the trees and the worn fence railing she stood on as she whispered across a field to a horse who was afraid of leaving the security of its pen. She drove down the road that led to the field and the large house.

It was easy to see that the property had been neglected, but not so much so that it might be uninhabited. Maggie parked in front of the house. It looked smaller than she remembered. She sat in the car and daydreamed about playing at her dad's store, the horses she rode, the horses she owned, the family she loved so much, and the people she'd cared about who'd died. As she drove down memory lane, looking past the weathered white gate toward the house of the mean lady, she smiled.

You need to let it all go. Things happen all the time. You don't just go hide.

Prompted by the long-remembered words of her dad, she got out of the car and approached the gate that protected a long walkway to the house. She opened the gate and walked down a path of weathered stepping-stones that led to the porch. She stood at the front door, deciding whether or not she should knock. At last, she did. Then she knocked again. And then a third time. She heard some rustling from inside and readied herself for what would assuredly be an awkward introduction.

An elderly woman, older than Grandma, dressed as though for church, even though it was a Saturday afternoon, stood a foot shorter than Maggie. The woman looked her over.

"Hello," Maggie started. "This is going to be a weird question, but do you mind if I ask it anyway?"

The woman looked Maggie up and down again but said nothing.

"I was curious to know how long you've lived here."

After a painfully long silence, the woman answered. "Long time. A very long time. Who wants to know?"

"Do you still own horses?" Maggie asked.

"I don't. And you still haven't told me who you are."

Halfway through Maggie's explanation, the woman invited her in. They spent the next hour talking about a dozen different topics: Ossining, horses, Maggie's family, the woman's background and the love she had for her property, and even death, when Maggie told her what had prompted the visit. It turned out the woman had lost her husband to cancer decades earlier.

The mean old lady was anything but. She and Maggie became friends and remained friends until the woman died a few years later. Maggie took her to several doctor's appointments, helped her with some financial matters, cooked a few dinners, and spent a few late nights comforting her with stories and conversation.

Maggie took death, the preparation for death, and the care needed to stave off death in stride. Sure, she was affected, but she felt she didn't have a choice but to jump in and attend to the people she loved who needed an extra pair of hands or a listening ear or a trusted friend.

Death happens. You don't just go run and hide.

When her sister died, Maggie eased the pain of losing her by taking long rides. When her friend from college died, it weighed on her heart for a long, long time, and she took many rides to help work through her emotions. When the not-so-mean-old-lady died, she rode her thoroughbred, My-T-Fine, through that mystical field of her youth, jumping high over the fence, as if unifying the fear of the unknown with the calmness of having broken its spell.

In between the tragedies and deaths and caring she attended to, Maggie always put herself back into her life's routine, sometimes with ease, sometimes through a process, but always while freeing her mind while on the backs of her horses.

Seeing Them Off

Grandma passed away when Maggie was in her midthirties. Maggie had been taking care of her for almost two decades, and she felt both acceptance and relief.

By that point in her life, Maggie was done with high-level competing; a few years prior, she had a shot at qualifying for the Olympics but fell short. Her life was still centered on the same few things, but Grandma's death created a void. Consistent with every other time she had a break between caring for one person and then being in a position to do the same with the next, she filled the void by providing more care or support to other in-need family members, working a little harder, and, of course, becoming more active in the selling and buying of horses, training more, working at the stables more, and jumping at more competitions. But the voids never lasted long; the ebb and flow between being around family, taking care of someone, work, and horses was an active cycle.

Maggie never felt she was burdened or obligated or held back in any way, but that was the pattern. Rather, she believed that the times she stepped in to care for someone were opportunities for her—and the opportunities never seemed to go away. Not long after Grandma died, Maggie had the opportunity to care for her dad's mother, who was suffering from a fight against cancer, and then a few years later, her mom.

Maggie's mom had pancreatic tumors, which led to several surgeries and procedures, and an endless stream of related illnesses. When Maggie was forty-two, she decided to move back in with her parents to help her dad care for her mom. Their house was still a fairly busy one, and there was simply too much for her dad to manage without assistance.

At first, the challenges of being back in her parents' home full-time were centered around trying to get her mom to allow Maggie to help her. Her mom had been the heart and center of a busy home. She went to church. She navigated the emotional highs and lows that came with a long marriage, having five children, and being the glue that kept a large extended family together. She volunteered at the historical society, and she maintained close friends.

Maggie's mom had been so proud of the fact that she was strong and capable and in control of the major aspects of her life, and it was incredibly difficult for her to see control of those things slip away. As her mom's health deteriorated, managing everything as before—and in as capable a fashion as she had for so long—became an unreasonable endeavor. Maggie's parents settled into new reduced-in-scope patterns that governed their lives. Over the next several years, Maggie and her dad took a larger share of the load as her mom's cancer and the related health issues became more severe.

Cancer can sometimes be managed, until it can't. Cancer had come and gone and come again for her mom during those years. When things progressed to the point where it became evident that her mom wasn't going to get better, Maggie prepared for both the physical and emotional demands that would surely come: She joined a gym so she could build her upper-body strength in anticipation of needing to lift her mom. She began to go to all the doctor's appointments with her mom and her dad so she could better understand all the details surrounding the illness. She talked to her mom—as much and as often as her mom was open to talking. They cried together—about all they were facing, about her dad, about death, about the people they had already lost, about how the family was coping, and most importantly, about all the emotions, the afterlife, and the meaning of it all.

The Bell

Growing up, everyone knew that if a bell rang, it was either time for supper, time to come in from the dark, or time to help Mom with chores. The bell became a family joke, a topic of teasing and remembrance through the generations who had gathered in Maggie's home for more than fifty years. One day, when her mom was noticeably anxious about her deteriorating health and her need to ask for help, Maggie offered her mom a bell.

"Oh, my gosh," her mom said. "A bell?"

"It wasn't just for dinner. You used to give this to us when we were sick, too. You remember? All we had to do was ring it, and you came. You and Dad taught me so much, through so many transitions. You taught me to remove the weights around my mind and heart. You showed me how death is a part of life. You were the rock during so many tough times for us. How could anybody who loves you not comfort you now? How could I not be happy for you to ring for help?"

Months later, cancer invaded her mom's liver and kidneys; it had metastasized throughout her body. Soon after, she was gone. Once again, Maggie was forced to remember she needed to live *her* life too. So many people had died. So many people she had tended to through their difficult times. She was there for so many people, and yet, at some point, she always moved on. That was life. That was the way of the world. *You need to let it go*, she thought. *Things happen all the time. You don't just go and hide.*

After her mom died, Maggie went to the stables more, she rode more, she worked more, and she trained more. Soon after Maggie settled into her life again, her dad began to need help: The tumors they had found in his stomach were diagnosed as malignant.

Maggie's Epilogue
....

Maggie didn't express abundant emotion during our talks. She was quite a matter-of-fact type of person. But that didn't mean she hadn't processed the emotions around death and dying that had claimed so much of her life's experience.

"If I were you, I don't know if I could've been so involved with taking care of so many people," I said. "How do you do it without getting depressed, losing optimism, or feeling so melancholic?"

"Cancer—or any type of illness or injury, like being shot or alcoholism or whatever—is part of life," she replied. "They're not the most important parts, though. How someone chooses to spend their life is the important part. My parents told me once not to always wish for the problem to be gone, because if losing the problem means losing the person, they're going to be gone for a long, long time. I've just learned to accept that we fall, and we have to get up—until we can't."

I asked what she was going to do when her dad passed away.

"I'll ride and work for a few more years. I'll go to the stables and jump and maybe retire to Florida—there's a big horse community down there."

"What I meant was, what are you going to do when there's nobody left for you to take care of?"

There was a long pause. "Well, now. That will create a problem, won't it? I guess I'll have to focus on taking care of myself more."

I doubt she will. I'll bet someone will come along and preempt her going down what to her would be an unfamiliar, selfish road. My guess is, she continues to care for others; that's who she is and how she has chosen to live her life.

Meaningful Encounters

I'd made it through Texas. Day twenty-three—from Baytown, Texas, to Sulphur, Louisiana—was a beast, a long, hot, windy Texas-sized exclamation point to more than a week's worth of monstrous rides and legendary encounters.

I stood in the shower, cringing from the initial pain of hot water running down the rash on the backs of my legs—a rash that had tormented me for two weeks. I was famished, sapped of every ounce of energy I'd need, save for the little I required to soap the day's grime and dirt and bugs off my skin and out of my hair, and I was as stiff and sore from the day as any before it. As I gingerly stomped on my cycling bib, jersey, socks, and gloves, cleaning them as I cleaned myself, the soreness from riding 135 miles in just over fourteen hours—and the accumulated result of biking more than two thousand miles in the three weeks since I took off—rippled through me, accompanying every movement of every muscle as though every cell in my body had gone twelve rounds with a brass-knuckle-wearing opponent. But as I was both the promoter and the willing assailant of that fight, I took an odd satisfaction in the weariness. I was winning the fight—even if *just* winning it—and by doing so, I was earning the right to go to battle each subsequent day. And, as always, there were only two things between the end of one match and the start of the next: a lot of food and a little sleep.

The only non-fast-food restaurant open in Sulphur was Joe's Pizza and Pasta, and Chad and I made it there moments before they locked the door. We enjoyed—well, he enjoyed, I attacked—a couple of plates of Sicilian style pasta, a whole pizza, a table-sized salad, and several baskets of garlic bread. The owner came by to check on us, and the subject of the bike ride came up. Several minutes later, our waitress joined in the conversation, then another waitress, and another. By the time I finished licking the plates, the restaurant was empty, save for Chad and me, the three waitresses, and the owner.

As we waited for the check, Chad and I made plans for the following day. He was scheduled to see me off, then drive the car to New Orleans and fly back to Los Angeles. I'd be self-supporting for only two days, but they were going to be long ones, so I wanted to carry as little gear as possible.

The owner came by and told us her family had gone through several encounters with cancer, and she wanted to pick up our check as a way of thanking us for what we were doing. We tried to dissuade her. After all, it was a small family restaurant that likely couldn't afford to be comping huge meals, but she insisted. As we were getting up to leave, the three waitresses came up to us to say goodbye.

"Can we take a picture with you?" one of them asked, handing me an envelope.

"Of course. What's this?" I asked them.

"Well," another said, "we wanted to do something to help you. It's not much, but we pooled our tips together to donate to your cause. Y'all are doing a good thing, and every one of us has been touched in some way by cancer."

It was easy to imagine how hard the lives of those waitresses might have been; they were all working nights, perhaps with families or second jobs, maybe dealing with medical issues or acting as caregivers or dealing with challenging personal lives. Imagining those things, I was almost moved to tears when I opened the envelope they had given me and there was sixty-three dollars in it—a full night's tips for three hardworking people. As much as they must have needed that money, their desire to support what I was doing was far more worthwhile to them.

I felt as if I rarely lost sight of the goodness in people in respect to the Cycle of Lives project, but I was also never far away from the proof behind those feelings; the truth was offered every day by people like those I met at Joe's Pizza and Pasta. Support—principally from strangers—balanced and reflected my efforts against all the emotional ups and downs and the accomplishments and struggles each day. And in weighing all that out, my ride was turning out to be successful and fulfilling and meaningful. As I lay in bed later that night, I thought of the book participants and what might possibly define their different successes. Each, whether by financial, emotional, relational, health-wise, self-valuation-related, or other means of measure, had a vivid sense of their failures and successes, *because each had cancer as their balancing point.* Most everyone I talked to said that cancer hadn't defined them or fully explained who they were—it wasn't the weight; it wasn't the counterweight. Instead, cancer was a fulcrum, a pivot point, a means by which they could reflect on their fortunes and misfortunes, their fulfillments and their failures, their happiness and their despair.

I fell asleep thinking of Neil, a *Cycle of Lives* book participant, who financially and otherwise was immensely successful. Financially, Neil might've been on the exact opposite end of the spectrum from those women at Joe's Pizza and Pasta. The collective magnitude of funds he had given and raised for a multitude of causes was quite significant, but when levered by their experiences with cancer, the emotions that were evoked from those experiences, and the significance of their generosity, those waitresses easily amassed as much weight as Neil did. They were moved to action just as passionately. Their impact was just as meaningful. The existential weights brought on by contemplating life and death, the realities of cancer, and the emotions experienced as a result of any amount of that kind of trauma are unwavering in their ability to equal the scales for everyone.

Neil

Relationship to cancer: Caregiver

Age: Fifty-eight

Family status: Was married to his late wife Kimberly for close to thirty years. Neil has five children, aged eight to twenty-six. He lost one child when she was eighteen months old.

Location: Chicago, Illinois

First encounter with cancer: As a teenager, via a close family member.

Cancer summary: Neil's wife was diagnosed with advanced brain cancer when she was fifty-four years old. She had surgery, radiation therapy, and chemotherapy, but the cancer couldn't be eradicated. She died eighteen months postdiagnosis.

Cancer specifics: Advanced glioblastoma

Strongest positive emotion during cancer experience: Relief

Strongest negative emotion during cancer experience: Grief

How we met: When I worked in financial services, I often befriended wholesalers, the professionals who provide products and services to our clients. After reading an online post about the Cycle of Lives project, Amanda, a longtime wholesaler friend, called to tell me about Kimberly and Neil. I was captivated by their story and asked if she could connect us. Several weeks later, I got Neil on the phone and asked if he and his wife might be interested in talking with me.

"I don't know that we would," he said. "Kimberly's cancer is not curable, and I think with all we're going through, now's just not the right time for us. I wish you luck."

About nine months later, Amanda called me again. Kimberly had passed.

"When I was back in Chicago for Kimberly's services, I spoke with Neil and also Kimberly's sisters," she told me. "They'd be open to talking now. It's been a few months since Kimberly died. They think Kimberly's story might help people. I think talking to you might help them, too."

Over the next year, I spoke often with Neil, two of Kimberly's sisters, and Kimberly's mother. Sometimes they would cut our conversations short when talking became too painful. I don't know if sharing their story with me helped them at all. But as I learned about Neil and Kimberly's lives, I felt a growing certainty that their story would help others.

Kimberly's Smile

N eil and Kimberly were destined to fall in love. Although they were very much their own people, and many facets of their respective personalities were very different from each other, they shared a startling collection of coincidences along the paths of their lives that demonstrated just how similar their experiences were. Those experiences would end up providing the foundation for their remarkable, lasting commitment to the other.

Similarity of circumstance and experience does not, by itself, generate enough fuel to burn the fires of love for all eternity, but they can provide the right amount of kindling to ensure sparks turn into lasting flames. Kimberly and Neil's meeting was not so improbable. After all, they lived in the same building in Chicago and were both dynamic, outgoing people. But their real beginning was brought about by a happenstance, one that could only be told as the story of a glorious love affair.

Similar Beginnings

Neil was born in 1957 and raised in Hillsboro, a quiet, conservative town in central Illinois. It was one of the endless small communities sprawling the distance—and located about halfway between—Champaign and Chicago, where Midwestern parents raised their families around school, church, sports, and meals. It was the kind of place where strong foundations, and stronger values, were impressed on the souls of its people.

Similarly, Kimberly was born in 1957. She was raised in Lafayette, a quiet, conservative town in northwest Indiana, another of the same small communities sprawling the same distance—and located about halfway between—Indianapolis and Chicago, where Midwestern parents raised their families around much the same things as those of the Hillsboro type. After all, Hillsboro and Lafayette, towns of about the same size and only two-hundred-odd miles away from each other, were founded in the same year, early in the 1800s.

Neil's mother and father had met in high school and married right after they graduated college. His parents raised Neil, his two sisters, and his brother in a comfortable, safe, active household. Although the bonds between siblings varied in tightness, the depth of their feelings of belonging and personal promise exceeded any measure.

Much the same, Kimberly's mother and father had met in high school and married right after they graduated college. Kimberly's parents raised her and her three sisters in a comfortable, safe, active household. Although there was a four- and then eleven-year age gap that separated Kimberly from her two youngest siblings, the bonds of sisterhood were wound tightly, woven strong by the family's values and love for each other.

Their families weren't wealthy, but they never had to struggle. Like every family, each family had endured heartbreaks through the generations. Neither family strained under the weights of separation that might, in less committed families, have torn its members apart as they pursued their own paths.

Growing up, both Kimberly and Neil heard stories of past losses and witnessed early deaths of family members caused by cancer and other illnesses. They each were only a generation away from witnessing a suicide in the family. As a result, they shared the same understanding that happiness, security, and fulfillment were not guaranteed. They'd seen how their families stayed centered on their values despite emotional hardship. Early deaths were openly grieved in each household; even the heartbreaking suicides were quietly acknowledged.

It might've been because of their parallel upbringings, or their open and deep relationships with their respective families, but both Neil and Kimberly were driven to succeed at whatever they tried. They each had an unflappable desire to make the most of their lives. Each was at the helm among their siblings. They were both book-smart and quick-witted, confident in themselves, their relationships, and their life paths.

Neil studied mechanical engineering in college but found out he didn't have his dad's engineering mind, so he switched to computer science and business. College was just a two-hour drive from home, but Neil used the distance to establish his independence. After college, he followed a few friends to Chicago. He landed in Lincoln Park, an upscale section of the city known for attracting young, well-to-do professionals who spent long days working in the research and analytics rooms of investment banks or in the libraries of the city's best law firms and late nights bouncing between the hottest bars and restaurants.

Kimberly attended Purdue University, where she majored in both marketing and project management. Even though the school was only on the other side of town, she chose to live on campus. She wanted a full, immersed college experience and independence. Eager to pursue a top-level career at an elite company in a vibrant city, Kimberly moved to the Lincoln Park section of Chicago and took a job as a public relations executive at a large media company.

Sidetracks

Neil was recruited into the systems division of a prominent commercial bank, but the social scene didn't draw him in. Soon after settling in Chicago, he married his college sweetheart.

Neil was sure his new wife would fit perfectly into the life he'd planned. She was great on paper: pretty, smart, popular. She wanted to start a family right away, and she came from a wealthy, religious family. She embodied everything Neil had envisioned for himself, and they saw no need to wait— life was supposed to go a certain way and at a certain speed.

There was one major problem for the newlyweds: They weren't in love. The wedding had been lavish, but it was all pageantry and no passion. By contrast, their divorce was unceremonious and quick. Neil explained to his friends and family that immaturity had gotten the better of him.

Besides the miscalculated marriage—an easily forgotten detour—at twenty-three, Neil's life was progressing well. He was pursuing his master's, he directed a ground-breaking initiative to transition the bank's operation to paperless, he had a close group of friends, and he'd settled into a Chicago frame of mind.

At twenty-three, Kimberly's life was also progressing well. Sears had recruited her to be a vice president in marketing; she enjoyed close friendships and stayed close to her family. As she became entrenched in the city, she became more aware of the needs of those less fortunate. She was building a name for herself in business, social, and community circles.

When they met, neither Neil nor Kimberly were desperate for love. But they were both dating, no doubt waiting to be struck by a sudden connection to their one true partner, the way their parents had been. Neil didn't want to make another mistake, so he dated women with little long-term potential. Kimberly, selective about letting anyone get too close, dated people who had little chance to touch any piece of her heart. By chance, Neil and Kimberly lived in the same building in Lincoln Park. But as fate would have it, neither had even *seen* the other until each was almost perfectly content with their singleness.

One rainy Saturday afternoon, Neil was doing laundry and reading a research report—he'd become fascinated with finance and was intent on becoming a corporate banker. He heard the door open and saw Kimberly walking in—she was stunning. He wanted to casually look back down at his report, but he couldn't take his eyes off her. Fortunately, she seemed not to notice, so he watched her every movement. Her skin was pale—but not too pale, with a slight tinge of pink to it—and her face and neck looked surreally smooth, as if he were seeing her through some sort of softening filter. He was hypnotized by her beauty and gracefulness. He followed the line of her dark hair as it wrapped from her temple around her ear and along her neck before sweeping back against her shoulder. He could see the flow of blood in her full-but-not-too-pouty lips.

When she finished loading the machines, she looked over at him. He clumsily tried to look away.

"It's not polite to stare at a woman's dirty clothes," she said. "Especially a woman you don't know."

"I didn't know I was staring. I thought I was reading."

"Then why is your notebook upside down?"

He laughed out loud when he saw it was true. "Okay, maybe I was staring. But at you, not your clothes. I haven't seen you around. I'm sure we haven't met. I'm Neil."

He walked around the table and reached out his hand. She grabbed it firmly, but he noticed how soft and warm her skin felt. It was all he could do not to sigh or shudder in comfort. He hoped he didn't look as flushed as he felt.

"No, we haven't. I'm Kimberly. You're new in the building?"

Neil nodded. "Almost a year. You?"

"I moved in a couple of months ago."

"Well, it's about time we met, then," Neil said, smiling.

She smiled back, crossed her arms, and leaned against one of the washing machines. "Things happen when they do," she said.

"I guess they do."

They talked for a few more minutes, but Neil was too focused on her face to pay attention to what she said. Neil was a confident guy, but the combination of her velvety coolness and her natural, unpretentious warmth shook him loose and made him wonderfully uncomfortable. It was hard to break away when the dryer buzzed that his laundry was done.

"Upside down. Funny. Really great meeting you," Neil said as he walked toward the door. "If I'm lucky, I'll see you around in another year sometime."

Her smile pierced him again—an ample, genuine, sexy smile—and her teeth glowed white, her skin a bit pinker than a few minutes earlier. He had to shake himself to turn away.

Several days later, Neil was walking toward his apartment building. He saw Kimberly coming out. She was with some guy, looking as though she were on a date. They were laughing at something as they talked. Neil stopped and watched. His chest felt tight, and his cheeks burned. They had talked one time for a few minutes, but as he stood there, it hit him that he'd been completely knocked out by her.

So much for that, Neil thought. *I guess some things don't happen when they do.*

The following Monday morning, Neil found a small pale-blue envelope leaning against his door. He looked down the hallway and then at the envelope again. He picked it up, headed down the stairwell, and walked to the

Armitage station, where he took the 7:55 purple line to downtown each morning. Neil leaped up the stairs to the platform just in time to see the train approach. Once inside, he settled into a window seat and opened the envelope.

Neil, I know it's a little forward writing you, but I just thought you should know that it was great meeting you, too. I don't think I'm ready to have you stare at my dirty clothes, but maybe we could talk more someday soon. You can leave me a note if you like. I'm in 140B.

Regards, Kim

P.S. The other day was a last date I was on.

On their first date, Neil and Kimberly discovered the many similarities in their experiences growing up. On their second date, they talked more about their feelings on life, the value systems their parents had instilled in them, and the family members who'd meant the most to them. After their third date, Neil knew Kimberly was unlike any woman he'd known before. She was confident but didn't come off as overbearing, she was determined but not closed-minded, and although she appeared self-conscious with how quickly she was opening up to him, she confided her desire to have a big family, live a meaningful life, and serve her community. She said that making that type of life—a big mark and a big family—would be like living on a cloud near heaven. She talked with such certainty and optimism, and with a seductive sparkle in her eye—as if she knew something nobody else did. Neil was overwhelmed, somehow knowing he'd regret it if he weren't the one to see those things happen with her.

They dated for two years, and although there were some ups and downs during their courtship—as a result of each's unflinching will and self-reliance—they decided to become one stronger unit rather than two separate ones. Their love was sometimes chaotic and overcharged, but they always came back to each other armed with a binding avowal: They knew, undeniably, that they were meant to be together. In the fall of 1988, when they were both twenty-six, Neil and Kimberly wed. Three years later, their first son, Jake, was born. Shane was born three years later. They had become a family.

The Closeness of Joy and Tragedy

After nearly ten years of marriage, Neil and Kimberly were in the midst of realizing many of the dreams they had shared together during their earliest of dates. Neil was a successful entrepreneur and businessman. Kimberly maintained their home, volunteered at a center that helped less fortunate families and at-risk youth, and was the center of busy family relationships on both sides. Their boys were healthy, active children.

Life is never perfect, however, and Neil and Kimberly had gone through rough and unhappy times—she was frustrated about giving up her career, and he'd developed an underlying current of stubbornness, distance, and lack of empathy about that.

On one hand, Neil knew that Kimberly was fulfilled and grateful for the life they had, but on the other hand, her emptiness and frustration made him feel unappreciated. Both Neil and Kimberly were passionate in their beliefs, which enhanced the extremes of both their good and their difficult times, but to make the challenging times worse, Neil was not very compassionate. As a result, their disagreements often lasted longer than they needed to, which robbed them of some of the pride and enjoyment they otherwise may have gotten out of their marriage.

In addition, there were constant reminders that life was no fairy tale. Neil's father died of liver cancer just months after retiring, leaving his mother a young widow. Not long after, Kimberly's father began a battle with cancer. Kimberly's youngest sister had developed an addiction problem, suffered from depression, and became estranged from the family. Kimberly's best friend, her sister Jackie, who was only a year younger, struggled with a rough marriage and a rougher divorce. Her other sister, Tracy, was forced to abandon a budding tennis career after suffering serious medical issues, which led to emotional issues as well.

Out of these difficulties, two huge changes emerged: First, Jackie, then Tracy, and then Neil's mom moved to Chicago—all within a few minutes of Neil and Kimberly's house. Second, in spite of their own problems, Kimberly and Neil became the core of their combined families. Their home became a bustling center of activity. It seemed that everyone in their families, in one way or another, relied on Neil and Kimberly for help and support. Neil and Kimberly, meanwhile, often relied on a trusted counselor to help them

navigate their differences. But a busy household and sometimes-stormy relationship aside, they were still building the meaningful life together that they
had promised each other.

In the summer of 1998, they welcomed their daughter, Brooke, into the
world. When Brooke came along, many of the positive facets of their lives
were enhanced, and most of the negative ones disappeared. Having a daughter
not only fulfilled Kimberly in a way she couldn't have communicated before
but also brought Neil a new understanding of Kimberly. She became different,
better, elevated in every way. As a result, Neil and Kimberly were able to talk
about their emotions rather than just act emotionally, and Neil developed
some previously unseen softheartedness. Brooke was a blessing for them, and
for the next eighteen months, they lived in a special place.

"Our address? It's Cloud 9, Wheaton, Illinois," Kimberly would often tell
her kids, sisters, and friends. "That's where we live."

But they fell off Cloud 9 in early February of 2000.

• • •

Kimberly was headed to New York with some friends to visit an art exhibit
celebrating the relationships between mothers and daughters. Neil dropped
her off at the airport with a promise to take Brooke, who'd developed a fever,
to the doctor's office on his way home.

"She's at 103 degrees, which is high but not so alarming that we need
to do anything extreme," the pediatrician told Neil. "She doesn't appear
lethargic or disoriented. Take her home, give her plenty of sleep, keep an
eye on her temperature, and call the office if anything changes. I'm sure
she'll be fine."

Neil put Brooke in her crib and went downstairs to work in his office.
About an hour later, his nine-year-old son, Jake, came home from school.
Neil told him to wake up Brooke and bring her downstairs before Shane was
dropped off so they could get a snack ready for everyone.

A moment later, Neil heard the scream. He leaped up the stairs and ran
into Brooke's bedroom, where Jake was crying and shaking her.

"Wake up, sister. Wake up!"

It took a second for Neil to process what he saw. Brooke was blue, unresponsive, lifeless. He sent Jake downstairs to make sure that if Shane came home, he wouldn't come upstairs, and then he lifted Brooke and ran her to his bedroom, where he breathed in her mouth as he called 911.

"My baby is blue. She's not breathing! I'm giving her CPR, but we need someone here now."

Four excruciatingly long minutes later, the paramedics arrived and carried Brooke to the ambulance. Neil squeezed Jake hard, then told him to go to the neighbors, and watch for Shane. He got in the back of the ambulance with Brooke.

"What happened? What possibly could have happened to my Brooke," he cried to the paramedics as they raced toward the hospital and continued CPR on her little blue body.

Kimberly had called home, and when no one had answered, she had tried Neil's cell phone and then the neighbors. The neighbors told her what they knew, and then Kimberly had called the hospital, who were able to put Neil on the phone. He told her every detail.

"My poor baby, my poor Brooke, and Jake. Oh my God. What are we going to do? Honey, what are we going to do?" she cried.

"Pray hard, honey. I don't know what else we can do. They're trying everything."

An hour later, Neil called Kimberly's cell phone. She was on her way to the airport.

"Don't say it," she begged. "What you called to tell me, I know it in my soul. Just don't say the words. Please, honey. Don't say the words."

• • •

Neil, Kimberly, Jackie, Tracy, Neil's mom, and a few of the closest neighbors were together in the living room, downstairs from where Brooke had died just hours before. Kimberly was wrapped in a ball on the sofa, knees to her chest, head down. Neil had his arm around her. Nobody talked; they simply arrived, walked in, and were there. There was nothing to say. Nobody dared look at anybody for more than a quick glance. For Neil, not catching anyone's eyes, as awkward as it was, was the only way he could keep his thoughts away. Even the tiniest amount of mental activity would probably have made him throw up and shrivel away. He couldn't afford to shrivel away, so he banished his thoughts.

After a few hours, or it could've been minutes, spent staring into the darkest abyss possible, Neil pulled himself back to where his body was and went upstairs to check on the boys. They were both in Shane's room, lying on the bed, back-to-back, with the lights out. Neil walked over and fell to his knees next to the bed. He tenderly patted their heads as they both cried into their pillows. Neil began to cry himself. The tears felt warm on his cheeks. He hadn't cried in years; he couldn't remember when the last time was. Then he became angry that he was crying, because crying forced him to think. The pain that he felt took over his entire body and was utterly indescribable. If he could have collapsed into nothingness and disappeared forever, he would have.

But the boys, Neil thought. *These poor kids.*

Neil couldn't disappear forever. For the sake of Shane and Jake, he couldn't just collapse. He began to sob harder, and he began to think more. He thought about how cold Brooke had felt, how he hated that he had to tell Kimberly her precious baby girl had died, how he was horrified for what Jake had found when he went to wake his baby sister, how he had no idea how he was going to help his family, and how desperate he was to figure out some way to make it all go away.

Thank God Shane didn't see Brooke. Thank God it wasn't him who found her, Neil thought. *At least he didn't have to see.*

The next few days were unbearably quiet in the house. Family members stayed, and various other people—neighbors and friends from college, work, and school—came and went. But time seemed not to move at all. The hours rarely changed because the minutes trickled, as if the cosmic clock were frozen. The world had stopped at the sound of Jake's scream, at the sight of the little blue baby upstairs. It was the end of happiness and joy and everything good.

Each day, people stopped by to help with Shane and Jake, bring prepared food and groceries, and help clean and do laundry. Neil knew they were there to show support, and even if he couldn't show appreciation, he was grateful they had people in their lives who would show up when there was so much anguish in the air.

For Neil and Kimberly, the days and nights were unbearably quiet. The days crept by slowly, but darkness's unending silence was a punishment that went on for an eternity each night. They were unable to do much besides sit and stare into the nothingness as the enormity of what had happened began to sink in. Neil would lie next to Kimberly as she cried herself to sleep. He desperately searched his heart for an answer to how his wife would ever move forward after losing her baby girl. No answers came, and he sometimes dozed off for an hour or two before being awakened by the weight he felt on his chest.

Maybe three days later—although it could've been five or eight, for all Neil knew—he, Kimberly, and her mom sat at the table, still not able to talk or look each other in the eye. They had been sitting like that for a couple of hours while the rest of the house was still early-morning silent.

Kimberly stood up. "I don't know," she said softly. "I should probably go brush my teeth now. That's probably what I should do."

Neil looked up at her. She stood there, as if waiting for either Neil or her mom to give some signal validating her decision. Neil reached over and held out his hand. Kimberly entwined her fingers with his, and he shook his head faintly. She gave him the frailest of smiles, one that only her husband of many years could have detected, and then walked away.

After she'd left the kitchen, her mom reached over and put her hand on Neil's.

"She's going to be okay," she told him.

That night, Neil slept a few more hours, and the next night, a few more.

Soon after Kimberly had taken the first step toward healing, she and Neil found out the cause of Brooke's death—*streptococcus pneumoniae*, a bacterium discovered in the late nineteenth century. It causes severe symptoms, including death, usually in infants. Clearly, the doctors had missed it.

Just a few months after Brooke's death, a vaccine for the bacteria was approved in the United States, reducing deaths by more than 80 percent. *Just months too late for Brooke.*

Knowing what had happened to their baby helped them heal, and like a mild springtime does to the winter ice, time thawed their frozen hearts, and the family began to move in step with the world around them.

Joy Returns

Trying to survive the death of a young child is something many families are forced to deal with, and the results are often devastating. In Neil and Kimberly's case, Brooke's death brought them new meaning. They lived more for the moment, for each other and their families rather than mostly for themselves. Through all the grief and unimaginable pain and trying to make sense of the disorder that Brooke's death brought to their sense of all that was right and wrong in the world, they came together.

And that's the way it went for them: When they encountered marital problems, they received counseling and returned to their strong beliefs and support system. When they decided to start Neil's new business, they relied on each other to fill the gaps created at home. After they lost Brooke, they grieved together, turned to each other, and continued to go to counseling together. When the world was thrown into chaos in the wake of 9/11, they coordinated their lives so Kimberly could volunteer more and Neil could double his efforts at work so his business would stay afloat. When Kimberly's father died of cancer soon after they lost Brooke, they helped each other deal with the pain of another death. When Kimberly got the news that she was pregnant at forty-one, they came together even more and planned with optimism for a new chapter in their lives. Through all the peaks and valleys, closer together was always their end goal.

The emotions were palpable as Kimberly and Neil watched the doctor perform an ultrasound. "Imagine if it's a girl," Kimberly said. "Do you think the boys—can Jake—be okay with her?"

"He can. Together, we can do whatever we need," Neil said.

"Well," the doctor said, "isn't that interesting."

"Interesting?" Neil asked.

"It's not a girl, I'm afraid, but it's not exactly a boy either." There was a short pause as the doctor moved the wand around Kimberly's belly. "Yup, you see here: It's *two* boys. Twins."

She put the ultrasound wand back in the holster and pressed a button next to the screen. An image printed on thermal paper. The doctor showed the image to Neil and Kimberly.

"You see, here's baby one, and right there, that's two."

• • •

Months later, Luke and Harry were born. Life got better for everyone in the family and stayed that way for several years. They may even have begun to find their way back to Cloud 9. But when the twins were seven and Kimberly was forty-nine, a dark cloud fell over their lives.

One never forgets something as traumatic as the death of a child, but a dozen years had passed since Brooke had died, and many years since Kimberly's and Neil's fathers had died. Death wasn't something they thought of regularly, but they were hypersensitive to the idea that sickness and death could come at any time. As a result, they were extra attentive to their four children, taking them to see doctors at any obvious or perceived concern. And since they were both conscious of the fact that cancer had claimed relatives in both their families, they both knew anything unusual should be checked out at once.

Sometimes they'd wait a few hours, sometimes a few days, between "not feeling right" and feeling as though something should be attended to by a professional. They'd notice something, keep it inside for a brief period of time—hours or days, depending—and then it would either go away or they'd go see their doctor without further delay. They had no appetite for lingering denial or avoidance after what they had been through.

Kimberly had complained to Neil of not feeling right for several days, but when she developed several symptoms almost overnight—a fever, lethargy, acute pain in her lower abdomen, dizziness, and an overriding sense that something just wasn't right—it was time to go to the doctor.

Kimberly set an appointment with her primary care physician. Neil was scheduled to go out of town that day, so she went alone. Neither of them said "Let's make sure whatever's going on is not cancer" to the other, but they shared a knowing glance before he left.

But it wasn't cancer. As soon as she was out of the appointment, Kimberly called her sister Jackie, the one person she could tell something to before telling Neil.

"I was at the doctor," Kimberly said. "Oh my God. I mean, I haven't been feeling so great, and I thought, you know, I'm *forty-nine* for Christ's sake."

"You're not . . . ?"

"Pregnant? Yes, I am," Kimberly said. "I'm *forty-nine*, Jackie, what the hell?"

They had a long talk. They discussed every aspect for hours, including the possible problems of having a baby at that age, what tests they had for older mothers-to-be, what each of the kids might think, how Neil might react, and the possibility that Kimberly might be pregnant with a girl this time. It would mean so much to her and Neil after all they had been through.

Seven months later, they brought Faith—a beautiful, healthy baby girl—home from the hospital. Neil and Kimberly's life went from remarkable to perfect. Faith brought happiness and joy to their lives neither could've imagined. She was like an unexpected fringe benefit, a perfect little dividend for the years of standing together through the joys and travails of being part of a family whose members were unbreakably committed to each other.

Neil's mother already lived in Chicago, and after Faith was born, Kimberly's mom moved there too. Christmases, Thanksgivings, and birthdays seemed to double in size. Their house was alive with activity like it had never been. Neil's business was thriving. The boys were all doing well at school—Jake at college, Shane in high school, and the twins in elementary.

Kimberly was involved in both a community development project she formed to help revitalize one of the troubled neighborhoods near Wheaton, and in the organization she and Neil had started in Brooke's memory to raise funds to benefit children in the surrounding communities.

Becoming Someone Different

As Faith went from diapers to onesies to first-grade dresses, there was one dynamic that plagued an otherwise wonderous stretch of years: Kimberly and Neil had, again, despite their work to the contrary, become distant with each other. They disagreed over things that ordinarily wouldn't have bothered either one, they argued almost daily, and their relationship felt strained like it hadn't in many, many years. As much as he hated himself for it, Neil fell into a pattern of thinking Kimberly was the cause of the problem. He knew he could be stubborn and sometimes aloof—and not everything was all her fault—but she was changing, she was becoming someone *different*, and he didn't like it.

Things got so bad that, as they had done in the past, they sought counseling. After all, for twenty-five years, they'd been used to working hard at their relationship, which sometimes required outside help. They had always been committed to doing whatever they had to do to get through the rough patches, and though they had never encountered a patch as rough as the one they were struggling through, they knew they'd work together to figure things out.

But Kimberly started to become angrier and more short-tempered and less willing to work together. Neil tried to rationalize that perhaps Kimberly was going through menopause, or maybe she was feeling the strain of Faith starting school. Whatever it was, she was turning into a person who wasn't very pleasant. At the same time, he was becoming more distant and less tolerant of Kimberly's outbursts. Soon, even their long-term marriage counselor expressed concerns about whether they could continue on together. In a few short months of intense and escalating episodes, they had come close to erasing a quarter century of promises to each other.

Neil was almost resigned to figuring out a plan of coexistence until Faith was out of high school and then presenting it to Kimberly, when one day, Kimberly went completely over the edge of reason. She and Neil fought as they had never fought before—about nothing comprehensible, rational, or even intelligible at times. It took so much out of her that after an all-night yelling session, she collapsed on the bed, crying, shaking, incoherent, and in an almost seizure-like state. Neil sat next to her, feeling desolate and helpless.

"What are we going to do?" he asked out loud.

Kimberly looked up at him, her eyes unable to hide her devastation. She reached for his hand and gave him the answer he secretly wished she would have offered weeks, even months, earlier.

"I need to be put in a hospital. I'm not right. Neil, I know I'm not right. I'm going crazy." She gazed up at him, eyes still churning out water that long should have dried up. "It's me. I need help," she said.

Neil knew she meant it, and he knew she was right. The next day, Neil and Kimberly drove to a world-renowned mental institution in the city, and together they committed Kimberly for full-time professional observation and testing.

The hug between them was cold, but there was also an undeniable tinge of warmth still there—they were, deep down, still the couple they had always been.

Two nights later, the phone on the nightstand rang. Neil fumbled to pick it up. The clock showed that it was 3:20 a.m. It was the head physician at the institution. Neil's heart stopped cold.

"You need to come here, right away," the doctor said. "We've all been notified just now of some results that came in. There's not a minute to waste."

As Neil tried to shake the sleep out of his head, the doctor went on to explain the center's protocol was to do a full range of physical testing and analysis, and as part of that process, they performed an MRI on Kimberly's brain. The MRI revealed a massive, tentacled tumor. They'd need to perform major surgery as soon as they could prep Kimberly and gather the best team to assist the surgical oncologist and neurosurgical team that had already been called. There was no doubt about it—time was of the essence with a situation so dire.

Neil called Jackie. "None of this is going to make any sense, but I need you to come here. I have to leave right now," he explained. "Kimberly went in for observation. You know she hasn't been herself lately, to say the least. They told me they need to attempt to relieve pressure in her skull and remove as much of a complicated tumor as they can. Jesus, Jackie, it's the size of a baseball, in a dangerous place in her brain. I'm leaving the house this second. Everyone's still asleep."

An hour later, Neil was sitting next to Kimberly. She was sleeping and sedated. The lead doctor had told Neil a few additional details. He discussed the initial plan for surgery, who was coming on board to perform the procedures, and what the likely next steps would be. He assured Neil that they had access to the world's best team, giving Kimberly the best chance of success. He also asked Neil to acknowledge that he understood what was happening, though they'd have to figure out what course of action to take once they had relieved the pressure in her skull and removed most of the tumor. He explained that there was a good chance the surgery wouldn't go well, that there was a great risk of many dangerous complications, including death. Somehow, Neil had to tell his wife what was happening.

As Neil sat there, holding Kimberly's hand, waiting for her to awaken so he could talk to her, he was numb. He could only think of how he'd felt years before, when he'd had to call Kimberly and tell her Brooke had died. Kimberly had begged him not to tell her what she already knew. He'd thought that it was the most impossible thing in the world, but this might be worse. How was he going to tell her these words now? As he tried to think of what to do, Kimberly opened her eyes. She looked at him with the beautiful, sparkling brown eyes that had lost their depth and love over the previous months.

"What is it?" she asked, searching his face. "What's the matter?"

"Honey," he started, "I don't know how to say what I need to tell you."

He figured out a way. When he was done telling her everything that he was told, tears ran down her face. She smiled a wide, glowing Kimberly-smile and squeezed his hand.

"Thank God," she said. "Thank God, it's a tumor and not *me*."

Half a Lifetime's Deep Connection

That first phase of surgery was two surgeries. They needed to relieve the pressure on Kimberly's brain by placing a temporary drain to release the buildup of cerebrospinal fluid. Next, they needed to do a surgical biopsy to determine the type of tumor. The biopsy would be taken while Kimberly's neurosurgeon completed the craniotomy—removing a section of her skull—in preparation for the second phase of the surgery, where they'd remove as much of the tumor as possible without affecting healthy brain tissue. Kimberly was in the operating room for fourteen hours.

Glioblastoma can be a devastatingly aggressive and severe cancer. Kimberly's particular tumor was known as a "primary tumor," a quickly appearing, aggressive, malignant tumor that was going to be very difficult to treat, because it had intricately woven itself into inoperable parts of the brain. Since it was being fed by an ample blood supply, the tumor had a huge appetite for invading healthy cells. In addition, the tumor itself was made up of several different types of cells, which made it very difficult to devise a treatment plan.

Kimberly would need to undergo radiation therapy, general chemotherapy, and targeted chemotherapy. There might be additional surgeries. The prognosis was dire—Kimberly's chances of long-term survival were in the single digits. The odds for her to live longer than a year or a year and a half were just as low.

Neil and Kimberly talked often in the days following the surgeries—when

Kimberly was up to it. There were plenty of tears between them. The future was grim, and the seas were going to be very difficult to navigate. But the awful reality of their situation was countered by an immediately recaptured unity and belief in half a lifetime's deep connection—a connection that enabled them to successfully steer through the many storms their brazen life brought. Besides, Kimberly had never been a pessimist.

Neil and Kimberly couldn't hide what was going on from the family, yet they didn't outwardly focus on the negative aspects of what was happening, either. Kimberly never complained. She and Neil never gave any indication to others that they didn't believe her treatment would cure her, regardless of their knowledge that she had very little chance to overcome the disease and regardless of the discussions they had between themselves about what would happen after she was gone.

When Kimberly spent time with her mom, she talked of the future. When she spent time with her boys, she talked of the years ahead. With Jackie and Tracy, she talked about how they'd all be grandmothers together one day. With her friends, it was all about the stuff they'd do when things became easier for Kimberly. Talking about tomorrows was a way to help get past the difficulties of each day.

The time Kimberly spent with Faith and with Neil was different.

Faith was Kimberly's baby girl, her angel, the gift that put the family as close to being back on Cloud 9 as possible. Dealing with Faith was heartbreaking for Kimberly and Neil, and they walked a delicate line between giving her enough information so she would be prepared should Kimberly not recover, but not so much information that she'd be traumatized. At seven, Faith couldn't understand much about what was going on, other than that her mother was sick. They couldn't very well put fantasies in her head about the future, but they also didn't want to force her to face the unedited present. Kimberly and Neil knew that everyone, save for Faith, could see that Kimberly was dying.

As much as Neil would have given everything to be able to see that future come to pass, he was presented with the unavoidable reality that, at fifty-seven, he'd soon be the sole parent to their five kids. The twins had just started high school, and Faith was only in the second grade. Neil knew he'd need to make huge changes. Kimberly had run their household for three decades while he'd built successful businesses. She was the social organizer, the family planner, the coach, the doer of homework, the fixer of problems, the go-to source for all things motherly and domestic. Kimberly was the referee for family battles and the shoulder for people to cry on. She took on the role of the "toughie" so Neil could be the softy—except when she needed to be the softy. She filled the cupboards and the bellies of her family and the empty spaces under the Christmas tree. She did it all.

Neil was going to have to learn to be a better *parent* and not just be a dad. He was going to have to work less and learn how to communicate better. He'd need to become more involved in his kids' emotional lives and more compassionate and present each moment of the day. Knowing he needed to change and actually changing were two different things. Fortunately, for a while he had Kimberly to help prepare him for his metamorphosis.

Kimberly's chemotherapy was unimaginably tough, and radiation was debilitating. The targeted therapies—hormones, inhibitors, corticosteroids, anticonvulsants, protein enhancers, and more—had their heads spinning with both hope and despair, along with many other side effects. Through it all, Kimberly and Neil did their best to fight and stay positive for as long as they could. And Kimberly spent as much time with her family as possible.

Belief and determination can last only so many rounds against an opponent as unyielding as advanced glioblastoma. The reality that Kimberly's fight was ending came almost as quickly as it had begun—things turned bad swiftly. Kimberly didn't want to give up or leave her family. She didn't want to miss seeing her children grow older; to miss one day of taking care of her little angel, Faith; or to miss continuing to accumulate the years with her true soulmate. She wanted to continue to build something meaningful in the community. Most of all, she didn't want to stop being at the center of a wonderful and vibrant universe, the place she and Neil had built together, the place she'd always dreamed of being. But she wasn't given those opportunities.

Eighteen months after that night when she'd felt relieved to know she had cancer, her battle ended. With her family having said their final goodbyes—all her boys, her mom, Neil's mom, her sisters, and even Faith—Kimberly died peacefully while Neil held her hand and whispered in her ear about all the wonderful things they had done and about the beautiful life they had built together.

Neil's Epilogue

I had the pleasure of talking to Kimberly's sisters Jackie and Tracy, her mom, and Neil many times over the course of the time it took to understand what they had all been through. I was touched by each of their experiences. It's not often an outsider gets to learn so much about a person, told from so many different perspectives, and I was enthralled to hear each person tell stories and describe emotions and recall experiences in their own unique ways. By the end of our talks, I had a real sense of who Kimberly was and how much she meant to those who knew her best.

For all of them, Kimberly was the consistent, unchanging center, the rock of the family, the unflappable one, and the person whom others adapted to. She was the cause of, or took on a major role in helping the people around her go through, their own substantial changes; her attention and impact affected the dynamics that shaped who they became. Kimberly was the not-so-secret cipher, the key that solved the formulas of their lives. If life was an artist, then she was the brush, not the paint.

When Kimberly moved to Chicago, everyone in her family followed one by one, leaning on her for support, gathering around her as the center of their family. They changed their lives to fit into hers. When she was working on her community revitalization project, she convinced community leaders and corporate partners to change their normal protocols and adapt to her vision of how things could be accomplished. When Brooke died, she showed her family how to recover, rebuild, and emerge happy again. When Kimberly knew she was going to die, she helped Neil learn how to be a more present, compassionate parent.

After learning about Kimberly's role in helping others change and adapt to change, the story her family told me about the butterflies became even more poignant.

When Kimberly was recovering from the massive and traumatic surgery she'd undergone just after her tumor had been discovered, one of the first things she told her family when she woke was that she'd dreamed of monarch butterflies. In her dream, thousands of butterflies floated against a cobalt sky, their orange-and-black wings fluttering just hard enough to send them meandering above an endless field of blooming daisies on a warm summer's day.

"They were so free, so casual, so soothing," Kimberly said. "Like all of them together lifted my soul and . . . allowed me to float away." Her family stood next to her, watching her struggle to form the words.

A few moments later, Faith pointed out the window. "Look, Mommy. Look, a butterfly. It's right here looking at us!"

Everyone turned toward the window, and as they did, the butterfly flew away gracefully, giving the family a moment of beauty at a time when there was so much fear and unrest. After that day, each time someone saw a butterfly, they mentioned Kimberly's butterfly dream.

About a year and a half later, as Jackie sat on the steps of a church waiting to go inside for Kimberly's memorial service, a monarch butterfly flew down and landed on her shoulder. The family was all around her, and with hushed voices—so as not to scare the butterfly away—remarked how it was a strange coincidence that a butterfly would land on someone's shoulder, on Jackie's shoulder, at that exact moment. The butterfly flew away just as Jackie got up to walk into the church.

Later that day, back at Neil and Kimberly's home, where tables and chairs had been set up outside to accommodate all the people who came by to give their respects and offer support to the family, Kimberly's sisters and mom and a few friends sat silently. A butterfly, like the one that had sat on Jackie's shoulder earlier, like the one that Faith had seen in the hospital room's window, like the ones in Kimberly's dream, flew down and landed on Tracy's hand.

Jackie retold the story of Kimberly's dream, how a butterfly had appeared outside the recovery room window, and how earlier outside the church, a butterfly had sat on her shoulder. As she did, while everybody watched Tracy's hand, the orange-and-black monarch stayed still. Then a friend told a story about Kimberly, then another, and another. People got up and left, others sat. The table was sometimes overwhelmed with laughter and sometimes silent with a flood of tears. The stories went on for hours, and the butterfly on Tracy's finger stayed the whole time.

Perhaps people look for coincidences to help themselves deal with loss, or maybe there are mystic strings that tie what we can see to the things we take on faith, but something magical happened with Kimberly and the butterflies, and that magic etched a permanent remembrance on the minds of the people who witnessed it.

Butterflies emerge as the result of an extraordinary metamorphosis. They're forged from their caterpillar selves through a delicate and miraculous transformation. Perhaps the butterflies were there to remind the people Kimberly had touched of the significant role she played in their own evolution. Or maybe, just maybe, they were something more.

Four-Mile Bridge

I woke from a deep sleep motivated to set out for the day ahead. I put on the still-damp clothes I'd trampled clean while showering the night before. I was eager to get moving, because I knew day twenty-four, a 151-mile, flat, sticky, humid stretch between Sulphur and Port Allen, Louisiana, was going to be another beast of a ride.

Chad stayed with me for as long as he could, but by noon, I was on my own, rolling along endless spans of highways that paralleled an incessant, loud flow of traffic a couple of feet to my left and a very real, stinking green swamp about ten feet to my right. All day long, I was certain that at any moment, if a car didn't swipe me into the nasty everglades, an alligator would chase me into the path of the speeding cars. As a result, my grip on the handlebars was viselike, my attention was unfailing, and my legs mashed purposely—I couldn't span that many miles quickly, but I wasn't about to linger, either. After all, dark would fall at some point, and I wanted as little road ahead of me as possible when it came.

In the midafternoon, Chad called me from the airport to check in on me and warn me of some issues he spotted on his drive to New Orleans. "There are a few areas with no shoulder," he said, "so you'll probably want to wear your lighted vest. There aren't any tricky turns or construction or anything. But there's a bridge at about mile one hundred twenty-five that looks a little sketchy."

"Sketchy?" I asked.

"It's pretty tight, not much room between the road and the railing."

"How long of a bridge?"

"Well, I didn't start measuring it until it hit me how hairy it was, but it might be close to two miles long, I'd guess."

Chad was an engineer. If he said close to two miles, then it was close to two miles.

"Two miles of sketchiness? I can handle that."

"I don't think there's a way to bypass it, so you'll want to be careful."

"Got it. Lighted vest, proceed with caution, deal with two miles of hairiness," I said.

"Oh, and something called *microbursts* are delaying my flight. Watch out for those, if they make their way to you. I'm looking out the window, and *those* are freaking hairy."

Hours later, as the sun began to disappear behind me and cast its golden-hour red, orange, and yellow hues on the massive cumulous clouds forming in the distance ahead of me, I stopped to take a break and prepare my safety gear. The sky was beautiful but also eerie, as the entire distance between the base of the clouds and the horizon below them was a dark greenish-gray—the color of a distant and ominous-looking thunderstorm. Or microburst. I was heading right into the throat of it.

As darkness smashed the daylight down and into the earth far behind me, the storms roared and snarled miles and miles ahead of me, taunting me to keep biking forward. I had no choice but to show my nerve, as I was at least twenty-five miles past the last little town I'd gone through. I had set the route up to traverse east along US-190 instead of I-10, because I wanted a break from all the heavy traffic. US-190 isn't an empty highway, but there aren't many towns along it big enough to attract travelers.

As I approached the one-hundred-mile mark, roughly two-thirds of the way to my destination, darkness had completed its inevitable dominance over light, and the blackness ahead was interrupted only by short flashes brought on by the faraway lightning. I pedaled on, but doubt crept inside me as the low, long rumble of distant thunder reverberated off my bones, shuddering my entire body in a way the bumpiest road of the ride couldn't have matched. Since I was pedaling into a headwind (of course), cool droplets of water began to pepper me. Soon, the droplets turned into a steady rain, and then the steady rain turned into a shower. I was soaked and biking on the thin ribbon of shoulder of a two-lane highway. By the time I hit mile 125, I was eleven hours into the day.

I wouldn't have noticed I was even on the "bridge," as the road didn't so much rise above the ground as the ground simply gave out below the bridge, except that one minute there was a shoulder on the road, and the next, there were literally inches between the right side of the right lane and a four-foot cement barrier that marked the edge of the causeway. A thick metal railing spanned the top of the barrier, and a small curb, about six inches up from the road and extending an equidistance from the side of the wall, ran along the base of the barrier. A couple of spins of the wheels onto it, and I became ensnarled in the sketchiness Chad had warned me about. I pulled over and balanced myself by putting my foot on the curb. I could easily touch the barrier, so I held the railing as I looked over my shoulder.

If cars come barreling onto this bridge, I thought, *I'm screwed. If trucks do the same, with the rain, I'm completely fucked.*

There was no turning around, no waiting, no alternate route, no plan B. I was going to have to bike across. But I needed a strategy. There was no way I could stay on the highway if a vehicle came from behind; there wouldn't be any clearance—well, there would be if vehicles traveled in the left lane, but not if they occupied the right lane, and for a couple of thousand miles, I'd seen every single vehicle outside of every big city occupy only the most right lane, if not half of the right lane and half of the shoulder. So I'd have to stop, unclip my shoes, get off the bike, step on the small curb, lift my bike up, lean the lower half of my body against the barrier, lean my waist against and over the top of the barrier while holding my fiftyish-pound bike close to my chest, wait for the vehicles to pass me, then set the bike back down, jump on it, pedal like mad to make some ground, continually look over my shoulder for oncoming headlights, pull over, and do it all again. To make the situation more harrowing, I was running on fumes, my judgment was not razor sharp, and the heavy rain added some challenges.

It's only two miles, I thought. *With all the jumping on and off the bike, I probably have fifteen minutes to get over the bridge.*

The first vehicle's lights began to bear down on me. I unclipped, lifted my bike, and leaned against the barrier. When it whizzed by, I felt a rush of wind and was simultaneously splashed with water that shot up from the road and sprayed behind the speeding car. Then another car went by, then another. When I was finally able to put my bike down, I clipped into the pedals and took off. I looked over my shoulder every couple of seconds, and soon after, I stopped and jumped on the curb again. Two cars zoomed by. Then I biked again. Then a group of four or five cars screamed by—all in the right lane, all speeding, all spraying water all over me.

This continued for about six or eight minutes, and then I saw bigger, brighter, higher headlights behind me. It had to be a truck. I jumped off the bike, hopped on the curb, and leaned so severely into and over the barrier that any slip and I'd have fallen over the edge and into the Atchafalaya Natural Wildlife Preserve (read: alligator-infested swamp) below me. When the big rig passed, it sounded and felt like what I was afraid it might: a seventy-mile-per-hour, seventy-five-thousand-pound, eighteen-wheel monster—and it barreled by me not more than a foot away. The bursting stream behind it pressure-sprayed the color right off my face.

"Are you kidding me right now?!" I screamed at the truck, my heart tearing a hole in my chest, my arms and legs shaking from the strain or the fear or both. "You can't move over one lane? Are you serious? Can't you see me? I'm wearing fifty freaking lights on me. What the *hell*!?"

I must have been a sight: dripping wet, jumping on and off my bike and out of the way of the oncoming right-lane-hugging traffic, huffing and puffing as I raced forward, blurting out obscenities as I desperately measured the distance between me and a rearview mirror or a swerving trailer or a texting driver, screaming futilely at trucks and cars to answer me.

At last the road opened up, the shoulder reappeared, and the pandemonium subsided. I wanted to pull over, but the rain was so intense that I needed some cover to attempt any type of recuperation. I made my way to a gas station a few miles up the road, and when I pulled under the canopy, unclipped my shoes, and swung my leg over the bike seat, I almost collapsed. Instead, I hobbled the twenty feet over to a bench that abutted the wall next to the convenience store's door and crumpled onto it. A few minutes later, confident I hadn't died on that causeway, I went inside to grab a Red Bull and a snack.

"You need a drying," the woman behind the counter said as she reached under her register and handed me a roll of paper towels. She studied me for a moment. "Were you choosing to bike in this storm?"

"Yeah." I smiled. "I just came over that bridge. It was the scariest two miles of my life."

"You came that way, over Old Four-Mile Bridge?" she asked.

"*Four* miles?"

So much for Chad's engineering degree.

"Yeah, that bridge is four miles from there to here. Why didn't you call the sheriff?"

"The sheriff? Why would I do that?"

"You can't ride over that bridge. It's too dangerous. The sheriff will escort you across."

"Well, being as I just came across it, it's a little late for me to make that call."

"Right. Right. Either way, next time, you should call the sheriff, although he might not have believed someone would want to cross at night with this weather. Did you really do that?"

"Pretty stupid, huh?" I asked.

She grinned. "Better 'not smart.' I wouldn't rightly say 'stupid' to a stranger."

I went outside and sat on the bench and waited for the rain to lighten up. A half hour later, I continued on my way to Port Allen. I was too wiped to give it much physical effort, but my mind continued to race. I experienced something on that bridge that I don't think I'd ever felt before—a kind of isolation, a desperate loneliness. I wanted to turn to someone for help, but there wasn't anyone to turn to. There wasn't anyone who would see me or hear me. Nobody could have protected me if anything went wrong. But I chose to continue. Regardless of the circumstances, I had no choice but to continue.

I thought of a few different book participants who'd tried to explain their own times of desperate loneliness, solitude in the face of fear, and inability to turn to someone for help. I felt as if I'd caught a slight glimpse into the levels of anxiety they must have had and the overwhelming feelings of seclusion and panic that must have overtaken them at times. The source was incomparable, but the resulting effects might have some semblance of similarity. I passed the last couple of hours of the ride thinking about the loneliness and the isolation and the disquiet that afflicted so many of the people I'd talked with, perhaps none more than Dave.

Dave

Relationship to cancer: Survivor, secondary caregiver, advocate, professional

Age: Forty-one

Family status: Married

Location: Rochester, New York

First encounter with cancer: Twenty-five years old

Cancer summary: Diagnosed with testicular cancer at twenty-five, Dave had an orchiectomy and radiation therapy. At thirty, he was diagnosed with a different type of testicular cancer, had an orchiectomy of the other testicle, and underwent nearly two dozen radiation therapy treatments, along with hormone therapy. When he was thirty-five, Dave lost his father to cancer.

Cancer specifics: Testicular cancer, germ cell. Testicular cancer, nonseminoma.

Community involvement: Senior executive at Gryt Health, responsible for driving digital innovation that connects research and care to the cancer community by building a peer-to-peer connectivity platform. Dave served on the board of Stupid Cancer for several years. He is a keynote speaker at multiple cancer functions and acts in various capacities as an advocate for the young adult cancer community.

Strongest positive emotion during cancer experience: Inspiration

Strongest negative emotion during cancer experience: Anguish

How we met: One of my book participants, Terri, referred someone she thought would be perfect for this project. He was Matthew Zachary, the founder and chief executive officer of Stupid Cancer, the country's largest organization serving the young adult cancer population. While Matthew's story was intriguing, he didn't have the time to participate in the project. Instead, he invited me to be a guest on the Stupid Cancer podcast. A few minutes after wrapping up our interview, my phone rang.

"Hello. My name's Dave Fuehrer," a man said. "I happened to be in the studio just now and heard the show. I'm fascinated by your project, and I'd like to learn more. Would you have time to talk?"

We set up a call for later in the week. I wanted to do some research on Dave before we spoke. I found out that he was a two-time cancer survivor, an entrepreneur-turned-executive at Stupid Cancer, a former world-class competitive bodybuilder, and a huge advocate for the young adult cancer population—particularly with respect to survivorship and fertility issues. While scouring the internet, I found more facts than narrative, but I came to our talk armed with enough information to at least know who I was speaking with. After exchanging a few pleasantries, I told Dave what I'd found out about him.

"There's not a lot of detail out there on me, I think, but you have a few of the highlights and lowlights, for sure," he said.

"What was it you wanted to talk about?" I asked.

"I guess it's more of a *why* than a *what,*" he said.

"Sounds interesting. *Why* are we talking, then?"

"I was struck by your openness on the show and was wondering if you might be willing to answer some personal questions about your transformation and your commitment," he said.

I was certain Dave wanted to talk about how I gave up smoking and went from being a couch potato to competing in endurance events, since I'd talked about both of those on the podcast, but he went in an entirely different direction.

"I'd like to know about June," he said. "Tell me about your sister."

I was caught up short. I hadn't been expecting to talk on the spot with someone I didn't know about such a private matter. The tables had turned. *I* was usually the one asking strangers about their sisters who had passed away from cancer. I felt uneasy. Over the years since her death, I'd thought often about June but hadn't really talked to anyone about her.

"What was she like?" he asked.

I told him how June was such a likable and sincere person. How it broke my heart she didn't get to see her kids grow up. I told him about the way we leaned on each other as kids and how we had admired and respected each other as adults. How, even in the face of an undeniable death sentence, June shamelessly displayed strength and optimism.

Then we talked about the upcoming bike ride. I mentioned how I hoped my experience with June and her cancer journey might help me deal with some of my own emotions while I interacted with strangers and book participants on the ride.

"That's enough about me." I laughed. I was unprepared to delve too deep into my own issues. "Why are we talking again?"

"I'm on a bit of a journey myself," Dave said. Then there was a long silence. He attempted to clear his throat and paused. I wasn't sure what was happening—if he was stuttering or had a tick. It sounded as if he might even be holding back tears. I waited for him to continue.

As we came to know each other better, I learned that when Dave paused abruptly, followed by silence broken by intermittent throat clearings, it wasn't a tick or a stutter. He'd stop when he felt overwhelmed by emotion. Then he'd need to take a minute or two to work through the sobs and tears that he fought to keep down. That first day, not knowing what was happening, I matched his silence and waited. After what seemed like a long time, he spoke again.

"Mmmmh . . . I'm sorry," he said. "You seem so in tune with the depth of the emotions involved. That's something very new to me."

I was surprised. Based on what I'd found online, it had been some ten years since his last bout with cancer.

"Have you not dealt with the emotions of what you went through—what you're *going* through?" I ventured.

"When I heard you on the podcast describing people who didn't deal with their emotions, it really hit home," Dave admitted. "Not too long ago, I started on the journey you seem to have already navigated. I'm somewhere between points A and B—like you said, where A is when cancer enters your life and B is today—only for me, it took a *lot* of years before I was able to even acknowledge point A."

"Why's that?" I asked.

He paused again. "Do you have more time?"

Medals

Fear and Confidence

Dave's pager buzzed. His father's number scrolled across the small display. He wanted to stop and call his dad, but he didn't have time. He was late and he was lost. Dave always spoke to his dad before a competition, and this one was a big one. No matter that he was twenty-four years old or that he'd been competing for five years, he wanted to hear his dad's reassuring voice. Talking to his dad always made his mind calm before entering the chaos of the competition—and calm was what he needed to pose effectively. He found the theater and pulled into the parking lot. He had less than an hour to prep. He ran in to the building. There was a payphone in the hallway leading to the backstage area. He found a quarter and dialed his dad's number.

"Hey, Dad. I got your page. Thanks for thinking of me. I don't have any time to talk. It's totally hectic."

"That's okay," his dad said. "I just wanted to remind you that you know what to do. You're prepared. Now, go inspire people."

The idea of inspiring people had been planted in Dave's head by his father ever since he could remember. Dave was attempting to become a world-class bodybuilder. If he continued to advance through more qualifiers, he'd be invited to the New Jersey state championships. Dave wasn't sure that winning bodybuilding competitions inspired anybody, but he liked that his dad thought it would.

Dave made his way through to the registration booth, unpacked his sports bag, and sized up the competition. He was at the peak of his weight class, but it didn't hurt to see who else might look ready—and it never hurt to hear his dad's confidence boosters. At first glance, nobody looked close to as strong as Dave felt. Fortunately, he drew a high number, which gave him extra time to engage his final eating strategy, change, pump, and oil up. He knew nobody had a chance against him.

Although Dave overflowed with confidence, a trickle of doubt, some mysteriously borne underlying current of anxiety that never went fully away and created a life's long battle against a terrorizing fear of failure, still ran through him at tense moments, such as when preparing to go on stage. Dad's voice worked to calm him, but Dave had a special ritual to—at least temporarily—exorcise the fear: turn to the crowd and find *her*. A few minutes before his group was to go out, Dave peeked out at the spectators from offstage, looking for the face of the woman he was there to win over.

Most competitors at bodybuilding competitions focused on impressing the judges; others on impressing the competition. Some were so self-absorbed, they seemed only there to impress themselves. But not Dave. He wanted validation. He *needed* it. What better way, he'd long since determined, could he accomplish that than to impress a woman? It didn't matter that he didn't know which woman—she was always out there. It didn't matter that he didn't know what she looked like until minutes before jumping on stage. It only mattered that he found her in the crowd.

Dave squinted through the glare of the stage lights. He scanned each row, his eyes racing from left to right, trying to find the cute blonde or brunette or red-head that he'd focus on during posing. Finally, he spotted her. She was stunning. She had long brown hair parted in the middle and flowing over her shoulders. She was toned, although it was difficult to see if she was a lifter. Dave preferred to think not; he liked women who were toned, not built. She had a Latin face; beautiful, soft, full lips; dark eyes; and an aura of grace about her. The glow that separated her from the others might've been cloudiness caused by the glaring lights, but Dave preferred to think the glow was something he alone saw.

That's her, Dave thought. *No doubt about it. That's who I'm going to impress tonight.*

The rush from the last-minute sugar intake—three bites of a peanut butter and honey mixture sprinkled with glycerol—coursed through Dave's body, hardening his muscles, pumping his veins, and spiking his energy. He was ready to show off all his hard work, but he was especially eager to show it off to *her*.

His group walked on stage and faced the judges. His body was still and ever so slightly flexed for the symmetry round, but his eyes focused on the woman. She was looking toward the stage, but Dave couldn't catch her eyes. The group turned to the left, then back front, then to the right. He couldn't twist his head to find her as he wasn't about to break a pose, but the anticipation of locking glances with her was maddening. The group turned away from the judges. Dave knew he was hands down the most pumped and lean and cut out there, and he knew that she *had* to be staring at him. When he turned to face the judges one last time, he caught her eye, and a shiver raced from the part of his brain that always sparked when locking a first eye-to-eye glance with a beautiful woman—and the shiver made him feel *stronger*.

During the routine of mandatory poses, Dave kept his gaze unfocused and soft. He moved from pose to pose, fixated on staying flexed through the transitions, imagining that his woman was so mesmerized by his definition that she was dreaming about what it might be like to be with him. Each time he maximized a pose, he imagined that holding the position allowed her to measure every inch of him, to dream about his tanned, strong features. But his time to shine, to win her over completely, would be in the freestyle session.

He was right. The music was perfect, his vascularity was perfectly timed, his routine was flawless, and the woman never turned away. Dave imagined she knew what was going on in his head, and he relished the thought. It was all so predictable and magical and emboldening—even if it was all contrived just to help him get past the fear and win.

Win he did that day, but he didn't get the woman. He scanned the crowd for her during the awards ceremony, but she was nowhere to be found. If she were there, maybe he would have talked to her; maybe he wouldn't have. Either way, she'd served his purpose.

Shallow Waters

Growing up, life for Dave was ideal. He had well-rounded, loving, inclusive parents; an older brother he admired and got along with; and whether by the watchful hands of his parents or the simple fortune of the safe, quiet time and place he was born into, a trauma-free childhood and young adulthood.

Dave was born in the mid-1970s in upstate New York, to parents who met at a high school dance, married young, and enjoyed a healthy marriage. Dad had endured a brutal tour in Vietnam that included direct bombing on his barracks. He was the sole survivor of the attack and, after returning home, suffered from extreme nightmares and debilitating flashbacks. Still, he had an infectious optimism, persuading people that things would turn out well based solely on the fact that believing so would make it happen.

Dad was a chemical engineer, a meticulous notetaker, a tinkerer and innovator, and a process-driven, often stoic man. But he could also be emotional. He was comfortable displaying affection for his wife and boys. There was no doubt about who the man of the house was, but he encouraged open communication in the household. Dave and his dad were very close, their relationship based on mutual admiration and respect.

Mom was an educated and inquisitive middle school teacher who had many passions: breeding and raising Labrador retrievers, reading, learning, cooking—which she tirelessly pursued while also including her family in the juggling act. Although Dave's mom supported her husband's practice of taking the occasional outing alone with his sons, she took pride in doing most things as a family. "BNO" (Boys Night Out), "PNO" (Parents Night Out), and "FNO" (Family Night Out) were celebrated, but when home, doors were left open, meals were eaten together, and discussion was unabridged, relevant, and candid.

Neither parent wasted time, nor did they allow their boys to idle. As a result, Dave's youth was crowded with activity—school and learning were priorities. Sports such as soccer, football, and baseball were fixtures.

Dave was driven to excel in sports, but he wasn't obsessed with them; Mom and Dad had taught Dave that sports were about achievement and competition, not about testosterone and domination. Even as he competed through and beyond puberty, where testosterone and a desire to dominate hung as heavy and rank on the fields of play as it did in the high school locker rooms, Dave was motivated by the contest of sports, not the aggressiveness. Competition between boys can be a sweet thing to watch, but once boys become young men, much of that sweetness turns acrid, and Dave didn't like the stench of organized sports once he became older.

So in high school, when strength training became a more pronounced facet of organized sports, Dave made a shift; he traded in more traditional sports to explore bodybuilding. Not only did he find that strength training and conditioning came naturally to him, but he also discovered that bodybuilding empowered him, putting him in control of not just his body but his entire demeanor. As he became hyper-in-tune with his physiology, he could see and feel tangible changes in his conditioning and physique from day to day—even from workout to workout. As he learned how to shape his calves, back, arms—virtually every muscle in his body—he could feel the uncertainty and cloudiness of young adulthood dissipate. His general anxiety never disappeared, but muscles helped Dave mask the fear of failure. He learned that he could mold not only his physique but also his perspective and his ability to take charge of an intended path. Bodybuilding helped Dave develop confidence, self-reliance, and a kind of inner peace.

Dave watched while some of his peers experimented with steroids and other chemical enhancers, but he was drawn to the natural side of bodybuilding; his goal was conditioning and symmetry and curves and power, not bulk and size and abnormal form. By the time he started entering competitions, it became apparent that he could set lofty goals, as his height, genetics, and ability to absorb intense training was evident when compared to the people he competed against. He became obsessed. There was something magical, inventive, and creative in sculpting his body, because doing so also shaped his mind—and Dave became a savant artiste of his human form, thus the master artist of his identity.

In addition to successfully competing as a budding professional bodybuilder, Dave gained control of all aspects of his life: top grades at school came easy, relationships with his parents and friends seemed to flow naturally, he was super confident—especially around girls—and he developed a Zen-like demeanor. His mind was clear, his actions intuitive, and his fear of failure—of disappointing his dad—was a barely noticeable ripple in an otherwise calm world inside.

Dave saw that many of his friends' high school experience had them swimming in angst-filled waters, struggling to come into their own, unable to navigate the incoming tides of maturity, struggling just to breathe until they could make it to the other side. In contrast, Dave was making it through high school as if he were walking through ankle-deep water; there were no struggles, no turmoil, no flailing to stay afloat.

High school ended; college began. The stages got bigger, the classrooms became more challenging—as did his pursuit of women—and Dave continued to maintain a cohesive focus of body and mind through bodybuilding. As Dave continued to mature, he continued to feel in control of his life, but in the fall of 1990, waters around him started to rise.

Waist Deep

Self-delusion protects—or hides—who we really are inside, but the separation between who we are and who we think we are is still a space often measured by a thin one-way mirror. And for Dave, who was seemingly maintaining an upper hand on life, there were a few cracks in the glass. His success came without struggle or conflict. He seemed invincible in mind, body, and spirit. As a result, Dave started to lose some authenticity. His humble demeanor began to fade; he started to believe he was indomitable, extraordinary, immune to the blows that life dealt.

At twenty-five, Dave had completed his undergraduate degree; he was studying for his master's. He was a successful financial analyst for a major drug company, enjoyed strong relationships with friends and family, was in the best physical shape of his life, and had an active—and insatiable—sex life. Dave was *in command*. Success and achievement came easy to him, so he thought, because he was unique, because he had unmatched and exceptional gifts. He almost smiled at his doctor when she said what would ordinarily be a string of heart-stopping words.

Dave thought he had pulled a deep muscle during competition—the probable cause of the sharp pain that appeared mid-pose during a meet in Massachusetts. At first, he ignored it, but the pain became excruciating on the drive home. He went to see his doctor the next day.

"I'm sure I pulled something, but I just have no idea what," Dave said.

"Where's the pain?" she asked.

"Kind of in my left testicle but higher up, inside—and it's pretty intense."

She asked a series of questions, administered the standard turn-your-head-and-cough test, and examined his abdomen. "I doubt you've experienced a hernia or a pull," she said. "It's not usual to have a high level of pain with no swelling. I'm going to do an ultrasound on the area."

Dave waited in the examination room, the pulsing pain in his testes not causing any emotional concern.

She came back and asked him to lie down and relax. "I'm seeing a mass . . . here." She pointed to the screen with one hand while pressing the ultrasound probe between the base of his penis and his left testicle. "You see? That's not normal." She moved the probe, capturing varying angles. "The mass. It's asymmetrical. You see that—how right here it's uneven in shape?"

"What's that mean? Did I tear something? Is that bleeding?"

"No, it's not blood. There's no swelling. It's likely a tumor of some sort. I'm sending you to another doctor, and they're going to need to do a biopsy. It might not be serious, but it could be. There's no waiting."

The slight smile that appeared on Dave's face was not in response to her words but rather a gut reaction to the idea anything might obstruct his strength of body or mind enough to be labeled as serious.

A few days later, Dave found out he had germ cell testicular cancer. The course of treatment would be to remove his testicle and then be administered a series of radiation therapy treatments in the immediately adjacent area. Because he was young and strong and had caught the cancer early, his prognosis was extremely good.

"With cancer, there's always concern, but I'm confident we'll eradicate the cancerous cells, and you'll go on to live a long, healthy life," his oncologist said.

"Less one testicle," Dave offered.

"Yes. But there's no evidence it has spread. You can expect to live a normal, active life—even sexually—after treatment."

• • •

Dave often looked in mirrors—the ones on walls, not the figurative ones inside—and when he looked at himself before, during, and after surgery and radiation, he saw himself as he always had: strong, healthy, capable, masculine. Surgery and follow-up treatments were simply procedures; he didn't think of them as procedures *for cancer*. Doing so would have been too ominous, too real, too human.

Dave told his parents what was going on, but he wouldn't allow them to be concerned, because there was nothing to be concerned about. He had a girlfriend—not so much out of love but convenience—but he downplayed everything. After all, he never thought of the two of them as being so close that he needed to be *that* open with her. He didn't ask for rides to and from the hospital because he knew he wouldn't need them. He could drive himself, even if he was sometimes blinded by pain and tiredness. He didn't tell friends what was going on because he treated the cancer as just another obstacle to overcome. He didn't miss but a few classes and only several days of work, because he wasn't about to let his life be interrupted. In fact, he didn't even cancel a few lingering dates, girlfriend and cancer or not. He postponed them, certain that claims of a busy schedule would buy him enough time to recoup his manhood and prove what he needed to prove to himself.

Over the following weeks and months, visits to the hospital came and went, surgery was successfully performed, and stitches were removed. Dave dragged himself from appointment to appointment and to work and school, and even to the gym to do workouts when he could. He remained almost the same Dave he always had been—with one exception: At every stage of recovery, his intensity increased. Within a few months of diagnosis, Dave finished treatment. He came out of his cancerous episode stronger, more determined, and more intent on succeeding. He completed his master's at the top of his class, excelled at work, won the New Jersey State natural bodybuilding title, and captured the hearts—and bodies—of countless women.

So much for serious, Dave thought. *Serious is a freaking lightweight next to me.*

A Rising Tide

As Dave approached thirty, life became a deeper ocean to navigate; the increased stakes of a more consequential existence tested his ability to captain the ship through the rising tides of getting older, moving past competition, and wanting to settle down and build a family. The added pressures also continued to try to exploit his long-ingrained insecurities about not succeeding in life. But he helped mask those insecurities by continuing to work hard and pursue women. He also started to become a regular drinker. Work, wine, and women all helped him to avoid looking too far inside. Then he met someone who, when viewed through Dave's distorted lens, was perfect for taking the next step.

Dave's girlfriend was a strikingly beautiful, well-to-do, high-maintenance woman—qualities that provided Dave with challenges. She was used to getting what she wanted, so he could constantly feel success by trying to please her. Thus, he was able to move past chasing women. She was everything he thought he'd wanted.

Before and after marrying, they had their ups and downs, but Dave's income sustained a modestly lavish lifestyle—one that satisfied his expectations, even if it fell a little below her standards. Any strain from his wife's need for a more abundant lifestyle was quelled by Dave's frenetic pace of working hard and doing all he could to maximize career opportunities. Besides, they were always the best-looking couple in the room, their social calendar allowed them to show themselves off regularly, they had a beautiful house and fancy cars, and the sex was frequent. Whether he glanced at the mirrors in his bedroom or at the ones inside his psyche, all looked just fine.

But during a routine follow-up appointment with his oncologist days after his thirtieth birthday, Dave was given a massive blow—a much harder blow than he'd ever have admitted to receiving: He had cancer again.

This time, Dave had his wife and his parents at his side during the diagnosis and subsequent treatment, but he still refused to show them, himself, or anybody else any weakness or need, because he didn't feel unglued or needy. He had cancer. So what?

Just another storm to pilot around, Dave thought. *I'm the fucking captain.*

Getting testicular cancer is not exceptionally rare, and although rarer, getting testicular cancer in a subsequent testicle is not unheard of. But getting two different, unrelated testicular cancers is extraordinarily uncommon. The first had a fairly predictable outcome, but because of the rare circumstances behind getting a second—this time nonseminoma testicular cancer—a board study was needed. The agreed-upon treatment would involve a second orchiectomy, radiation therapy, and an intense regimen of hormonal therapy.

As before, Dave willed himself through the treatments, although they were much more brutal the second time around. He continued to work—although with a foggy mind and a reduced energy level; to stay close—even if not truly honest and open—with his parents; to be optimistic about, and in control of, his marriage; and to believe—even if done so with heaps of self-denial—that the world and all it could offer were still his to capture.

It took a year, but the doctors treated and eradicated his cancer for a second time. This time Dave couldn't deny the side effects. The surgery, the recovery, almost two dozen radiation treatments, and the intense hormonal treatments had slowed him down considerably. As a result, he gained sixty pounds. In addition, his color was off, he lost most of his hair, and his face looked older and puffy. His libido was sometimes strong, sometimes nonexistent. Exhaustion and disconnection were always lurking by the end of each day. But Dave fought through those things, and he found calmer seas. During those days between not being himself and then slowly becoming himself again, there were emotional and psychological side effects as well. But for Dave, they were still well hidden behind the mirror. The nonphysical side effects mostly revolved around his marriage.

Dave knew what losing a second testicle meant: He wasn't going to be able to father children. He and his wife had talked about that reality and agreed they could be happy without kids. But from the momentary calm within the eye of the cancer hurricane circling around them, they didn't address the depths of that sobering reality. Dave's doctors never addressed fertility issues with him—they simply never brought it up.

But one day, much like encountering an unseen rogue wave or bashing into an unexpected reef, his ship was upended and smashed into pieces.

"I'm leaving you and finding another life," his wife said. "I want more."

"More what?" Dave asked, stunned.

"Everything. I want more things. I want more love, more honesty, more connection. I want kids. I want a *real* husband."

"Just like that?"

"No. It's not 'just like that.' You just can't give me what I want anymore. I don't know if you ever could."

You don't know, and you certainly can't identify in yourself, what you refuse to learn in life. Although devastated, it didn't take Dave long to conclude that a wrecked marriage didn't mean the end of the world. Sure, he knew he never had a true emotional connection (if such a thing even existed) with his wife, and he hadn't been perfectly faithful. And although some people might think he was shallow and self-absorbed, and although he hadn't succeeded at the levels he'd hoped for by then and experienced setbacks he hadn't overcome yet, he also knew, regardless, he could handle anything, even being left adrift to find some footing and start over.

Failures don't inspire people, he thought. *Not being a real man doesn't either.*

Dave refused to believe anything except that through sheer will, determination, and ability, he could prove his continuing control of everything. Losing his wife, his house, his intended future, even his dignity, was painful, but pain could be eased.

And over the subsequent months, Dave worked hard at easing his pains, covering up his failures, and finding his way back onto the comfortable footing of a somewhat dissolute and amoral path. He doubled his efforts in his career, which helped get him back on his feet financially. He hit the gym, which helped him grow stronger. He partied and frequently drank too much wine and whiskey, which helped him avoid self-analysis. With the help of Viagra and various hormone replacement supplements, he went back to trying to conquer young, free, superficial women, which helped sharpen his self-image. Then came a visit to the dentist.

Sinking

The usual crispness of an October day in New York can sometimes be softened by a warm breeze, the last breaths of an unexhausted summer, hanging in the air long enough to wrap people's thoughts in a blanket of relief, protecting them from the chaos of shortened days and the primal uneasiness of an impending winter. But on a certain unusually softened fall day in the city, Dave only noticed that he didn't need to bring a coat to the dentist; deep contemplation wasn't in his wheelhouse.

"How are we doing today?" the receptionist at his dentist's office asked Dave.

"Pretty spectacular. It's beautiful out." Dave gave her one of his classic suave smiles. "Much like in here."

"Oh, boy, you're still a charmer, aren't you? Twice a year with you. Have a seat, and we'll call you in shortly."

Dave smiled again at the receptionist when he was led in for his cleaning. *If you only knew,* he thought. *Maybe one day you'll find out just what a charmer I can be.*

Dave sat in the technician's chair, listening to the hygienist's stories, forcing out a one- or two-syllable grunt when he could. She scraped at Dave's teeth with various tools and then used her curette to pick around his gums. She then reached for the motorized tools. Each time the ultrasonic scaler tickled his gums, he felt the faint, cool, metallic taste of blood. *Bloody gums?*

Something seemed off. Was he supposed to remember something about bloody gums? He felt a tiny itch inside his brain, one he had no idea how to scratch.

"You're bleeding a lot. Has it been a while since you were here?"

"Uh-uh," Dave grunted.

"Hmmm . . . you're flossing?"

"Uh-huh."

"Make sure when you're flossing, you go forward *and* backward. You have to work the gums really well. Less inflammation and bleeding, you know."

"I-ow."

"Well, good. I'll have the doctor look at you before we're done, anyway. We're almost finished. I don't see any signs of cavities. Nothing was too sensitive?"

"Uh-uh."

"That's it. Rinse really well," the hygienist said, handing Dave a small paper cup filled with diluted mouthwash. The itch inside grew, making him uncomfortable, cold—almost shivering cold. He felt nervous and unsure. He closed his eyes and swished the minty liquid around, trying to concentrate, to picture running down the hallways of his mind, looking for the file cabinet that held the answer that might scratch the itch. *Bloody gums? I'm supposed to know something about that.*

Dave spat the liquid into the bowl. It came out in an uncoagulated mixture of light blue mouthwash, blood, and white spittle. He wiped his lips with a tissue, unable to find any relief for the prickling in his brain. He opened his eyes when the doctor came in.

"How are you?" the doctor asked. "Been a while. No?"

Dave sat up. "Not that long, I think. Maybe six months."

"All good?" the doctor asked the hygienist. He washed his hands and put on gloves.

"Yes. A little bleeding, but . . ."

"You flossing regularly?" the doctor asked.

"Yes."

"Well, let's take a look." He grabbed a mirror and small metal probe and deftly manipulated the tools around Dave's mouth. "Everything looks good. Nothing unusual." He jumped up and took off the gloves. He flipped through Dave's chart. "No receding, no decay. You don't get many cavities, do you? When's the last time we did X-rays? Let's see . . . is that right? Five years ago?" He shrugged and looked at the hygienist and Dave. "Five years?"

The hallway lit up. *No ... no X-rays. I always made up an excuse why I couldn't, didn't I?*

"Well, five years is too long, even with you having a healthy mouth," the doctor said.

The file cabinet appeared. Shivers ran up from the small of Dave's back and down his arms. *I can't take X-rays.*

"Let's take a full set today," the doctor said. "I'll be back to review them with you after."

I can't take X-rays. Dave could feel the blood flowing out of his head. He stood and started to feel faint, dizzy. His pupils opened, and the lights in the room brightened. He was never cold, but right then he was freezing, shaking. He tried to hide everything, but he felt that he might fall down. He was confused—frightened, even.

The doctor popped his head back into the room. "Oh, just to be sure, you haven't been exposed to any radiation in the last five years, have you?"

The file drawer flung open, and a blast of white light exploded inside Dave's head. His eyes filled with tears, and his mouth dried up. He looked at the hygienist for help, but he didn't know what he needed help for. Then he frantically swiveled his eyes toward the doctor but only saw the open doorway behind him. Dave's legs were heavy, but not too heavy to move, and he tried to mumble something as he ripped the blue towel from the alligator clip around his neck. He couldn't see through the tears. He couldn't talk. He couldn't think. He just knew he had to go, to get air, to get away, to not take X-rays, to run, to run out of there. He made it to the waiting room and through the door to the hallway, then ran down the hallway, controlling nothing but direction—not his legs, his breathing, the sobs that burst from his chest, or the blinding flood of tears that poured out of him. He ran out of the building, out of breath, legs crumbling beneath him. He stumbled to the ground, missing by inches the bench he had somehow almost made it to, and he fell into a heap of exhaustion and weakness.

"I can't have X-rays! I can't have them," Dave cried loudly.

You don't know what you don't know until you know it. Until that minute, when the warm October air fought to comfort his cold body as he lay against the bench, drowning from an unimaginable and unseen weight he had carried for so long, crying as he had never cried in his life, Dave hadn't *known* that he'd had cancer.

Gasping for Air

For weeks after that inevitable day of cognizance, Dave sank further and further into the depths of his reality. Somehow, he'd discovered his way home that day, although he wasn't aware of his surroundings or aware of his outward self; he was lost inside his own head, every conscious thought obliterated by a waterfall of realizations—each second's flow an unstoppable force of truths. That one-way mirror inside had instantaneously shattered, forcing him to look at his raw, undeniable inner self for the first time ever—and he became overwhelmed by fear and anger and regret and shame.

He spoke to his mom and dad often in the subsequent months, sometimes alone, sometimes together. The pain of facing his shallowness, denial, and obliviousness was excruciating; he felt weak, unsure, confused about what to do and how to move forward. He knew he had hidden from his fear of failure, and everything that crashed in on him pointed to him being just that: a failure. He'd felt so self-assured his whole life. He'd known things would turn out well for him along a mostly predictable and manageable path. He'd been the master of his destiny. He'd been at the helm, navigating the journey despite the well-buried insecurities. The only doubt in life was *when* he would accomplish his goals and objectives, not *if* he would.

Sure, there had been some high and not-so-high points, but they were inconsequential when compared to the truth of his cancer. Once the barrier between the real Dave and the vain, hollow, superficial Dave was removed, insecurity and doubt coursed through him; his former self was a pile of dust blown away by the winds of self-realization—and only questions remained.

"What am I going to do? What can I possibly look at for hope?" he asked his dad. "They took away my manhood, my ability to have children. Couldn't they have taken a minute to tell me how to preserve that part of my life? It's going to be impossible to be happy—to make someone happy."

"The difficult we do immediately," his dad said. "The impossible takes just a little longer. You've always been so quick to handle every hard thing that comes your way. You'll figure things out. Just breathe. Look at this as a starting point. Make a plan for the impossible from today on."

"But I feel like I'm gasping for air, like I'm drowning, Dad. I could've died, right? I could have not beat cancer both times, and what would I have accomplished in my life? What? I wore a few medals and put a few notches on my belt—what good were those things anyway? I've never been open or honest or *real* about things. That has just hit me so hard, and I have no idea what to do."

"You will, Dave. Trust me. It starts with believing in yourself—"

"But I don't know who I am anymore. You understand what I mean?"

"I do," his dad said. "Sometimes I wake up in a panic, hearing the whistle of that bomb getting louder and louder, and I see everything around me blow up and everybody blow up, and it feels so desperate and real, and my heart races, and it's all I can do not to scream. But then I feel myself, and I'm okay, and I see your mom next to me, and I'm okay, and I realize all that was in the past, and I'm okay. You can do that now too. It's all in the past."

Dave's Epilogue

Soon after Dave began his journey of self-discovery and healing, he found out his dad had cancer. Not long after, his dad passed away. Near the end of his dad's care, Dave met Renee, a sweet, smart, strong yet soft, honest, emotional woman. She was the attending nurse at the cancer center that cared for his dad. Dave called her after his dad died and asked her for a date; something magnetic had drawn him to pursue her. They fell in love and married not long after.

Less than three months after his dad died, Dave walked away from the corporate world and joined the executive team at Stupid Cancer, the nation's largest organization focused on catering to the young adult cancer community. He has since gone on to found and run Gryt Health, a provider that connects people affected by cancer to both their peers and the care community at large.

"I had swept everything about cancer away without a thought," Dave told me. "And when I left the dentist that day, I felt so alone. When I lost my dad, I was devastated and alone. But Renee came into my life, and Stupid Cancer came into my life, and I started to learn I wasn't alone. I learned about real love. I learned there was a community of people like me, people who needed support and friendship. They were searching for others who would understand the things they were going through. I understand them, and they understand me."

The first time I spoke to Dave, he told me how transformative speaking on stage at Stupid Cancer's annual gathering had been for him.

"I prepared some notes about a few initiatives we were working on, and I stood in front of eight hundred people—people like me who'd beaten cancer or were fighting cancer, who might soon die from cancer. People who'd dealt with loss and abandonment and a system that failed them on fertility issues and left them alone to figure out how to move past cancer. I started to talk, and the emotion overtook me in a way I can't explain. I folded my notes up and broke down on stage. I was a wreck. Somehow, I managed to get a hold of myself, and I managed to talk about what it meant to be able to open up and to be honest about the impact—the *profound* impact—cancer had on me. And I talked about how I'd never acknowledged its effects, let alone dealt with them, until years later. I don't know what I said, but I admitted how I needed to heal and how important they all were in helping me do that, because they understood me, and I understood them. I felt all the pain and loss and suffering, and I had as much healing to do as they had to do."

Dave explained how much he had learned about himself since that day at the dentist, how he'd had to face the person he was and the way he had treated women. How he'd based so much of his life on meaningless ideals and had hid behind denial and alcohol and a twisted sense of machismo. How he had evolved emotionally more in the past couple years than he had in the previous thirty-odd years. He told me how truthfulness, honesty, love, and vulnerability cleared the way for him to mend himself and rebuild his ship.

I told him it was impossible to ever imagine what he must have gone through—what he was still going through.

"The difficult can be done immediately," he said. "The impossible just takes a little longer."

Any Amount

"Four-Mile Bridge" was thirty-odd miles behind me, but I was still shaky from the experience. Fifteen hours had passed since I'd started out that day, and I desperately wanted a shower, some food, and a bed. The only thing between the end of that hellacious ride and those three joys was the woman behind the hotel's check-in counter.

"Mr. Richman?" she asked, greeting me with a friendly smile.

"Yes. Not too many people left to check in at this hour, I'll bet," I said.

"Definitely not—besides, none of them are on a cancer ride across the country."

I gave her a confused look.

"My manager left a note about you and said that we're not to charge you for the room," she said. "We're really glad to have you."

She went on to tell me that her grandfather, whom she was very close to, had passed from liver cancer only weeks before. We talked for a few minutes, and then she offered up the only real solution on food—the Burger King around the corner was the last place in town still open. She asked how she could donate to the Cycle of Lives, and then we took a picture together.

Meeting her was just what I needed. Like so many times before, I was reminded about how eager people were to take a breath and share their experiences with cancer. And, once again, my own experiences were humbled by the difficult realities that seemed to face everyone I ran into. I rode my bike through the Burger King's drive-through, and ten minutes later, I was in my room, making my way through a Double Whopper, large fries, and Dr. Pepper.

The phone rang. "Mr. Richman, it's Candice, from the front desk."

"Of course. What's up?"

"I was wondering. I hate to bother you, but I went on your website and gave a donation."

"That's very generous of you," I said.

"It's just . . . do you know if that's a monthly amount or a one-time donation? Because I can't afford to give each month."

"It's only a one-time donation. It's really thoughtful of you. Thank you so much."

"That's great. Okay. Goodnight, now," she said.

As I went back to my perfectly delicious, not particularly nutritious meal, I checked the notifications on my mobile phone. Candice had donated what, to her, was enough to hurt—and she needed it to be a one-time event because she didn't have room in her budget for a monthly gift. For the second night in a row, I was overwhelmed by the generosity of strangers.

As I lay in bed, ready to pass out, I thought of the difficult miles I'd put in, the heat, the wind, the causeways, the open stretches of southern Louisiana everglades, the swamps, the big rigs, the couple dozen instances of avoiding death along Old Four-Mile Bridge, the anxiety, the fear, the lightning and thunder of vigorous microbursts, and the generous act of giving any amount, when that amount meant so much to the giver's ability to put food on the table that month. Then, as I drifted asleep, I thought about some of the people I'd run into who had disclosed a struggle in life they experienced over finances, including one of the book participants, James.

And I thought of how lucky I was that people cared about what I was doing.

James

Relationship to cancer: Caregiver, professional

Age: Fifty-seven

Family status: Married with two children

Location: Laguna Beach, California

First encounter with cancer: In his midtwenties

Cancer summary: As a physician, one of James's first patients was a poor, uninsured father of four who was diagnosed with terminal brain cancer. He uses that experience, along with his own upbringing, to advocate for people who do not have access to the medical system. In his current position as a chief medical officer of a major national health-care company, he advocates for inclusive care and treatment standards.

Strongest positive emotion during cancer experience: Passion

Strongest negative emotion during cancer experience: Frustration

How we met: When my wife, Erin, worked as in-house counsel at a major health-care company, she often spoke with sincere admiration about many of her colleagues. One in particular, Dr. James Cruz, the chief medical officer for the California health plan, was one of her favorites.

"He's a true advocate for doing the right thing," she told me. "I don't know if he knows anyone you might talk to for the book, but I'm sure if he does, he'll want to help."

Weeks later, I connected with Dr. Cruz. We spoke on his way home from work. James Cruz had a soft, comforting voice, and from the first moment we spoke, he seemed engaged and relatable. I briefly described the project and asked him if he knew of anyone who might make an interesting participant for the book.

"Well, fortunately, I haven't been in private practice for a long, long time," he said.

"Fortunately?" I asked.

"The world of medicine today doesn't make it easy on physicians," he explained. "I do miss caring for people, but the bureaucracy is maddening to navigate."

"It must be even tougher from where you sit."

"You'd think so, but it's not. I don't care about corporate politics. My energy is spent trying to actually effect change. Trust me, many, many people could benefit from the system changing. This way, I can have a much greater impact than just seeing one patient at a time."

"For this project," I told him, "I'm more interested in the emotional side of things than the actual care and treatment of people."

"There's not much room for emotion in medical care anymore," he said matter-of-factly, "although I guess there might be in some areas. There used to be."

I asked if he had time to explain what he meant.

"It takes me an hour-plus to get home. I've got time on the drive, if you'd like," he said, then spent the next hour providing me a colorful overview of his past. Although there'd been no opening to discuss potential referrals, I was fascinated by his stories. By the time he pulled up to his house, we'd agreed to speak again.

I talked with James many times on his commute home, and I never did ask if he knew anyone else I could interview—his story was too important to pass up.

I Love My Life

··

J ames had been in private practice for four years when he met Mr. Porras. The dozens of patients he saw each day fell into two main categories. The first were people who suffered from minor problems that required basic remedies and simple treatment plans. The second, and much smaller category, were patients who had serious or complicated issues that required a complex, collaborative process of diagnosis and treatment. As James dictated the details of Mr. Porras's initial appointment, it was clear that he was definitely in the second category.

"Referral from Dr. Richard Creighton. Unknown circumstance of patient's initial consult with referring. Mr. Porras, Hispanic male, forty-two years old, no known medical interventions. Appears patient has not sought prior attention for multiple ongoing and escalating symptoms. Unknown family history. Employed as a janitor. Spouse unemployed. Uninsured."

No insurance, he thought. *Without insurance, Mr. Porras is in deep trouble.*

Dr. Cruz held the recording microphone in his hand, his fingers preparing to tap the record button on the neck of the microphone, his thoughts alternating between dictating the specifics of his evaluation and contemplating the plight Mr. Porras must have had so far in life, and the hopeless battle he'd likely be up against.

"Mr. Porras complains of severe neck pain, reduced mobility, persistent cough, exhaustion, confusion, temporal cephalalgia accompanied by related vomiting and vertigo. Initial observations—"

James paused his recording. He sat back in his chair and looked at his dark-walnut-framed medical school diploma on the wall across from his desk. He often stared at the diploma, not to reassure himself that he was qualified to practice but because it was a tangible sign of how fortunate he was. If he'd been born ten years earlier, or if his parents had been less involved in his education, or if any number of slight differences in his life's circumstances had occurred, he might have had an entirely different reality. If life had given *him* a few different twists and turns, he might be a Mr. Porras—stuck in a world where manual labor was the only option and where he was subject to inequitable systems, like the very medical system Dr. Cruz worked within, that offered no solutions for, and often not even the chance to get attention toward, very tangible and real life-and-death issues. Patients like Mr. Porras were at the mercy of a discriminatory and unbalanced health-care system where they were more often ignored than treated.

"Initial observations are such to order ultrasound-guided FNAB on what appears to be a three- to four-centimeter nodule. Possible genetic prevalence for medullary thyroid carcinoma or multiple endocrine neoplasia? Laryngoscopy reveals inflammation. Drew for spectrum testing. Order thyrotropin prior to thyroid scan and possible RAIU."

James knew from the first moment that he began to examine Mr. Porras that testing would find at least one tumor, but the real question was whether there was also malignancy and possible metastasis. There was more to dictate, but he'd get to it later—other patients were waiting. But Mr. Porras stayed on his mind all day. He seemed to be a decent, humble man—one who'd never been to the doctor before. Now, he was probably very, very sick. He had four children and a wife he was trying to support, working as a janitor, and he was scared and lost. James knew life wasn't going to be easy for Mr. Porras—he was going to need to see a lot of doctors.

I could have been him, no doubt about it. I could have been him.

Life: Developing

Before James's parents divorced, life was about only two things in the Cruz household: work and family.

Work, depending on who in the household it applied to, could have been described many different ways. Work was one's job, a second job, military service, schoolwork, chores, community service, and basically any and all things that were done almost all day, every day, with the singular purpose of contributing to life's ultimate goal of constant advancement toward a greater good for oneself and the community.

Family could only be described one way: Family was the dozens of collective Cruz and Cruz-related members who were measured by the continuity of their inclusion in his grandma's circle. If one wasn't seen from time to time at his grandma's house on Sundays, one wasn't considered family.

The drive to Grandma's house wasn't far for James's family, but it wasn't fast either; the road was too chopped up and dusty to easily negotiate in James's family's rusted-out 1956 Ford F100 pickup truck.

James's grandpa was definitely not part of the family. He'd come to America under the bracero program in the late 1940s and met Grandma, whose family was also back home in Mexico. They married and had three kids but went their separate ways while still young. Although James's dad lived with his father during a stretch of his youth, James's grandpa was a distant, field-hardened, and narrow-minded man who drank too much with the money he worked too hard for. Few friends—and even fewer family members—sought his company.

James's grandma, on the other hand, was charming, funny, and chaotic; she sang and played piano and loved being surrounded by people. Grandma's tiny house was always overflowing. James and his family would join the uncles and aunts and cousins and great-uncles and great-aunts and all the other family who came to help Grandma cook, or who had stayed there while they worked a few local days on the nearby farms so they could give Grandma the extra money they earned, or who just made it a regular practice to be around family. They did all the things that big Mexican families did when they got together: cook, eat, fix things, cook some more, and plan birthday parties, weddings, baptisms, and quinceañeras while they laughed, told stories, and gave advice to younger ones among them.

Talk often began light and then intensified as the sun descended in the sky. The family talked about Cesar Chavez's exploits, the Black Panthers, the Vietnam War, protests, boycotts, and the struggle of their family—and all Mexican American families—to realize the ever-elusive American dream. The darker the skies became, the heavier the tone of the conversation. Out of those deeper exchanges, James and his brother and the cousins nearest in age to them were given the cherished bits of advice, guidance, and opinions that had been learned and adopted over the previous decades through countless days of hard labor, uncertainty about the future, and unwavering adherence to deep cultural ideals and beliefs.

"Always respect your mother and father," an uncle would tell James in conversation.

"No Cruz gives up. You always finish what you start," another would say as an aside.

"Always, always put family first. That is what determines what kind of man you are," his aunt would pronounce.

"Your father works hard for you and your brother. Hard—to give you opportunities and choices," another said.

"No matter the pains for yourself, what you do for others is what matters," his grandma admonished.

James's generation was expected to do better in life than their parents. They were not going to have to work as hard, and if they did, it was going to be in the classroom and not in the fields. They were the beneficiaries of change. They didn't need to clear the obstacles and endure the dangers of navigating a new country in new times—trails were being blazed for them so they could travel further in life. James's adolescence was defined by work, family, talk of a better future, and constant reminders that values, morals, and worthwhile purpose were the building blocks for his material and spiritual advancement.

But the narrative changed slightly after James's parents divorced. *Work* meant the same thing—James's father was not going to waver from life's one overriding principle—but *family* came to mean different things, depending on whether James was staying with his mom or his dad. Family became defined not just by the eccentric, dynamic, and complicated group of dozens inside the circle on his dad's side but also by the much smaller, nondescript, noncohesive one on his mother's.

James relished belonging to a big family. He liked feeling a part of something meaningful, watching and learning from the spirited and active interactions of the scores of people on his dad's side. His parents' divorce disrupted that for him—it certainly resulted in missing out on too many Sundays at Grandma's. But James didn't focus on his parents' issues. Instead, he looked to each for what they could give individually. Thus, James's post-divorce childhood was not filled with negativity but rather affection and closeness—more so with his mom—because she was in a place where she was free to be more sensitive and demonstrative with her children than James's dad would ever have settled for under his roof. As a result, James's motivation in life was borne not just from the weighty life lessons he learned while watching and listening to his dad and the other Cruzes as he grew up but through the patience, understanding, and guidance of a loving and expressive mother.

Those balanced tenets—putting family first, becoming educated, working hard, pursuing significance, openly caring for loved ones, and showing sensitivity—were not just admonitions heard and appreciations learned by a young boy; they were alternating bricks cemented into the pathway of his youth by both the father and the mother he admired so much.

James learned the concept of striving to accomplish more from his dad. He and his siblings were the first in the family to graduate high school. He learned respect for authority through the lessons his dad taught him from his service in the Air Force after high school. James strove to achieve at school because he saw that a few aunts and uncles had attended college, and he watched his dad work as a grocery clerk during the day and study at night for many years to achieve his own college degree and become a youth counselor. James was taught that education, because it would guide one to work in a profession that

might serve others, was more important than the more selfish and inconsequential pursuits of sports or arts or leisure.

To an equal degree, thanks to his mother's soft and loving temperament
around the home and when interacting with others, James developed a caring,
sensitive, attentive disposition. So it was no surprise to either parent, because
of what each knew they were imparting to their son, when in the eighth grade,
James declared he wanted to become a doctor.

Life: Planned

By the time James finished high school, he was attending premed conferences
so he could learn what was ahead of him. He started at Sacramento State
College right after high school, then went to the University of California,
Davis, to complete his undergraduate degree. At twenty-two, he began medical school at the University of California, San Diego.

While James enjoyed the studying of diseases, he preferred learning how
to care for people. He was intrigued about how to diagnose and determine the
problem, then tailor a specific treatment plan based on each patient's unique
set of factors. He gravitated toward the more holistic side of the profession
and decided to become a general practitioner.

After working a few years with a small medical group where the empha-
sis was on medicine as a business, James opened his own practice, intent on
offering meaningful care and meeting patient needs above all else. Up to his
eyeballs in debt, and with no understanding of how to run a medical practice,
James opened his doors and welcomed the opportunity to work with patients
who might otherwise receive less personal care.

• • •

Months after coming to see James, Mr. Porras was diagnosed with stage IV
metastatic anaplastic thyroid cancer. It had spread to his neck and, a short
time later, to his brain. It was terminal. James and Mr. Porras spent quite a bit
of time together over the next several months, and Mr. Porras came to rely
on James to help him with many facets of his care until he required hospice
at the end of his life. James had an affinity for Mr. Porras, not just because he

could see how his own life could have turned out so different but also because he understood how many patients like Mr. Porras didn't have the chance to receive adequate care.

Mr. Porras was the sole breadwinner for his family, which included his wife and their four children and her mother. He continued to work two jobs through unimaginably difficult circumstances, because there was no other choice but to work, and he commuted two hours each way on the bus for his appointments—sometimes as many as four per week. He spoke little English, had no formal education, and had nobody but James to turn to for his medical needs.

James was deliberate, attentive, and patient when interacting with Mr. Porras. He had to be, because no other physicians took time to give him any care. More so, James was certain that few other physicians would have understood Mr. Porras, or someone like him, the way he did. It was impossible to give that type of care and attention to everyone; he had a practice to run. Most patients weren't in need of those things. But some were. James struggled to balance his desire to make a meaningful difference in the lives of his patients with the reality that he could only affect one patient at a time—sometimes only one patient at the expense of having enough time for the others. If he wanted to have an impact on delivering better care to more patients, he'd need to change the focus of his career. So he decided to leave his medical practice and became a medical director for a small hospital.

James lost very few patients while he was in private practice. Mr. Porras was the first of a small group, but he was also the most impactful patient Dr. Cruz had cared for, regardless of mortality. Even had Mr. Porras not died, he still would have represented many things to James. He remained etched in James's memory as a constant reminder of the needs of those less fortunate and as a simple and pure representation of one of James's most intimate truths—that he was only a few fortunate happenstances away from working in the fields of his youth, struggling to make a living and support a family, uncertain about the future, and ill-equipped to deal with things such as catastrophic illness. There were endless numbers of people like Mr. Porras out there, and but for the grace of God, he could have been one of them.

Life: Unplanned

Some doctors possess both the desire and the ability to form a real connection with the people they care for, while others don't want to or can't understand the need to develop an emotional bond with their patients. James knew that one factor alone—making a connection—probably had the single biggest impact on the doctor-patient relationship. He learned that from taking care of patients like Mr. Porras. Being comfortable with his own emotions allowed him to be understanding when patients expressed their feelings—and he always tried to stay aware of the fact that people processed things in unique ways and reacted to things differently. If he created a safe environment for his patients and allowed them to freely express themselves, he believed that some of the shock and uncertainty involved in people's diagnoses, treatments, and care could be overcome. If he was able to demystify things and empower his patients—by taking the time to *talk with them*—then he could remove most of the anxiety, uncertainty, and distress they felt.

James knew that his ability to form a bond with patients differentiated him from the majority of his peers, and he believed real and lasting change could only be brought to health care—and health care desperately needed all kinds of change—by thinking and acting in new ways. By being a minority— even a dissenting—voice, not only as a Hispanic male but as a doctor and an executive who, unlike many of his peers, considered the little guy, he could address the need for compassion, concern, and a thoughtfulness that might lead to change.

James's professional life, as measured either as a physician or an executive, was driven by his empathy and self-awareness. Those qualities, along with that strong desire to effect change at a meaningful level, gave James the belief he could advance his agenda of improving health care for those who don't have many options. James envisioned a future where he'd achieve ever more dynamic positions and thus be uniquely positioned to further his lofty agenda.

Those same qualities—empathy and self-awareness—defined him during the most challenging times in his personal life as well.

Life: Harmony and Discord

When James married his first wife, life couldn't have been better. He'd launched his new practice. He had strong relationships with his family and friends. He felt in the right place emotionally to begin to start his own family. Most of all, he looked forward to sharing a purposeful, grounded, and complete life with a partner. He was optimistic about the future and enthusiastic about each day. For the first few years of his marriage, his life was what he hoped it would be. But after their first child, Adam, was born, his wife began to change. She became emotionally volatile, less joyous, often overwhelmingly gloomy and sorrowful. Becoming a parent did more than simply change his wife at the margins—it transformed her into someone else. That person wasn't one bit the woman he'd married. After their second child, Anthony, was born, things got much worse.

Anthony was born with Leber congenital amaurosis, an untreatable and rare genetic eye disease, which led to complete blindness when he was very young. James's wife, whose negative emotions had intensified over the previous two years, had almost completely broken down and was unable to perform the most basic of daily tasks, parental or otherwise.

A year into his role as a hospital administrator with two young children, one of whom was severely disabled, and a wife who refused any psychological or medical attention, James had no choice but to seek a divorce.

The divorce proceeded slowly and was hard on their young boys. James knew he needed to get full custody—not only was his wife ill-equipped to be a parent, but she was incapable of caring for a child with a severe disability. He also knew it would be pretty near impossible to be both a full-time single parent, especially with special circumstances, while also pursuing a high-level career, but he saw no other choice but to try to do both. Fortunately, the judge gave his full consideration to the psychological evaluations performed on both James and his wife, and James was awarded full-time custody.

Over the next several years, James's life was a blur. Caring for the boys meant that he often had to bring them with him to work, because he often worked long days. He also had distant commutes and had to travel for business. His youngest son's special needs were expensive, intensive, and time-consuming, which added to the stresses and helped cause James to move from one job to the next. Although some moves led to positive opportunities, others involved professional setbacks—but that was the reality of the path his life had taken.

Over that same time, the divorce proceedings continued. Having lost the custodial rights to their children, his estranged wife attempted to gain anything she could from James, whether she went after his money, which he'd amassed very little of; his income, which was relatively unstable and inconsistent; or his psyche and character, which she attacked in exasperating and harmful ways. She wanted to try to get what she could get from him. More accurately, she wanted him to lose anything and everything and hurt him in one way or another.

Five agonizing years after separating, the divorce was final. It came at a heavy price. By the time he thought he and his sons could finally move past the fights and threats and ups and downs and emotional carnage that accompanied a brutal divorce, James could do anything but relax. Yes, the divorce was final. Yes, he had a restraining order for him and his kids against his ex-wife. But he also had no assets; a two-hour commute each way to a consulting job that barely paid the bills; almost daily issues to attend to involving the boys' schooling, special needs, and care; and no end in sight to the wreckage from the recent chapters of his life.

Life: The Low Point

One Friday afternoon, in the middle of June, Adam was at baseball camp and Anthony was at a camp for blind children. The house was empty of enough food for a full meal. James needed his paycheck so he could buy groceries and cook dinner that night. Getting to work, picking up his paycheck, cashing it, and getting back would take at least three hours, but there was no choice. He had to go get the paycheck. When he went to start his car, the gas gauge showed empty. James put his head on the steering wheel, closed his eyes, and took a long, hard, heavy breath in.

What am I going to do? he thought. *What in the world am I going to do?* And then a flood of thoughts released inside as he slowly exhaled. *Look at you, you made it. From where you came, you're a doctor—top of your class at medical school. You have two beautiful boys, parents who are proud of you. Your own mother went to nursing school because she was so proud and inspired by you becoming a doctor. Mr. Porras had it so much harder than you ever will, but he persevered like a man who was so much larger than the experiences life had given to him.*

You got unlucky and are having some rough times. Who doesn't? You didn't make all the best choices or get the best breaks, but look at what you can do. You got your whole life ahead. You believe in yourself. Your kids believe in you. Get out of the car, find some change, go get some gas, get your paycheck, and come home and cook dinner and spend time with your boys.

James got out of his car and walked into the house. He started to smile to himself.

So, what? I have to look for change in the sofa? Big deal.

He started laughing as he turned over the pillows on the couch. In total, he found ten dollars throughout the house—enough money for gas so he could pick up his paycheck. Dinner that night was spaghetti and meatballs, a movie, and laughing with his boys. It was a beautiful summer night.

James went to work that Saturday for a few hours and began to plan his next professional move. He had a health-care system to change, a slew of Mr. Porrases to help, and he was grateful for the chance to make a difference for others.

James's Epilogue
....

After his consulting stint, James once again became the medical director of a medium-sized hospital. In that role, he was able to institute policies that furthered his belief that there was room in the health-care system to attend to the needs of all patients, regardless of their circumstances. But it wasn't until his next position as the chief medical officer for the California health plan of one of the country's largest health-care organizations specializing in Medicaid that James found himself in a position to effect real change, both in substance and scope, for people living at or below the poverty line.

We talked about patients' hierarchy of needs and how less fortunate people didn't have some of the resources that many people take for granted, such as the ability to sit at a computer and search for information about a particular disease, the opportunity to take time off work to deal with a medical situation, access to the kind of transportation necessary to attend to a complicated set of treatment parameters, or the money to supplement one's care with such basics as healthy food, proper clothing, heat and air conditioning, and stable living conditions.

We talked about how undocumented people were afraid to seek preventative care or seek attention for anything but the direst of medical needs, which, in the end, created a much greater strain on resources than if they felt they could have sought early intervention; how the more educated people were, the sooner they sought care for their medical needs; how the insurance system would not strain under the pressure of uninsured patients in crisis if only doctors and hospitals would accept all patients; and, how doctors needed to develop more compassion and understanding of the difficulties that some of the people who came to see them had to deal with.

We talked about those general observations and the hard work he and his teams did while trying to advance initiatives and policies that could help both the patients and the caregivers.

We also talked about how he met his second wife, how happy they had been in almost ten years of marriage, how their children got along so well, and how James often found himself acting like his own father in pushing all four kids to strive for excellence so they could achieve more than he had— including his blind son, who was a college sophomore pursuing a degree in computer science.

In one memorable exchange, James summed up his thoughts on life:

"I think about Mr. Porras often, how he was fortunate to find perhaps the one doctor who understood him and cared for him the way I did, regardless of the costs," he said. "How fortunate I was to see firsthand how someone could handle the things he handled, and how he did so with such grace and a humble and appreciative attitude. I think of what might've happened to his wife and kids and how much more horrible his last couple of years could have been had he and I not crossed paths. How I might not appreciate as deeply as I do the need to create a system that could enable Mr. Porras to deal with his thyroid cancer before it became terminal. I think of how much I owe my parents, how lucky I am in so many ways. I have a career I could only dream of having—one where I institute material change in the lives of patients and in the care they receive. I have a family I love and who loves me more than anything. I love my life. I love that I can still taste the dust of those Sunday rides in the truck, can still recall my uncles' voices teaching me what makes a meaningful life. I try to never forget where I come from. I even sometimes still reach under the sofa cushions for change to remind me of how far life has taken me. I can't say it enough, I love my life."

Not in Alabama

··

When I awoke for day twenty-five, after that insane fifteen-hour day, it took an hour to work the pain and fatigue out of my muscles and joints enough to get back on my bike again. Luckily, the thought of being only ninety flat miles away from New Orleans and seeing Erin again (she'd flown back out to support me for a few days) helped me gain the emotional fortitude to overcome my revolting body.

Halfway through the day, I came across the bridge that was supposed to take me over the Mississippi River so I could make my way toward the city. As I approached the monstrous mile-long structure, still reeling from the prior day's harrowing experience, I noticed the bridge had only two lanes and an inches-wide shoulder—there was no room to ride right of the right lane, and there was also no curb to hop on to get out of the way of oncoming cars. I stopped my bike and stared at the road ahead as I watched the heavy traffic squeeze onto the narrow crossing. There was no sense calculating the chances of attempting to bike across. No doubt I'd get run over if I tried. Besides, there was a huge sign to the right of the beginning of the bridge warning "No Bicycles, No Pedestrians." Had I not had a Four-Mile Bridge experience already, I may have taken my chances anyway—but I'd learned my lesson.

It took an extra couple of hours, but I ended up riding a dozen miles down-river; took a safe, traffic-free ferry across that muddy giant; and then happily rode the long way into New Orleans. The previous night, I'd taken a selfie on the bridge so as to give some closure to Erin should that have been my last hurrah. Taking a picture on the barge across the Mississippi was blissfully less dramatic.

Day twenty-six was a stunningly beautiful day. I was approaching the three-thousand-mile mark and was excited to get into Florida so I could see the Atlantic Ocean. But as I made my way along and just over the one hundred miles of pancake-flat, serene Southern highways, past beaches, marshes, marinas, deltas, and bridges, and through iconic and history-heavy towns

such as Pass Christian, Biloxi, and Gulfport, Mississippi, it was impossible
not to slow my tempo, quiet my mind, and consciously breathe in the beauty
and the grandiosity that unfolded mile after mile in the states just west of
Florida's panhandle. I was intoxicated by the moist air of endless peat bogs. I
was soothed by the contemplative awe that washed over me while I observed
two-hundred-plus-year-old estates proudly line the highway and look out
over the Gulf. I was hypnotized by a constant chorus of cicadas and crickets
that emanated from both the ground and the trees, whose music provided a
constant, stereophonic reminder that the Deep South is rooted not just in the
soil but in everything that occupies it.

Cycling from the Pacific to the Atlantic and up the East Coast, especially
in the zig-zag way I'd laid it out, was an epochal event, and as I put more of
the country behind me than I had to conquer ahead, the weight of my journey became more pronounced. There I was, fifty-three years old and biking
toward a distant line, one that was going to mark the end of a journey that
was turning out to be revelatory in many ways about others. Yet I still felt I
was in search of so many answers to questions about myself. Over the course
of the ride—and before the ride, during the many long discussions with the
book participants—I began to understand more about how others were finding peace or tending to the issues that had wounded their souls.

But I was finding little remedy to my own ills. No matter how optimistic
I was, no matter how energetic and driven and rightly purposed, my heart
still had an irregular beat, a weightiness, a pressure on it that darkened me.
I was not at peace about June's passing, and I continued to be bewildered by
the people in life who so collectively and absolutely disappeared from mine
after she died. Trying to understand how my mother could toss me aside in
such a definitive way so many decades before still held a piece of my brain
hostage. The strain of grappling with myself for answers that probably didn't
exist to the questions that never completely went away wore on me. Even
though so much in my life was right, a part of me was still engaged in an
ultimate fight against an unseen enemy—the elusive antagonist inside—the
part that enjoyed no acceptance or reconciliation. I pedaled along, day after
day, state after state, discovering so much understanding about others, yet
the air inside of my own bubble was still so confusing and turbulent.

As I approached Moss Point, Mississippi, as if in deference to the contemplation going on inside of me, the skies turned nasty. A vicious storm
had formed some twenty miles ahead. The wind whipped, the skies began to
spit, and monstrous booms vibrated the world around me, chasing freakishly
shaped trees of lightning, one after the other, snapping the air excitedly. I
pedaled on, unsure of what to do. It was as if the road was a long black tongue,
intent on curling me into the head of the storm, ready to engulf me, ready to
toss *me* around in contemplation.

Maybe if I battle that, I thought. *I might be shown some answers.*

But as much as my imagination wanted to believe such a thing, I knew
the storm hadn't been created as a sign, some kind of mystical portal through
which I'd be shown the secret solutions to the things that pained me inside.
Using my better judgment, I decided to pull over when I could find safe cover.

"No way you could imagine how violent that storm is. I'm coming to get
you," Erin said as I called her for help. She was already driving back toward
me. Now *that* was a sign. Sometimes, someone is more equipped—literally
or metaphorically—to brave the storm than you are. I didn't know if Erin
had any answers for me, but I sure was happy she was headed my way. I'd
feel safer—both metaphorically and literally—driving with her than traveling
through all that turmoil alone and unprotected.

• • •

I left Moss Point on day twenty-seven, excited about seeing "99 miles, Moss
Point, Mississippi, to Pensacola, Florida" on the day's route map.

Florida.

I made my way to Interstate 10, biked up the on-ramp, and continued
east, toward Mobile, Alabama. About an hour into the ride, I saw a not
uncommon sight ahead—a patrol car. As I got closer, I could make out the
patrolman. He was leaning in, talking to the driver of the car he must have
pulled over. He must have caught a glimpse of me, because he then backed
away from the vehicle, faced me, and pointedly looked in my direction, arms
crossed. When I was a few yards away, he stretched his arms out, indicating
for me to stop.

"Do you happen to know where you are, sir?" he asked.

"Yes, sir. I'm in Alabama, about twenty miles outside of Moss Point," I replied.

"I mean, do you know that you are on my interstate highway?"

"Yes," I said. I understood from his tone that his questions were being asked with annoyance and sarcasm.

"What exactly *are* you doing on my interstate highway?"

"I'm biking. Across the country, actually."

"Do you know what the minimum vehicular speed is on my highway?" he asked.

"No, sir. I don't."

"Forty-five miles per hour. You reckon you were maintaining a vehicular speed of at least forty-five miles per hour?"

I smiled and shook my head. "No, but I've been on the interstate practically from the very start back in Los Angeles."

"Not in Alabama you have not been," he said.

"Oh, I definitely was. For the last day and a half."

"You might *think* you have been on my interstate for the last day and a half, but I repeat: *Not* in Alabama you have not. I suggest you safely exit as per the next off-ramp," he said and pointed down the road. "Then I'd suggest you find a safe, lawful manner with which to continue your bicycling from California, sir."

I had traveled three-quarters of the way across the country on busy highways, and although it wasn't really allowed, and it was definitely not the most peaceful way to travel the miles, it was, by far, the most direct route most days. I exited, as instructed, and after about an hour traversing one turn after another, attempting to stay somewhat parallel to my intended route, I got back on the highway and continued into Mobile.

I ran into many highway patrol officers on my ride. All of them—perhaps except one—were enthusiastically supportive of what I was doing, but none were as memorable as that particular officer who owned Alabama's Interstate 10.

The next book participant I'd see on my ride, Karen, worked for the governor of Florida, dealing with some form of transportation issues. I looked forward to telling her about the transportation issue I'd had in Alabama.

Karen

Relationship to cancer: Survivor, advocate

Age: Forty-three

Family status: Divorced mother of three

Location: Tallahassee, Florida

First encounter with cancer: Twenty-nine years old

Cancer summary: Diagnosed with thyroid cancer at twenty-nine, Karen endured radiation therapy and chemotherapy to eradicate the cancer. At forty, she was diagnosed with an aggressive form of breast cancer, requiring a double mastectomy, radiation therapy, and chemotherapy. One lymph node was affected, and radiation therapy was prescribed in the hopes of preventing the cancer from spreading. Several of her family members also have fought or are currently fighting cancer.

Cancer specifics: Papillary thyroid cancer, stage II; triple negative breast cancer, stage III; metastasis to lymph nodes

Community involvement: Volunteered for and was a board member of Ronald McDonald House Charities for more than ten years. Karen participates in cancer walks and organizes events to fundraise for families facing medical crises.

Strongest positive emotion during cancer experience: Cheerfulness

Strongest negative emotion during cancer experience: Fear

How we met: In my search to find people with inspiring and compelling stories I could include in this project, I contacted several cancer centers. The people at Moffitt Cancer Center in Tampa, Florida, were particularly helpful and encouraging. I spoke to someone in the public relations department who suggested I speak to a woman undergoing treatment at their center for an aggressive form of breast cancer.

"Karen is pretty unique," the public relations representative told me. "She's a stubborn fighter and a ball of energy. She's always smiling, talking, and upbeat. She's an active and vocal supporter for the center and our patients. And she *loves* to talk. I think she might be able to help you."

In my first conversation with Karen, I spent about five minutes introducing myself and the project, and she talked for the rest of the hour. Karen touched on her cancer, experiences, family dynamics, optimism, and love for life. By the time I hung up, my head was spinning. Karen's cadence was faster than my ability to take notes, and she jumped from topic to topic so quickly I wasn't sure I had caught it all. We scheduled another talk for several weeks later.

After our second and our third conversations, I was still a little confused. I enjoyed talking to Karen, but I couldn't quite put my finger on an aspect of her experience that stood out—one that would distinguish her from other people I'd talked to. I couldn't make any deep connection to what she told me, because while Karen was always animated, she wasn't *emotional*. She had opinions and she talked about emotional things, but there was a disconnect between her ability to describe what she was going through and her ability to tell or show me how she *felt* about the experiences she described so vividly. That lack of connection between her experience and its emotional impact left me wondering how I'd be able to share her story with readers.

After four discussions and no direction, I almost gave up. But then it hit me: Karen was the same as every person I'd talked to so far—she hadn't yet processed or reckoned with the emotional price of her experiences. Emotions had run through her, and she could identify and label them, but she hadn't *dealt* with them. She wasn't intimate with them. Karen was, in many ways, a quintessential example of why I wrote this book. Her story is the story of everyone whose natural tendency is to avoid, suppress, disregard, and neglect the emotions cancer brings.

Strength in Turmoil

Take Your Son or Daughter to Work Day

Karen worked directly for the governor of Florida, in a role created to deal with both complex state transportation safety issues and related social media awareness campaigns. When her office held its annual "take your son or daughter to work" day, Karen brought Bailey, a high school sophomore and the oldest of her three kids. Besides being proud to show off her daughter to so many important people, Karen knew Bailey might one day want to work in government, politics, or maybe law. Karen's goal was to increase Bailey's awareness of the kinds of careers her daughter might take into consideration when she began planning for college. Karen's goal was not to increase Bailey's awareness of life-and-death issues. Nor did she intend for Bailey to be witness to one of the most terrifying moments of her life. But that's what happened.

After a few brief introductions to her coworkers, Karen and Bailey went to Karen's office, took out a legal pad, and drew up a plan of action for the day—subject to adjustment, based on when the governor could find time to meet with them, as he'd promised. When Karen's phone rang, she answered, expecting the governor or one of his assistants.

"This is Karen," she said in her usual bubbly tone.

"It's Dr. Wilcolm's office. The doctor asked that we call you and see if there's any way you can come in today. The biopsy results have come back, and he needs to go over the test results with you."

"I really can't today. I can come later in the week," Karen said before her breathing froze.

"The doctor was hoping you could today," the woman said. "He'll arrange his schedule to accommodate your availability."

Karen's heart dropped. A couple of weeks earlier, she'd found a lump on her left breast. The lump was small, but with her history of thyroid cancer, there was no viable "wait and see" approach. Dr. Wilcolm had performed both a breast and lymph node biopsy. The fact that he wanted to see her right away meant the news couldn't be good. She couldn't show her fear or talk candidly to the doctor's assistant with Bailey sitting just two feet from her, so she took a deep breath and put on an even bigger smile.

"I'd love to come by today. It's just that I have my daughter with me, which makes it rather difficult to scoot out of here. Is it urgent?" She was hoping to get reassurance that her instincts were wrong.

"Rather," the assistant said. "The doctor wants to block a half hour for today."

Karen tried her best to keep the smile going, but Bailey motioned for Karen's attention by directing a questioning look at her. "What is it?" Bailey asked.

Karen asked the doctor's office to wait. "Probably nothing, but I have to meet the doctor, and they say it can't wait," she told her daughter. "I'd need to leave or take you with me. It won't take long." Karen went back to the phone. "Can I come in right now? We have a lot planned for the rest of the day."

Karen made a quick call to the governor's office and found out he wouldn't be free until the afternoon, which helped ease her stress a little. She didn't want Bailey to miss the opportunity to meet her boss.

"I'm sorry, but we won't be long," Karen told Bailey, whose face dropped into seriousness. "Don't worry, it's just routine. I can leave you here if you want—"

"Of course not. I'll come with you," Bailey interrupted.

Karen was certain Bailey could sense her fear. She had to know from hearing the conversation that it wasn't just a routine visit, but Karen couldn't think of any words that were available between a mother and her sixteen-year-old daughter for a you-have-to-come-in-right-away-and-find-out-if-you-have-cancer drive to the doctor's office.

Fortunately, the doctor's office wasn't far, because Karen was uncharacteristically quiet on the drive and probably couldn't have kept her thoughts to herself for very long if Bailey had wanted to talk—she was certain she looked as flushed as she felt.

Karen sensed the uncomfortable tightness in the nurses' body language and *knew* bad news was waiting for her. She knew it in her core. She'd known it since the first tiny little twinge of pain showed up in her breast when she and Bob were making love weeks before. But until the very moment when she and Bailey arrived at the doctor's office and the nurses avoided making eye contact, she hadn't allowed herself to give it any conscious attention.

Bailey put her arm around Karen's waist. "I'll come in with you," she said.

"You sure? It's probably nothing," Karen lied. Her mouth was dry, and it felt as though her voice was suddenly two octaves too high.

The nurse who had come to fetch Karen settled the question. "The doctor would prefer to see you privately," she said.

Bailey nodded and sat down. She grabbed her mother's hand, forcing Karen to turn back toward her, and when she did, Bailey threw a you-got-this look at her.

Why do my kids have to be so damn smart? Karen thought.

The nurse led Karen to the doctor's private office. "Have a seat. The doctor will be right in."

Karen felt like tapping her toes, but her feet wouldn't move. She felt like strumming her fingers on the armrests, but her fingers had turned to cement. She wanted to close her eyes, but her eyelids wouldn't budge. She wanted to scream, but her lungs were being crushed under the weight of a hot-air-balloon-sized bubble of anticipation. A few hour-long minutes crawled by, and the doctor finally came in.

"We've quite a bit to discuss, Karen. I'm glad you came so quickly."

"My daughter is out in the waiting room. I hope this won't take too long."

"I understand. Later, we'll determine our specific course of treatment, which can't be today, anyway," he said briskly. "But we need some time to talk about what's happening. That shouldn't wait."

Karen clenched her teeth, bracing for the specifics.

"I'm sorry to say, the tests came back positive—both biopsies," the doctor said and then paused, awaiting some type of response. But Karen was frozen, and the silence became unbearably shrill. Finally, he continued. "You're probably thinking, *What does that mean?* Well, we have more tests to do, and we'll consult with other specialists, but I'm afraid our options are going to have to include at least surgery, chemotherapy, and radiation. Radical surgery."

"Radical surgery?" Karen asked.

"Yes. The cancer is advanced and has spread to your lymph nodes—fortunately, to only one. But I think there is no other option than to take an aggressive stance against it."

In a flash of reality—brought on by hearing the words that had only been well-suppressed notions—the hot-air balloon exploded, and with it a blast of thoughts burst loose inside Karen's head. Winds of chaos spun around, sucking immediate and random thoughts into the vortex. She fought to find a place calm enough to talk. The sudden commotion in Karen's brain made it just about impossible to say anything coherent, but she managed to force words out of her mouth. "May I have a few minutes alone? Is there a room or a closet where I can go by myself for just a minute?"

"Come with me," the doctor said. He held her elbow as he led her to a small room, perhaps a patient room, or it could have been an emptied closet. He went to turn the light on.

"Please, don't," she said. "Just a minute of quiet."

He closed the door, and she crumbled to the floor, softening her fall so no one would hear her collapse. She shut her eyes against the burning tears that erupted out of her. She held both hands to her mouth to suppress the scream of despair that fought to escape. She felt a hammering inside her chest, and she held her breath in an attempt to slow down the pounding.

Radical surgery . . . aggressive stance . . . radiation. Karen heard the doctor's voice in her head. Then, somewhere deep down, she heard her own. *What am I going to do? My life is over. I'm going to die. I know I'm going to die.*

Five Minutes of a Life

Karen curled herself into a quasi-fetal position on the floor.

Such a short life, she thought. It made her think of her mother's womb, the one she'd shared with her twin brother. She would often joke that she grew up so tough because she had to fight for space from her very first moments. She was a fast runner because she'd raced to be first out. She'd been a baby only a short time ago.

I'm always in such a rush.

She might not have been in such a hurry to enter the world if she'd known that her father had left her mother many months before she and her brother were even a noticeable bump.

He left. Who does such a thing?

It made things so difficult for her mom, caring for two babies on her own, but by the time Karen understood that she had no father—and she might never know who her father was—her mom was in no mood to talk about it. Her mom was a strong, proud woman who had become toughened by her late twenties; she was too overworked and exhausted from struggling as a completely single mom to worry about such things.

There was another way, an opposite approach.

Karen was an innately happy child; and a resilient one. Even through tough times and living in a home absent a lot of extras, she helped care for her brother and let him care for her, and they always seemed to find safe and happy—if not somewhat lonely—places along the pathways of their youth. But as the teenage years approached, the differences in temperaments between her and her mom strained their relationship. She began to lean on other people for comfort and guidance. People like Grandma.

Grandma.

Grandma was such a sweet woman. Mom had moved the family next door to Grandma's. Karen often wondered, if she had not lost her grandma to cancer when she was in college, what kind of impact she would have had on her own daughter. But she had come to learn that being a sweet person doesn't mean you can guide the people around you in any substantial way. As Karen readied to leave for college, she thought fondly of Grandma and Mom, but wanted more than what either had had. Her independence urged her to move on, in search of her education, friendships, and the hope to form her own close family, the kind you see in books, with a mom and a dad and a house full of children. She had so much to see and learn and discover.

Learning . . . college.

Karen entered college armed with a strong sense of independence and self-reliance, but she craved close relationships. She spent less time with her mom and brother by then, she imagined she wasn't going to talk to Grandma much, and nobody she knew in high school was going to her same college. So she searched for anything and anyone that would help her to shape her own identity. During her first months at college, she joined every group she could find. She was strong enough to avoid the people who were after her for the wrong reasons, but she didn't shy away from attention. Her openness helped her make friends quickly. She dated, went to parties, and became academically and socially immersed in college life. She met her first real boyfriend, and she discovered the joys and the fears and the uncertainties of intimacy.

Intimacies . . .

Her mind was sparked with intrigue and a yearning to understand the human condition, so she studied psychology. She left college intent on spending her life exploring people's private emotional experiences, learning and appreciating the depths of people's motivators and limiters, and broadening the understanding of her own life's experiences to gain more insight into her own mind and heart. But she never pursued that passion.

Understanding the heart . . .

When she met Keith, the man she thought she'd live the rest of her life with, she was in the best place she could imagine. She was healthy and happy, she had close friendships, and her self-image was positive. She felt strong, capable, and grateful. She was in the right mental and emotional place to share her life with someone. A brief courtship with Keith led to a proposal and a romantic wedding—life was unfolding the way she'd hoped it would.

She and Keith bought a large home that could be filled with kids. She soon became pregnant with Bailey, then Ashton, and then Grayton. Her kids were all perfect.

But curled up in the closet at the doctor's office, she remembered that life wasn't.

Before Grayton was conceived, she had a short battle with thyroid cancer. Being diagnosed with cancer stopped her perfect life cold, but she had been just twenty-nine, caught the cancer early, and was told she'd have a near 100 percent permanent recovery. She didn't let the cancer hit her emotionally—she was living a full life and was intent on continuing to do so. She had a marriage and two kids. She was a runner and a triathlete. She was active in the community. She had a future to build. She fought through the cancer and quickly recovered.

Fights . . .

Over the years, she and Keith had had minor differences, but they never really fought until she decided that she wanted to go back to work; after all, she had been home for a dozen years raising the kids, and it was time to also think about herself. Soon she saw a darker side of him she'd never seen before. Amid a barrage of insults, accusations, and misdirected anger, she began to fight for the life they had built and for their three kids. But the fights took their toll, especially when it came to her husband, who seemed to have emptied his heart of compassion, love, and decency.

Giving up the fight . . .

Karen had long since stopped working outside the home after Bailey was born. Her lack of income didn't stop her soon-to-be ex-husband, a successful attorney, from taking the house, more than half of their assets, and most of their belongings. She let him win—she didn't want to bring their children into combat. She knew the kids were going to get their fair share of emotional shrapnel regardless of how the assets were divided.

Divorce took a hard toll on her, but faced with no other choice, she had to get up each morning and figure out how to adjust to her new life. She reentered the work force and rebuilt a safe and healthy home for herself and her kids. She shared custody, and although painful, the time away from the kids allowed her to focus on work, to get back in physical shape, and to spend more time with her friends. Over time, she began dating and met Bob. Finding new love helped her regain her optimism and joy in living.

I'm always full of energy. I always want to be happy. I want to live. And I want to keep doing better. I want to continue building stronger relationships with my loved ones and family. I want to reconnect with my college friends, give my kids more guidance, figure out a way to get along with their father, make more of an impact at work, go on more golfing vacations with Bob, run more, do triathlons again, eat better, keep looking young, enjoy my friends more, do more charity work, use my degree to build a practice, help Bailey pick a college, watch my boys grow up and get married, become a grandmother, live a long life, do meaningful things . . .

• • •

As Karen lay on the floor of her doctor's office, a violent storm of memories and emotions overwhelmed her. She felt fear, abandonment, solitude, vulnerability, self-pity, happiness, regret, comfort, jealousy, and despair. She felt guilt, weakness, embarrassment, insecurity, and shame. Then she felt a sudden eerie calmness, then fear of loss and complete disorder. Then she felt love and so much more love: for her kids, for being alive, and for all the happiness in her heart. Then all went quiet, and she breathed softly. She saw herself getting up off the floor, and she felt a tiny spark of hope and then optimism, followed by tinges of fear, then bits of strength, and then the conviction that she wouldn't give in to the fear and that she might be strong enough to stand.

So she did, and she wiped her face and slapped both cheeks and felt just enough like herself to leave that dark, hellish, but enlightening outburst in the closet behind her. She pushed the door open, walked down the hallway, and stopped at the reception desk. "Is the doctor still in his office?" she asked the two nurses.

"Yes, he is. Please go right in."

She was already past them, intent on going into his office. She put her hand on the doorknob, closed her eyes, took a deep breath, and then opened the door. "Thank you," Karen said to the doctor. She reached into her purse and pulled out a legal pad. She took a pen from the doctor's desk. "Okay, I'd like to make a list," she said. "What do we need to figure out? What comes first?"

The doctor pursed his lips, but Karen could sense the smallest hint of a smile on him.

"I understand," he said. "First, let me explain what's going on." He didn't sound condescending or as if he was placating her. She was emotionless as they spoke.

A half hour later, Karen drove Bailey back to the office. Bailey asked what had happened, but Karen wasn't ready to talk. She wanted more information before she spoke to anyone. She'd taken scores of bullet-pointed notes, but she needed to formulate more questions, start doing research, and make a prioritized to-do list before talking to her kids. This cancer treatment was going to be complicated and hellish, and she needed to try to wrap her arms around it quickly; there was going to be lots to do.

"We're going to be okay. We'll figure it all out," she said to Bailey. She gave her a long smile. "Let's get back to the office."

Even if I'm going to die, there's so much to do . . .

Karen's Epilogue

When I first talked to Karen, she'd just undergone a bilateral mastectomy, finished multiple radiation therapy sessions, and was enduring the last few cycles of chemotherapy. About a year into our talks, she underwent comprehensive breast-reconstruction surgery. During that year, Karen shared many personal photos with me and invited me to follow her on various social media sites. There was never a picture of her when she wasn't smiling—whether with her kids or her boyfriend, Bob; whether she was on the beach or in the chemo chair or on a gurney, recovering from surgery.

Throughout our many talks, I realized that her indomitable smile wasn't driven so much by happiness—she was often immersed in emotionally daunting and physically draining events—but by a much deeper feeling. Karen's unwavering smile was fueled by gratitude. Through all the nonstop talking about her outlook on life, and through all the bounding optimism, the positivity, and the high energy, Karen knew she was given the one gift that trumped all the rest: time.

Often while on long rides during difficult patches, I received inspirational notes from people who helped me keep moving forward as I struggled with the sheer physicality and contemplated the greater meanings of the ride, when I struggled to understand the journeys of the book participants and also find answers to my own life's struggles and meanings. On one of those days, Karen texted me a picture of a beautiful Florida sunset. She'd often texted me pictures of sunsets with some comment about how the day's ending came too soon or how she was proud that she hadn't taken for granted that she was given another beautiful day. Karen's sunset picture that day reminded me of a conversation we'd had about how grateful she was to have time.

"When I was deep into treatment, I was afraid to go to sleep," she said. "I was afraid I might not wake up. I wrote in my journals every night. Then I read or lay in bed struggling to keep my eyes open. For months and months during treatment, I tried desperately to stay awake.

"You see, before my breast cancer, I always woke up happy and excited for the day ahead. I had no problem going to sleep because I never stopped moving, and I accomplished so much. I fell asleep knowing that the next day would also be a glorious day. But each time I awoke after cancer, I was overcome with an overwhelming gratitude for having been given the chance to be alive, to have that one more day.

"Cancer shows you how little you control in life—how without time, without another day in front of you, everything is over. You don't fight cancer. You fight to wake up again, to be able to see your kids another day, to check off all the things you can muster the energy to accomplish, to watch the sunset, and to be given a chance to want to sleep so you can do it all again."

Only in Florida

As I pedaled closer to Pensacola, I was awash in emotions. I'd biked to *Florida*. Florida was so far from California, yet the two were tethered so closely in my head. Most of my life had been spent in California. Endless California experiences shaped who I was. But I was born in Miami, and several important, defining experiences of my life also took place in Florida. As I got closer to the state line, I knew that my personal connection between California and Florida was mostly the result of constant struggles with the dysfunctional nature of my family's history. And that aspect of my life, the family I had—or better yet, didn't quite have—had haunted me for as long as I could remember. Rolling into Florida forced me—no, it *offered* me the chance—to find some answers, or so I imagined.

I had spent a month powering myself toward Florida, relentlessly pondering the Cycle of Lives stories—all of which contained at least some elements of relationships between family. Over that time, I replayed immeasurable conversations in my mind that I'd had with the book participants to try to wrap my arms around these people's stories of dealing with the emotions of cancer. I'd spent a great deal of energy thinking about how most had tried to reconcile the emotions, *especially in relation to family dynamics*, that affected their life's journeys, and yet, when it came to ponderances about my own family, I was left shaking my head at the missing pieces that made it so my past and my emotions about family could not be reconciled.

June and I had been brought into the world by parents who were thirty-eight years in age apart from each other. They must have had much to hide, because they didn't talk about—or allow us to ask about—the crazy circumstances that must have brought them together. The rules of the house didn't allow for inquiry. I'd collect a crumb here and there—my mother's father was an abusive alcoholic, and her mother had allowed the abuse to continue until my mother ran away to Florida as a teen; my father's parents had been born in Russia and had fled the Bolshevik Revolution as children only to meet as teens in New York, marry, and raise seven children. I'd overheard that my father had been a doctor in World War II and a surgeon after, and at other times he'd been an inventor, a world-traveling professional gambler, a writer, and an entrepreneur. It was as if I were part of a five-hundred-piece puzzle with the edges and almost all the inside pieces missing. I was left staring at the many glimpses of my life that had no connection to one another.

I knew I was born in Miami. I met an uncle once in my teens who mentioned I had family in southern and central Florida. But my parents never took us back to Florida to visit my aunts and uncles—apparently, those relatives had distanced themselves from my dad after he married such a young woman—nor to see my mother's mother, who'd moved to Florida herself after her husband died. My mother and grandmother rarely spoke because of the trauma of my mom's childhood, or so I heard from my mom's sister, who was in and out of our lives during my youth.

As an adult, I have gone to Florida dozens of times, for both work and pleasure, but it was a bit hollow when I went because none of the trips offered me a chance to learn about my past or family. Each time I went to Florida, I felt as if there was more business to be done than just that which was aligned with the trip at hand, and each time I left Florida, it felt as if I'd somehow left unfinished personal business behind—even though there wasn't anything I could have done because I had no connection to the family I yearned to connect with.

In my midforties, while on yet another of my countless trips to Florida, I went for a run in the West Palm Beach neighborhood, where my mother taught school. I found out she'd moved permanently to Florida at some point, and I toyed with the idea of confronting her for having treated my sister so poorly during her cancer ordeals and for abandoning me for basically my entire adult life. But I decided it would be an exercise in futility; she wasn't about to turn into a real mother just because I was prepared to have her face me.

As I stopped to take a selfie at the "Welcome to Florida" sign, I was flooded with emotions. Florida had left so many marks on either end of my emotional spectrum. I was going to bike eight-hundred-plus miles into, down, across, and up the state, hitting many of the places that had become so familiar to me, visiting with book participants and a few of my closest friends who were spread out over a half-dozen different cities. I'd even be biking within a stone's throw of my mother.

I sometimes regret the past I never had and long for a present that can never be. But, even so, I'd always hoped for a future that might include some way to make up for some of what I'd missed because of my broken family. When June died, I knew that would never happen. I also knew that the future would have to start with my mom, and as excited as I was to bike through a state that had so much meaning for me, I knew I'd pass right through her town without even slowing down.

In truth, I was always mad at my dad for being old and dying so early in my life, and angry at my mom for living her life as though she never had me. As much as it pained me to admit it, I was mad at June for dying and leaving me without the one person who understood the loneliness that defined knowing you were the child of two people who shouldn't have had kids.

Of course, how and when June died was a horrific and tragic thing for her family, and as much as I wanted to dwell on my own loss and isolation, my pain would never overshadow the loss and isolation that her death caused for her husband and kids and close friends. So many people have things so much worse than me. I'm at peace not being a martyr in that way; I really am a very fortunate person in many, many ways, and I really have very little to complain about. But there's no denying that I sometimes feel unfairly abandoned and left to try to not drown in the dark truth that my past is often not a comforting place to visit.

I had finished day twenty-seven in Pensacola, less than twenty miles into Florida. Erin was set to head back to California for about a week. As I lay in yet another hotel bed that night closing the day's chapter with pointed thoughts, it felt oddly apropos that I was about to bike through most of Florida mostly alone. Sure, I'd be visiting two book participants, Moffitt Cancer Center, and several friends, but I'd be by myself for much of the one thousand miles I'd be biking in Florida. Even if you're not lonely in life, the road to the future can sometimes take you on lonely stretches through the past. I fell asleep still imagining that the roads ahead might somehow show me some long-sought-for answers.

I woke to a full-blown, horrible cold on day twenty-eight. In addition to the accumulated overall fatigue and super sore legs, I was stuffed up, felt lethargic, had a sore throat, and was lightheaded—basically, in perfect condition for a 114-mile day. I got moving quickly so I could start the day early. I was looking forward to riding along the beautiful Emerald Coast and through my favorite area of Florida—the Destin, Sandestin, and Panama City area—before finishing in Callaway. Erin had to leave early too, as she'd offered to fly out of Tampa, some five hundred miles away, so she could leave the truck where I'd have access to it halfway through my Florida route.

My friend Dave met up with me around Destin and rode with me for about the middle third of my ride—quite a feat since he hadn't ridden a bike in years.

As I rode into Panama City Beach—along the same stretch of highway I'd ridden on during the first Ironman triathlon I'd completed more than a decade earlier—I was reminded of how small the world is and also how quickly time passes while on it. The smells and lights and *feel* of the road were the same for me more than ten years later. It was hard to imagine that so much time had passed in a snap and so many life experiences had occurred, and yet it was as if I had blinked once and a dozen years went away. It sunk in how much of my life had been spent without the constant of *family* being there as I quickly blinked through life. Some places remained the same, some experiences repeated themselves; life was somewhat circular. But the center, the essence of me and the people I'd touched, was linear. Aside from my kids and the life I'd just embarked on with Erin, there was no collection of repetitive touch points to my past; there was no hub attached to the wheel.

I awoke feeling less sick the following day. Good thing, too: Day twenty-nine was going to be a bruiser—146 miles from Callaway to Perry. After doing a 6:00 a.m. interview for a local news station interested in my cross-country adventure, I took off. My friend Dave had convinced his wife he should accompany me for a day or two so he could offer support, and a few hours into the ride, I was happy to take a break (alongside a friend instead of alone, for a change) from the constant rumble of logging trucks lumbering a precious few feet away from me as they raced to move felled trees from forest to mill. When you're biking 146 miles on spent legs, you need things to go right, and the break was a needed one to plan the day out with Dave so we could make it through what was going to be one of my longest days with as few snags as possible.

I had planned to meet Karen near mile one hundred. She was going to drive an hour south from her home in Tallahassee to meet me for dinner. We both broke down in tears as we hugged, meeting in person for the first time after spending so many hours together on the phone. After a long dinner filled with laughter, crying, and endless talking about her kids, about Bob, and about all things cancer and otherwise, I got back on my bike and continued on my route. I still had fifty miles to go, and it was approaching eight o'clock.

East of Tallahassee—like, two hundred miles east—is Jacksonville. In between those two cities is a whole lot of nothing. But south of Tallahassee, where I was heading, toward Tampa, which is 250 miles away, makes nothing look like a lot. There's *nothing* but forest, swamp, and endless, desolate highways spotted with the very occasional burg, whose population can be counted without needing more than fingers and toes, at most, to keep count.

There was no moon that night. It was perfectly warm and comfortable. The roads were among the quietest I'd encountered; a car came about every twenty minutes. Dave had ridden up ahead to take a nap. I settled into a smooth, almost meditative zone, pedaling down the center lane, listening to music, staring up at the magnificent and brightly starred sky, hearing the occasional wild cry of an animal who was hunting—or was being hunted—in the forests surrounding me. I felt wonderfully alone and at peace with my surroundings. The dense trees to either side of me made it feel as though I were biking down a surreal outdoor hallway, the ground dark, the walls dark, the roof lit with a magical chandelier of stars.

I moved down the endless hallway, but my mind was stuck on that mental treadmill, still contemplating the dilemma of family. I went from book participant to book participant as my thoughts rolled around, replaying conversations, trying to piece together themes and various dynamics, and hoping to find some parallels, some clarity, some answers. I turned off my bike's headlamp and my safety lights. After a few minutes, my eyes acclimated even more to the celestial chandelier, and I gazed up in amazement, my legs continuing to power me down the dark hallway, the still, slightly damp, warm air filling my lungs, my breath steady and calming. The meditation took me deeper within myself, but there were no answers; there was no clarity.

An hour later, through the ethereal silence, an inner voice started to whisper, as if a singular distant point of light from the stars above had awakened something. The voice told me, as though it were the clearest of messages told, to stop trying to reconcile that aspect of my life, to stop focusing on the regrets of a past that I had no control over back when they were the present. My wounds would never go away, it said; they could either heal (and that clearly hadn't happened) or they could scar over if I'd let them. And my brain filled with the thought around one word: Everybody has wounds, *everybody*. The Cycle of Lives hadn't taught me anything if it hadn't taught me that *everybody* is dealing with—or has dealt with—some type of real trauma.

"Everybody," I said aloud.

I was on a quest to offer help on how people can deal with emotions around trauma, and I was acting as if I hadn't learned a thing. *But I had.* I had learned so much from the people I spoke to. I'd learned how they were able to move on, how they processed regrets in their lives, how they navigated their own lonely stretches. Suddenly, my mindset shifted from wanting to unravel the jumbled mess of self-centered nonsense around my own issues of loneliness, regret, and bitterness over a lost family. I began to think of all the other people whom I might help do some of their own unwinding by showing how many of these remarkable, often brave, fifteen book participants had dealt with their own issues around family.

Flashes of the scores of people whom I'd met along my journey who commented about what they or a loved one or a friend was going through played in my mind. I thought about their declarations of not being equipped to deal with their emotions, of not knowing how to communicate well, and of not knowing how to deal with the traumas they'd encountered. I suddenly became overwhelmed with a sense of purpose and pride, even satisfaction. I just *knew* that when the book came together, it would be able to help people. It could, literally, help *everybody*. The next hours went by in what seemed like minutes. I felt lighter, less tired, *freer*.

Then my phone rang. My phone was attached to a mount on my handlebars so I could access it and view the GPS, routes, and so on, and the caller's name popped up brightly on the screen: Unknown. It was either a junk call or my friend Jerry—he's my only friend who blocks his number. The light from the screen and the noise of the ringer snapped me out of my sereneness, and I pressed "answer."

"Hey, brother," he said.

"Jerry. What's up, my man?"

"What you doing?"

"I'm biking. What else?"

"Where you at?"

"The middle of Nowhere, Florida. I mean *nowhere*. Like I'm in *The Twilight Zone*."

"You got a minute?" he asked.

"I got at least another hour."

"I know it's late—oh, wait, it's almost midnight there. You're still biking? What the hell?"

"Tell me about it. Long day. I'm getting close, though."

"I just left dinner with my dad and sister, and I just had to call you," he said. "You should have been there, doctor." He liked to call me "doctor" because of my initials: DR.

"Yeah, why's that?"

"I never would have thought it. They *talked*—about things they never talked about."

"Their cancers?" I asked.

"Yup. I sat there soaking it in. I mean, they talk, but they'd never *talked*. You know? About what was inside because of what they went through. They just aren't like that. You saw at the brunch. But I think your talk, meeting you . . . I don't know. It did something to them."

"That's amazing. How did it go?"

"They laughed. They cried. They just went at it. I didn't get a word in. I didn't need to. I can't thank you enough, doctor."

My eyes started to fill with tears. I coasted to a stop, right in the middle of the highway. I felt the blood flow throughout my body, my heart pump with emotion. I feasted my blurring eyes on the magnificence of the brilliant stars filling the sky, and it softened the thousands of dots above. "JP, you have no idea what's been going through my head the last couple of hours. It's unreal that you just called me right now with that." I didn't know if he could sense my emotions or not, but I was close to sobbing. There was a long pause.

"You still there, brother?" he asked.

"Yeah, I'm still here. And I've got a pretty unbelievable story for you, too, but now's not the time to talk about it."

We said our goodbyes and hung up, and I continued to pedal—more like float—down that magical stretch of highway. By the time I reached Perry, it was near one o'clock in the morning. I'd put in more than seventeen hours, and by the end, I was deliriously tired. I passed out hard and fast that night, as spent as I could've ever imagined possible, and yet before my eyes closed, I felt as though I'd accomplished something much more than a long day of biking.

Six hours later, I began day thirty, a 114-mile trek from Perry to Crystal River. Dave stayed on to support me, which allowed me to continue without carrying my supplies. It was hot, and we made a half-dozen stops so I could rest and rehydrate. My body was carrying the accumulated weight of a month's worth of extreme physical effort and needed more frequent rest breaks. But— aside from my devastated, aching body—I felt oddly refreshed inside, the result of the previous night's revelations. I knew I couldn't completely stop my mind from working on the personal issues I'd set out to better understand, but I decided to let go of the weight of my own problems and emotional baggage over family so I could continue to more freely contemplate and attempt to understand the book participants' problems and emotional baggage.

Joshua had been on my mind all day. He was going to bike the next day and a half with me and was currently driving up with his wife to meet us for dinner in Crystal River. Parts of his cancer story were exceptionally gut-wrenching, but they were overshadowed by other traumas he'd endured—many revolving around family.

Joshua

Relationship to cancer: Survivor, advocate, professional, secondary caregiver

Age: Thirty-seven

Family status: Married

Location: Tampa, Florida

First encounter with cancer: Twenty-seven years old

Cancer summary: At twenty-seven, Joshua was diagnosed with a severe sarcoma in his abdomen. He endured a newly developed full protocol of aggressive, long-term treatment, including six surgeries, more than two dozen radiation therapy sessions, and more than 1,100 hours of treatment during twenty-seven cycles of chemotherapy. He is now more than five years cancer-free. Joshua also helped care for his mother-in-law, who died of brain cancer.

Cancer specifics: Ewing soft-cell sarcoma, nonmetastatic

Community involvement: Volunteered at Moffitt Cancer Center, where he received his treatments. He currently works for Moffitt as a financial analyst and continues to volunteer in patient advocacy, community outreach, and fundraising areas.

Strongest positive emotion during cancer experience: Hopefulness

Strongest negative emotion during cancer experience: Loneliness

How we met: Joshua was referred to me early in my search by someone affiliated with Moffitt Cancer Center. I wanted to address issues such as fertility and mortality from the perspective of a young adult man. From what I'd read about Joshua online, his story of overcoming cancer—and how doing so profoundly shaped the direction of his life—was intriguing. I was eager to talk to him and learn more.

We began a conversation, and I found Joshua to be soft-spoken, thoughtful, and open. We spoke about his cancer experience, but when we began to explore his childhood, things turned very dark, very quickly. I came to find out that the emotional undercurrents of his cancer journey had been shaped by much more moving and consequential events in his life than merely those surrounding his illness. My natural inclination was to avoid getting too personal, because I could sense his pain and the extremely personal nature of the things he talked about. But Joshua was always willing to push forward into areas he hadn't touched on before. As a result, over the course of our conversations, we developed a deep trust that allowed Joshua to feel comfortable and safe while he shared one somber experience after another. Most times—even when discussing the most desolate subjects—Joshua did so with an unhesitant willingness to expose himself. His story was equal parts disquieting and captivating, and as one incredible ordeal after another was brought to light, the tragic narrative of his life unfolded.

I met Joshua in person for the first time about six months into our talks. If I hadn't come to know what a positive, uplifting person he was, I might have dreaded the heaviness of meeting someone who'd gone through so much. Instead, upon meeting we embraced each other.

Machismo

··

T he concept of memories is far beyond the grasp of a seven-year-old. A seven-year-old doesn't have the cognitive awareness or the developed reasoning to sit down and contemplate a string of memories that lead from some point in the past to the present day in the hopes of gaining insight into what led to the present circumstances. A seven-year-old doesn't know how to identify memories that might have foretold that something could have had a chance to take place. A seven-year-old simply understands that something *has* happened. They don't know *why* something happened. And no way, ever, in a million years of thinking about that something would a seven-year-old have the first clue as to how to make sense of any of it.

• • •

When he was five, Joshua spent a lot of time alone in his room because sometimes his mom would be mean to him or fight with his dad for a long time, and if he stayed in his room, then he could pretend those things weren't happening. When his mom was mean, Joshua cried. She got madder when he cried, and she told him to stop making her feel bad. But he couldn't help it. He tried not to cry, but he couldn't help it. His mom was mean a lot of the time and she yelled at his dad a lot, too. So he stayed in his room most of the time—especially if his dad wasn't home. Sometimes, he even played in the closet so his mom's yelling wasn't so loud.

His mom stopped yelling when her belly got big with a little brother inside. Joshua's dad said to her that the baby didn't like to hear yelling because it hurt his little ears, and then his mom told him and his dad how sorry she was. Then she just stopped yelling one day.

After his mom and baby brother came home from the hospital, it was the best time ever. Baby Johnnie was named after his dad and made Mom smile all the time. She talked so soft to the baby, and she would hold Johnnie in one arm and rub Joshua's hair with her other hand as they lay in the bed next to her. Joshua thought the baby was the best thing ever because his dad worked less after Baby Johnnie came home and his mom was happy a lot of the time.

Sometimes, his mom said stuff Joshua didn't understand about families, how hard life was, how nobody understood about all the things she did, and how she was always trying to make everyone happy. He especially didn't understand much when she talked in Spanish. He didn't understand why it was okay for *her* to cry but not for anybody else to cry. His dad would tell him that sometimes mommies cry because they feel so much love.

But babies cry a different way than everybody else. Joshua only cried when Mom was mean, but the baby cried whenever something was wrong with him, when he was hungry or tired or for no reason anybody knew at all. And Johnnie cried a lot in the day, even more when it was nighttime. His mom didn't like the baby's crying at all; it made her madder even than when Joshua cried. Even when he went into his closet, he could hear Mom screaming about how Johnnie needed to stop with all the crying.

Joshua was seven and had just started second grade when Johnnie had his first birthday. His mom had been in bed for so long, but she came out and made a special cake with syrup and sugar. She said it tasted like home. They sat at the kitchen table and laughed and acted silly, and his mom taught Joshua some words in Spanish. But after that, his mom stayed in bed all the time—she was too tired to do anything. Joshua didn't like that his mom was tired so much, that she didn't want to look pretty anymore, and that she didn't talk to anyone. But she didn't yell hardly at all anymore. She was too tired to even do that.

During the week, his dad took Joshua to school on his way to work and picked him up from after-school care. His dad and mom argued about him going to work some days, and when they did, his dad usually stayed home and took care of Johnnie, and his mom usually went back to bed. He knew his dad liked to take care of things because he would listen to his dad try to tell his mom everything would be okay, that he would take care of her and Baby Johnnie and Joshua, and that she shouldn't worry so much about everything.

One day, his dad dropped him off at home after school and then went back to work. Joshua was always careful to be quiet because he didn't want to wake Johnnie up if he was napping—or worse, wake both Johnnie and his mom up if they were both asleep. But the house was quiet when he went inside. Very quiet. They had to both be asleep. He went to his room and turned on the television. After a while, he heard Johnnie crying in his crib. His mom had to hear the baby, but he didn't hear her go to quiet him down.

He listened and waited. And waited. When Johnnie didn't stop crying, he left his room and went upstairs to find Mom. He went first to his brother's room. Johnnie was sitting up on his knees and holding the bars of the crib. His face was red, and he whimpered when he saw Joshua, but he stopped crying. Joshua grabbed the binkie that had fallen on the floor and put it back in Johnnie's mouth. Joshua went to go see about his mom. He tiptoed toward her bedroom. The door was open a crack, and when he pushed it open more, he saw that the bed was empty. A few times, he'd crept upstairs and peeked in to see his mom asleep, but he'd never seen the bed empty and made. He went inside.

Maybe she was in the bathroom showering and hadn't heard Johnnie. But there was no sound coming out of the bathroom. He put his ear to the closed door, but he couldn't hear anything. Joshua reached for the handle. It scared him so much to think about turning the door handle, but he didn't know where his mom was. She probably wasn't in there, and boy, would she be mad if she caught him, but he had to check. He bent down and saw no light coming from under the door. He turned the knob and pushed the door open a little. Nothing. He looked over his shoulder, scared his mom would come up behind him, but nothing happened. Then he opened the door all the way, and he stood there, frozen, unable to understand what he saw.

Joshua couldn't hear himself breathing heavily because his ears went quiet. He couldn't feel his heart pounding in his head because the only thing that worked were his eyes, and they were frozen. All he could see was one arm bent over the edge of the bathtub. He couldn't move or look away. He knew it was his mom's arm, but he couldn't see her because she was under the water, and the water was red and dark. But her arm was white, like a ghost, as if someone had painted on it. There was a long red line, a cut going from her wrist to halfway up her arm. Joshua pulled himself away to look down. He saw a thick red mess under the one shoe where he'd stepped on the rug of the bathroom. He pressed down, and the bloody goo squeezed up higher around his shoe. He looked at his mom's arm, at the dark water hiding her head and body, and then back down at his shoe.

He backed out of the bathroom and closed the door. He walked to the doorway of the bedroom, then stopped to look back. He could see four red steps made by his wet shoe. He didn't know if he'd be in trouble for that. Then he went into Johnnie's room and patted his brother's tiny, warm, soft head as he lay there, eyes open, sucking softly on his binkie. A while later, he heard Dad's car coming into the garage. He shivered, his face got warm, and tears rolled down his cheeks. He put his finger over his mouth to show Johnnie to be quiet, then he went out and sat on the top stair and waited for his dad to come up.

• • •

One morning, a few weeks after his mom's funeral, the doorbell rang. Joshua jumped. He looked at his dad, who was feeding Johnnie warm cereal. His dad motioned with his head, and Joshua got up and went to the front door. He pulled down on the handle, and the cold air came in. A man was standing there. The man was not very tall. He wore a big jacket, but he didn't have gloves on, even though it was super cold out. The man smiled at him.

"Hi," he said to the man.

The man continued to look at Joshua and continued to smile. The cold was making the man's eyes water.

"Who's there?" Joshua heard Dad say.

"You are Joshua," the man said. Joshua didn't know if it was a question or if the man was telling him.

"Yes," Joshua said.

Joshua's dad came up behind him with Baby Johnnie in one arm, and he put a hand on Joshua's head. "Can we help you?" Joshua's dad asked the man.

"Can I come in and talk about . . . well, do you know who am I?" the man asked.

Nobody said anything for a second. Joshua looked up at his dad. He didn't like the look on his dad's face. He walked behind his dad and wrapped his arm around Dad's leg.

"I am the father," the man said. "I am Roberto, Joshua's daddy."

• • •

That was the beginning of a long custody fight between Joshua's stepdad, John, in Minnesota, and his biological dad, Roberto, in Puerto Rico. People came to talk to John: lawyers, people from the government, and family.

Joshua's mother had died right before Thanksgiving, and around Easter, Joshua's dad drove him to the airport so he could fly to Puerto Rico and meet his other family. Joshua didn't want to go; he was scared that they wouldn't let him come back. His dad had talked to him many times about the fact that he *had* to go—they had no choice about it. Joshua cried a lot, but when the day came for him to leave, he was more nervous than afraid.

The court mandated Joshua go for just a one-week visit during custody proceedings, but at seven, a week could have meant a lifetime.

In Puerto Rico, the man he met a few months before, Roberto, on that cold day just weeks after his mom had died, waited for him to come off the plane and then drove him to what he said was Joshua's grandmother's house. When they pulled up, Joshua saw the driveway was filled with four-feet-tall white chalk letters. "Welcome Home, Joshua," it read.

Joshua and the man walked toward the letters, and Joshua wanted to mess up the second word. He looked down at his shoe—it was a different pair of shoes because the one with the blood on them had been thrown away—and decided it wouldn't be very nice to kick the chalk letters, so instead, he stepped around them.

Inside, there were a lot of people—four adults, two of them older, who had to be the grandmother and maybe her sister, and at least five or six kids of different ages. They all stared and smiled at him. It made him feel very embarrassed.

There was an awkward silence, and then all the adults started talking at once, half of them in Spanish and half in English. Joshua remembered a few Spanish words his mom had taught him. "No hablo Español," he said.

Everybody laughed, and the lady who he soon found out was his grandmother squeezed him tight with both arms wrapped around him. "Pobrecito, no, no hablas Español," she said in a sweet voice. "Is fine. You only needing speak English. Aye, pobrecito. Ven." She grabbed his hand and led him to the kitchen. There was a cake—like the cake his mom had made for his baby brother's birthday—and soon everybody was eating and laughing and talking.

Even though it felt strange to be around so many people he didn't know, by that night, Joshua was less nervous and scared than he'd felt before coming to Puerto Rico. This "new family" was happy and warm and kind, and they seemed to care about him without even knowing him.

Waves of Pain

After an eighteen-month battle, John was forced to relinquish custody of Joshua to Roberto. It was incredibly difficult for Joshua to leave Minnesota and what he'd always known as his *real* family and move to Puerto Rico, but that's what the court ordered. Just after he turned nine, Joshua hugged his dad and Johnnie fiercely at the airport, the tears gushing from his eyes. Getting on that plane was harder than anything ever, even everything that had happened to him with his mother.

Within a few years, the pain of being separated from all he'd known had all but disappeared, and only good memories of the family he was forced to leave behind remained for Joshua. During those years, Joshua assimilated

into life with his father, his grandmother, and all the other Puerto Rico relatives. He learned about his heritage, came to know extended family members,
and learned about how his grandfather, a famous architect, had developed
many prominent landmark areas throughout Puerto Rico. He went to school,
learned Spanish, made friends, and grew up as normally as anyone would
expect, considering the very unusual circumstances that led him to Puerto
Rico. In just a few short years, he *was* Puerto Rican.

The family didn't often discuss Joshua's mother, and when they did, the
conversation never lingered there. None of his friends asked about his mother
because they hadn't known her, and there was never any cause for anybody to
ask. As a result, Joshua never talked about what he'd been through—there was
never the opportunity. Instead, he lived with his own thoughts about what had
happened. On dark, quiet nights, when his mind replayed his worst memories,
he tried to understand the torment and heartache that lay deep within him.
He never vocalized his feelings or dealt with how painful and confusing the
visions of her in the bathtub were to him. He never came to grips with his
mother's suicide—if such a thing were even possible—because the only place
he ever acknowledged it was in his mind.

Joshua kept in touch with his Minnesota family, and Johnnie even came
to Puerto Rico for a visit once, but his stepdad wasn't comfortable with the
idea of visiting, and Joshua didn't fly back to the mainland until after he'd
graduated from high school, when his family considered him a man and able
to make decisions independent of their input. The Puerto Rican family had
become Joshua's own family, but the pain of the custody battle made it so the
two families refused to interact, no matter how much time went by or how
much it would have benefitted Joshua.

After high school, Joshua was accepted at Ohio State University in
Columbus. He'd formed such strong relationships in Puerto Rico that he was
torn about leaving. But he was excited to pursue an education at a respected
Stateside school. His first stop on his way to Ohio was Tampa, Florida, where
his Minnesota dad and Johnnie had moved.

Joshua hadn't seen his dad in ten years, and it'd been six years since he'd
last seen Johnnie. But in no time, they felt like family to Joshua again. It took
all of about one minute, after a strong, familiar hug in the airport, for Joshua

and his dad and his half brother to be comfortable in each other's presence. Joshua was grateful his dad didn't dwell on anything negative—not on time lost, the pain of being apart, Joshua's mother, or any of it. Joshua left Tampa secure in knowing that this dad was his dad and this brother was his brother, and he knew those things would never diminish his feelings about his family in Puerto Rico.

By the time he was twenty-six, Joshua's life was on track: He had a challenging job as an analyst at a major national bank, he was saving money, he had a girlfriend, and he was surfing, spending time with his Florida family, and visiting his Puerto Rican family several times a year. Life was good, almost perfect. He did have nightmares occasionally, and although he knew deep down that he always kept a part of himself hidden from the world—because he could only trust himself with the deep dark secrets in his heart—life was full and fulfilling.

Pain? No Big Deal

One day while surfing, Joshua pulled a muscle getting on his board, right in the wrong place—between his legs, deep in his groin. It hurt like hell, but he was intent on finishing his set. Within a couple of days, the pain was mostly gone. He didn't surf for a few days, and although the pain hadn't completely gone away, he was able to work around it. If he moved a certain way, or didn't move a certain way, the pain was simply a dull ache—but every once in a while, he experienced shooting pains from deep inside.

Over the next several weeks, Joshua became aware of other issues. He sometimes woke up in a sweat with a painful urge to pee, but then he'd stand over the toilet and nothing would happen. If he did begin to urinate, it would hurt like hell, and only a tiny amount would dribble out. Other times, he'd pee and then have to go pee again fifteen minutes later. Joshua wasn't worried—he was young, he was active, things happen. Perhaps he had an infection.

For weeks, Joshua got more used to the pain he felt while urinating. The pain made him sweat a lot, and he was almost ready to go to the doctor, but he got skittish when one day he peed and his urine came out with a faint red color. Joshua didn't think infections caused bleeding. Maybe he ripped something inside when surfing weeks before. No way he was going to talk to anybody about peeing blood.

As soon as he was about to give in and see his doctor, the pain from urinating diminished a little. Relief from problems urinating, which had carried over into his sex life, was overwhelmingly comforting, but as soon as his issues urinating and becoming sexually aroused seemed over, Joshua started having major constipation and painful cramps in his stomach. Some days, the cramps were so severe that he skipped out of work early, drove home, and lay down on the floor. On those days, he didn't even have the energy to make it to his bed.

Joshua knew that something more serious was going on, but he couldn't just go to the doctor and say, "Hey, Doc, it hurts like hell to pee, and I can't seem to take a crap, and my stomach hurts so much I can't stand up. Oh, and I can't get it up a lot of the time, too." Healthy twenty-six-year-old men didn't have those problems. He decided to skip the doctor and just fight through it.

After a few more weeks, things had gotten so bad that he told his girl-friend to cancel his birthday plans and apologize to their friends. He said she should go home, and he'd call her when he felt better. She pressed him to find out more, but Joshua hadn't let her in on what was going on with him, and he wasn't about to go crawling for help.

"I just need a couple of days to sleep this thing off once and for all," he told her.

He slept for almost thirty hours. When he woke, he was dizzy, weak, and doubled over with pain, and his stomach was so distended he looked as if he were six months pregnant.

Screw it, Joshua thought. *I don't care if someone sticks a catheter in my cock, gives me an enema, or slices me open and takes out a baby. This freaking pain is too much.*

He drove himself to the emergency room.

It's a Big Deal

When he got the news, he thought about not calling anyone.

How do you call your dad, your other dad, your girlfriend, or your boss and let them know you've got cancer?

But he knew he couldn't wait too long to say something. It wouldn't get any easier. So he called his Florida dad first.

"Stage III, T2b, G3, M0, soft-cell Ewing's sarcoma, the size of a grapefruit, in my lower abdomen," Joshua said. "Or some shit like that. Basically, I'm fucked."

The emergency room doctor had determined that Joshua had a mass in his lower abdomen and then called in one doctor to do a CT scan and another to do an incisional biopsy to determine if the mass was cancerous.

"I don't know what to do, but I have to find an oncologist. Hell, I've got to find a regular doctor. And a blood doctor—a hematologist—and who knows what else."

"I'll be right over," his dad said.

"No, I'm in the hospital. They're going to send me home today. They said after I see an oncologist and a surgical oncologist, they're probably going to schedule a surgery pretty quick."

"Well, I'll come and take you home, then. We can figure it out together."

"No, it's okay. My car's here. I'll come by after I'm done."

That's the way it was with Joshua: He wasn't going to become a burden all of a sudden. He could take care of himself.

The next several days went by like a Florida hurricane: fast, furious, and with no way to assess the damage until the storm had passed. By chance, Joshua's dad knew of someone who knew a prominent oncologist in town. That oncologist was aligned with Moffitt Cancer Center, the leading cancer center in Florida—which happened to be right there in Tampa. Joshua underwent blood tests, several X-rays, another CT scan, a PET scan, a review of the biopsy, and more. His oncologist discussed the results with a few specialists, along with a team of doctors at the center.

The treatment plan would begin at once. First, a surgical oncologist would remove the tumor. Normally, they'd try to shrink the tumor with chemotherapy, but the doctors decided surgery couldn't wait. The cancer hadn't metastasized, but time was not on their side. Then Joshua would undergo area-specific radiation treatment around the margins, depending on how the surgery went. Next, he'd begin a chemotherapy regimen, which might include more advanced targeted therapy as an adjuvant to the intended treatment, again, depending on how things were going.

Joshua was too stunned and overwhelmed and unsure about most of what they were talking about to have any immediate questions. But as each piece of information the doctors gave him painted a little clearer picture of what was going to take place, he was able to ask a few questions about his prognosis and what to expect along the way.

"Fortunately—if that can ever be used when talking about a cancer as serious as yours—you couldn't be cared for at a better time or place than right now and here," the oncologist at Moffitt said. "We are developing some very advanced protocols, and we'll give you the best opportunity to maximize the efficacy of treatment every step of the way."

The doctors said it was difficult to know Joshua's chances of survival, let alone know exactly how his treatment would unfold. They only thing they knew with certainty was that they wanted to do surgery right away to remove the tumor, then follow up with radiation treatment and determine the proper chemotherapy protocol. The other "fortunate" thing about Joshua's cancer was that his case would be presented to a board at Moffitt. That meant he'd benefit from the best collaborative efforts available.

Joshua explained everything as best he could to his dad, then with a little less focus on the details to his biological father, and then in even less detail to his girlfriend and the few friends he called. Although emotions churned inside of him while talking to the few people he disclosed his situation to, not only had Joshua not processed his emotions enough to discuss any bit of what he was feeling, but he was not about to allow anybody to get too deep a look inside. He suppressed the darker feelings and thoughts, stuffing them down into the place where he kept the memories and feelings about the traumatic experiences of his childhood.

Surgery was scheduled a week after his initial diagnosis. Joshua took two weeks of PTO from work—he wasn't about to go on any kind of medical leave. He prepaid some bills, arranged for a buddy to check on his place while he "headed to a place where he'd be incommunicado for one week or more," and called his family in Puerto Rico to assure them he was going to be fine.

Uncharacteristically, Joshua asked his girlfriend to stay with him at the hospital. He hadn't told her any of the specifics. He didn't want her to be anxious and afraid for him—besides, there was a deeper truth: Too much talk might've led him down a path of emotional exploration, and he didn't want to tell her how scared, confused, angry, and ashamed he felt.

Joshua was admitted in the morning for presurgery preparations. He hadn't expected so much talk. The hospital staff was forever repeating the course of treatment, explaining the surgery, and requesting confirmation that he understood what was going on. Doctors and nurses kept stopping by with instructions, warnings, and requests for consent. He could see it was affecting his girlfriend—so much so that he started to become more worried about her than himself.

"I can see it on your face," he said to her after about the tenth person had come in to work on his body—or more often the case, his mind—with their constant requests that he understood the dangers of the procedure. "I know this sounds bad, but they're just being cautious. Probably afraid of being sued or something."

There was a long pause. Joshua watched and waited for her to respond. She clearly wanted to say something but was struggling. She looked down at her lap, unwilling to look up. Her lips pursed as though she were holding back whatever was trying to come out.

A dozen thoughts raced through Joshua's mind, most of them varying guesses at what might be running through hers. Finally, she broke the silence.

"I know you can see it. You see, I can't hide things. Not like you, Joshua."

He couldn't deny that.

"This." She pointed at the IV drip in his arm. "It's not me. I mean, this is not *my* life. I can't do this." Before he could talk, she stood, shook her head, and stared at him with distant eyes.

"This is not me."

She turned, opened the curtain surrounding his bed, and walked out.

Waking Up to a Nightmare

Joshua sensed people talking, and he felt movement, but he couldn't place any of the voices or grasp the twisted, broken language they spoke or remember where he might be. He felt as if he was hovering above the ground, wrapped up tightly, being pushed from place to place. He wanted to open his eyes, but he couldn't. He could sense the brightness around him—so bright that he might be blinded if he dared peek. Talking was impossible, his mouth was open, but his tongue was paralyzed, and his vocal cords felt cemented over. All Joshua could do was listen. Slowly, the voices became clearer, the words became more intelligible, and the heavy cloudiness in his mind turned into a light mist. Thoughts came to him, interrupted by five seconds or maybe five hours of blackness. It was hard for Joshua to grasp any sense of time.

"Pressure . . . Doctor's coming . . . Fourteen cc's . . . Over 92 . . . Joshua? Do you know where . . . Liquids for . . . t depends . . . The lab results . . . I think he is, yes . . . Joshua? How are you? Can you tell me your name?"

It took another minute, or another ten hours, but the mist lifted, Joshua's eyes opened, and he gained a little control over his senses. As things became clearer, he felt a dull, heavy, achy feeling in his lower abdomen.

"Surgery," Joshua said, answering some real or imagined question.

"Yes, you were. You're fine now. The surgery is over, and we're going to take good care of you. Doctor is going to come by and talk to you in a bit. Is that okay? Are you cold? Can you squeeze my hand?" the nurse asked as another worked around him, moving lines and raising bars on the bed, then pushing buttons on a monitor and making notes on a tablet.

Joshua's dad came in, then the surgical oncologist. The surgeon explained to Joshua and his dad that the surgery was difficult and intricate, but extensive preoperative planning and some good fortune allowed for complete resection. He was confident the first step was a success. He reminded Joshua that various developments may cause an alteration of course, but it appeared all went as well as they could have hoped for.

Joshua could see his dad force a smile. He tried to smile back, but his face didn't work, frozen by the weight of abandonment.

She walked out on me when I was facing a life-threatening operation?

Sure, a five-pound tumor, seven hours of surgery, thirty-odd stitches running along a vertical path above his belly button, and thoughts of impending radiation and chemotherapy were unfathomable, but how his girlfriend could have left him at that moment seemed just too far beyond his grasp.

Joshua was awakened the next day by a blinding, jolting pain at the bottom of his stomach, in and around the area where stitches closed up an incision they'd made so they could remove the tumor. It took every bit of strength and resistance to not give in to the bolts of agony that ran through him, but Joshua was able to pull up the surgical gown he was wearing so he could see the wound. He flashed back to the gash on his mom's arm, but thankfully, that image was covered up just as neatly as his own wound. There were only odd colors—shades of orange, red, purple, and a yellowish-green—peeking out from around the four-by-eight-inch dressing.

The nurses had told him they'd help him sit up later if he could handle it, and maybe walk him to the bathroom so he wouldn't have to use a pan.

If I can handle it? They might know about the pain from cutting away the tumor and stapling me shut, but they have no idea. "This isn't me." Are you fucking serious? Right now? "This is not me." Me either, babe. None of it's me.

That afternoon, Joshua was on his second lap around the hallway when the nurses stopped him. He had gotten up and walked out of the room on his own, but he was ghostly white, sweating from the effort, and delirious with jagged spikes of pain hammering into each fiber of his being. The agony wasn't just physical.

A Picture of Health Is Worth Thousands of Hours of Healing

During his recovery and ongoing treatment, Joshua took a stubborn, me-against-the-world mentality when approaching every aspect of his new reality. He'd never turned to anyone before—he wouldn't have known how if he had tried. Joshua didn't let anybody know when he had appointments for treatment. If he did, he'd lie to friends and his dad and say he had already arranged for a ride to the center, then he'd lie to the techs and nurses and say that he wouldn't drive himself home, but he almost always did, often deliriously tired, confused, and drugged up. No way was he going to let any-body have the chance to walk out on him again.

There were times when he was confined to the hospital, so pumped up with poisonous chemicals that entire days disappeared. But through it all, he managed to take time from work with very little formal leave. He leaned on his dad on only a few occasions—basically, when he was too weak to move to the bathroom or too ashamed to sleep in his own pee. He was forced to accept help (outside of the medical necessities like actually administering the chemo) only a half-dozen times, like the time he was drugged out from the chemo meds being dripped into him through his port, and he passed out cold in the hallway while trying to make it outside to smoke a joint to ease his nausea.

For a full year, Joshua endured the difficult path from diagnosis to cure alone. He chose to be emotionally and physically detached from the people in his life, and he resisted help from both professionals and friends at every step. But eventually, cancer humbled Joshua. It was like a relentless assassin in its quest to kill him. As his treatments continued into a second year, he realized cancer was equally as relentless in its quest to enlighten him about his choice to be so alone. So Joshua began to accept help, becoming grateful for assis-tance. He developed profound appreciation for those who cared enough about him to try to lighten his load. He may not have become an open book, but by the end of his treatments, Joshua allowed his friends and family, and a few of the more intimately involved caregivers, to help turn some pages.

Months after finishing treatment, Joshua quit his job at the bank to work at Moffitt Cancer Center. At first, he worked as a temporary accounting clerk and volunteer in areas such as organizing outreach to the young male Latino community to talk about testing and prevention—who better to speak to the kind of machismo that almost cost him his own life? When a position in finance opened up, Joshua took it—Moffitt was a place he felt he should ded-icate his life to.

He organized community events, coordinated media outreach, and even convinced the higher-ups at Moffitt to allow him to start a Puerto Rican outreach program intended to replicate their efforts to educate young adult males about the importance of seeking help for medical issues. Joshua wanted to make some type of impact on the community he belonged to. A side benefit was that his activities brought him to his home in Puerto Rico a few times each year.

Working at Moffitt fulfilled Joshua in ways he never could have envisioned precancer. He counseled patients, mostly young adults, some of whom were being cared for in the same treatment rooms where he'd spent many long and lonely days and nights.

Five years cancer-free, three of which were spent in a nonpatient capacity at Moffitt, helped put Joshua at a point in his life where he could open up about his cancer experiences. Although he was terrible at posting on social media, he felt he should put the news out to the world. He typed a "cancer-versary" message:

> *Five years today since my port was removed. In all, six surgeries, more than thirty radiation sessions, twenty-seven cycles of chemotherapy. Over 1,100 hours of treatment. Most of all, I beat down three proclamations that I had close to a ZERO chance of survival. I guess I beat some pretty insane odds. Thank you to Moffitt Cancer Center and the dozens of people who worked to rid me of cancer and give me the gift of hope that I'll live a long life.*

He pressed "post" on his message, tears of gratitude warming his cheeks.

Within minutes, he received a popup notification of a private message: "Congratulations, Joshua. I had no idea of your ordeal. I just found out today about some pretty bad news—not cancer, but serious. Your note put a needed smile on my face. Are you really living in Tampa?"

The note was from Rocio, a girl he'd had a secret crush on in high school back in Puerto Rico. He hadn't talked to her in more than ten years. His heart raced. What are those odds?

He started typing a response.

Joshua's Epilogue
••••••••••••••••••••••••

As fate would have it, Rocio was scheduled to fly to Tampa for surgery for severe endometriosis a few days after their initial online exchange. Her brother, a physician in southern Florida, had found a specialist who he thought would be qualified to help her. She'd been misdiagnosed for years and only discovered the real cause of her problems through the urging of her family.

Joshua and Rocio planned to meet the day of her arrival. He showed up to her hotel room with flowers for both Rocio and her mother, who had come to be with her. Rocio and Joshua got reacquainted over dinner that evening, and from that unlikely set of coincidences, dinner turned into another dinner with Rocio and her mother, then into Joshua visiting Rocio each day during her hospitalization and recovery. Their romance blossomed into a long-distance relationship and, soon after, a proposal and a wedding.

Two years after they wed, Rocio's mother was diagnosed with incurable brain cancer. During the subsequent months until she passed, Joshua and his mother-in-law became very close. Joshua was her emotional escort through cancer, and she was his chaperone to a lifetime's worth of needed emotional reconditioning.

"I used to joke that I fell in love with her mother and gained a wife," Joshua told me. "She was an angel. I'd never understood how beautiful and nurturing a mother's love could be—obviously—and her mother and I became very, very close."

A few years after her mother's death, Rocio still grieved, as did her father. Her father was a physician in Puerto Rico and remained completely despondent after the death of his wife. He needed his daughter's attention and care, regardless of her life in Florida and regardless of the fact that he'd been a vibrant, engaged, active sixty-year-old man just a couple of years prior. Rocio needed to be near her father and yearned to be back in Puerto Rico. She put her life with Joshua on hold and left Florida to go be with her dad.

As our talks continued, Joshua detailed the painful experiences he'd gone through and the difficulties that he was navigating at the time, primarily surrounding the emotional ups and downs his wife and her family had experienced. But he also explained how the perspective he'd gained along the way had helped him stay focused on making the best he could of every situation, regardless of how challenging the circumstances.

He agreed that for better or worse, he had many untold chapters ahead. He'd need to see how and if his wife could recover from her loss. He wasn't sure if she'd be willing to stay in Florida long-term. He hoped to continue to have an impact at Moffitt and within the cancer community. He worried about his ability to father children and Rocio's ability to carry a successful pregnancy. He knew cancer recurrence was a possibility, and he didn't know how much fight he had in reserve in case the cancer came back. He wondered if he could ever reconcile the losses of his mother, his mother-in-law, and the young adults he saw die at Moffitt. He didn't know if he could ever fully recover from the death and abandonment events of his life.

Mostly, he remained unsure if he possessed the capacity to move beyond his scars and maximize the human emotional experience, but trying to do just that was how he had decided to live the life he was given. Machismo was a thing of the past.

Turn Left, Then Go 1,200 Miles

D ay thirty-one was a short day: seventy-five flat miles from the beautiful town of Crystal River to Joshua's hometown of Tampa. Both Dave and Joshua joined me for the first dozen or so miles, then Dave said his goodbyes and turned around to make his way back to Crystal River and then to his hometown of Niceville. Fitting he should live in Niceville—his support was just so . . . nice.

Joshua and I made it to Tampa in midafternoon and rode straight to Moffitt Cancer Center, where Rocio was waiting for us. Joshua took me on a tour of the center, adding another dimension to his harrowing story of survival. He showed me the hallways he had walked after his surgeries, the courtyard he'd snuck out to in hopes of finding some marijuana-induced comfort from the intense nausea of chemotherapy, and the recovery rooms he'd spent so much time in as both patient and supporter.

Later that evening, we went to a legendary restaurant in Tampa, The Colombia, and talked the hours away over traditional Cuban food before heading to their house for a long night of sleep. It was the first time in more than a month that I hadn't slept in a hotel, and I slept hard and peacefully.

Day thirty-two wasn't as easy—my route had quite a few rolling hills spread out over 122 miles of warm, sticky central Florida—but it wasn't that difficult either, as I was energized by my eagerness to get closer to the Atlantic Ocean. I'd been able to map the day's route along extended stretches of bike trails. In fact, I rode on eighty miles of blissfully quiet, vehicle-free, nature-lined trails between Tampa and Sanford. I'd almost forgotten the joys of biking without worrying about getting run over every minute of the day. My disposition and, overall, my entire sense of accumulated emotional weariness had been somewhat lightened as a result of having regained a clarity of purpose—and of somewhat reconciling the feelings of remorse I'd carried around for so many decades—while biking down that late-night outdoor hallway a couple of nights before. With the additional calmness brought on by a stress-free long ride, the miles flowed by. I still took just over eleven hours to finish that day. After all, lighter disposition or not, my legs had become so entirely thrashed that there was no recovering overnight.

Day thirty-three was an important day. It was going to be long—124 miles—but it would be significant. There wasn't anything special about the distance, but there was about *where* I was biking to; I was going to reach the Atlantic. *The freaking Atlantic Ocean.* I rolled out of Sanford intent on having another stress-free bike-trail-navigating day (at least until I reached the coast some forty-odd miles away)—a perfect backdrop with which to enjoy the enormity of having pedaled across the entire country. But, as with so many times before, best laid plans and all—about fifteen miles into the ride, I flatted. *No big deal. Flats happen all the time.*

I changed the tube out, but as soon as I blew up the new one, it popped. Then another popped. Then another. After running my finger along the inside of the tire for the hundredth time, I found and removed the microscopic piece of metal that had penetrated the rubber tire just enough to pop the tubes. I fished in the saddle bag for another tube. Then my heart sank.

Oh, shit. No way.

In a panic, I emptied all four of the saddle bags. No tubes. Somehow, I'd gone through my entire stash.

All right, calm down. There's a bike shop somewhere around here.

I pulled up my location on my phone and searched the map. The closest bike shop was thirty miles away, in Daytona Beach. In fact, the closest anything was three miles away. I was screwed. I put the wheel back on the bike and had no choice but to walk the trail. An hour later, I reached a tiny town built around a mini-mart gas station.

I sat on the curb and weighed my options. I could walk the roughly thirty miles to Daytona Beach, but that would take six-plus hours, and there'd still be hours and hours of biking after. I could call a taxi—if there was a taxi service anywhere near. Or I could walk some distance until I was close enough to Daytona Beach to call for an Uber. And that was basically it. I walked into the mini-mart and asked if they had a taxi service in the area. I might as well have been speaking German. Then it hit me: Why not call for an Uber right there?

They don't have Ubers in the middle of nowhere.

I opened up the Uber app and tried it out. I marked my location and destination and waited while it searched. "Your driver is four minutes away," it read.

Four minutes? Now, that's some luck!

But I had a bike—a big bike—with a lot of gear on it. I looked at the type of car and didn't recognize the model. *Oh, well, we'll figure it out*, I thought, hoping the Uber wasn't going to be a compact.

Sometimes—and once again—help comes when and how you need it. Four minutes later, an SUV pulled into the lot with an Uber sign on the dashboard. The driver was an older Brazilian man who had just pulled off the road less than a mile away from where I called from so he could nap after visiting his son in Orlando. He told me that out of habit, he'd turned on his driver app instead of setting an alarm.

About an hour later, after telling my cross-country journey highlights to the mechanic at the shop as he changed both tubes out, I was on my bike again. I turned inland, rather than toward the coast, so I could make up miles for having been driven into Daytona, but soon enough, after looping back, I took my bike shoes and socks off so I could put my road-battered feet into the Atlantic Ocean.

My self-congratulatory mindset lasted all of about two minutes as reality hit me: I still had ninety miles of biking ahead of me to reach Jacksonville, and it was already well past noon. *It's not the destination, it's the journey, right?* I asked myself rhetorically.

I grabbed my shoes and socks, walked my bike back to A1A, and began the last leg of the trip—a 1,200-mile ride up the coast to Central Park, in New York City. As I biked the narrow shoulder up the Palm Coast, admiring the beach hut restaurants and nautical-themed antique shops, I noticed people putting out sandbags and boarding up windows.

Is there a storm coming?

I'd been so focused on podcasts and music that I'd missed catching up on news headlines; one can check out from the world if one wants—just grab a bike and pedal twelve hours a day. I called Erin.

"What time do you land, again? I think there's a big storm coming."

She was scheduled to fly into Tampa, 165 miles west of Jacksonville, where she'd left the truck more than a week before, and then drive to meet me in Jacksonville. She said she'd be at the hotel by about ten that evening, which suited my flat-delayed schedule.

"Do we need to make plans around that big hurricane?" she asked. "We might miss it, but possibly not."

Hurricane?

"I'm sure we'll be okay," I said unwittingly. I had never been near a hurricane, but it almost always seemed they were all overblown in the end—more news event than actual event. "Let's figure it out when we finally see each other tonight."

I paid little attention to the hurricane-anticipating, frenzied antics of the news station's reporters as I tuned in to the CNN broadcast online; I was too wide-eyed as I pedaled through the historic town of St. Augustine, then the golf mecca of Sawgrass and the mansion-laden towns of Ponte Vedra Beach and Jacksonville Beach. But by the time I reached Jacksonville proper, a steady and heavy rain had settled in.

Day thirty-four was a much-needed rest day—my third of the journey. Erin and I had planned to visit a close friend and mentor of mine and her husband for most of the day and evening. Although these friends lived in Los Angeles, they had a second beautiful house on the water in Jacksonville Beach, at which they often spent many weeks a year. After doing some sightseeing, we headed out for dinner to their favorite local restaurant, a seafood house that sat right on the Intracoastal Waterway. By that evening, the rain had intensified so strongly that conversation at dinner was more like a shouting match.

When I awoke on day thirty-five, I was ready for our new goal: stay ahead of Hurricane Matthew—a storm bearing down on the northern third of Florida with Category 4 power. Throughout the ten hours of biking the ninety miles from Jacksonville to Brunswick, Georgia, I was pelted with rain, buffeted by strong winds, honked at by nervous drivers, and slowed by the clumsiness of biking with a monster poncho on me. That night, we altered my route to go more inland, as Hurricane Matthew was no joke. I called my friends in Jacksonville Beach; their house had been demolished. The hurricane was as bad as predicted and the worst they'd seen in the area in more than fifty years. Matthew was due to boomerang back on shore in the Carolinas, right where I was heading.

Day thirty-six was supposed to take me along the seaside vistas into Savannah and then out to Hilton Head Island and on to Beaufort. Day thirty-seven was going to take me into Charleston and then north after that toward Myrtle Beach and into Wilmington, North Carolina. But some of those cities were planning to shut completely down, so instead, I remapped a more inland route north for the coming days.

I left Brunswick and made it to Hardeeville, just under one hundred miles away. Just like back in California, Arizona, New Mexico, Texas, and Louisiana—minus the heat but adding in heaps of rain—I had nothing but headwinds for days. It seems hurricanes spin counterclockwise along the East Coast, thus creating headwinds for any biker foolish enough to be traveling north during that madness. I trudged along, hour after long hour, assaulted by the elements, half of me delirious from exhaustion, the other half provoked into continuing because I had picked a battle against an angry Mother Nature and I wanted to see how it would end.

On day thirty-seven, the battle came to a head. I left Hardeeville and headed north and farther inland—more than fifty miles from the coast. For the first four hours, I zig-zagged along I-95. Most businesses were closed, and as the day progressed and Matthew's rage continued to grow, I slipped onto the interstate, as there was absolutely zero traffic. I found myself almost entirely alone, heading north on I-95, buckets—more like sheets, or sheets of buckets—of rain inundating the roads, my bike sludging through water that was, at times, more than a foot high. Walls of wind blew me around, forcing me to steady myself with a death grip on the handlebars. If my GPS hadn't been covered by my poncho, it would surely have displayed that I was going no more than five or six miles per hour, but I was mashing the pedals as hard as I ever had.

After having the interstate to myself for close to a half hour, a string of headlights approached me from behind. As the vehicles closed in, I noticed the lights were about a half-dozen Army or National Guard trucks. When they reached me, the lead transport truck slowed to match my pace, and the passenger window opened up. A young soldier, maybe midtwenties, screamed down at me through the noise of the wind and rain.

"Sir," he bellowed, "are you aware you're dab smack in the middle of a hurricane?"

I smiled wearily and screamed up at him. "Absolutely aware."

"Are you sure you want to be out in these weather conditions, sir?"

"I'm sure," I yelled. I had a schedule to maintain.

"Do you need anything, sir?" he shouted.

"No. Thank you, soldier," I hollered back.

"Well, okay. If you're sure, then. Carry on, sir." He gave me a thumbs up, rolled up his window, and motioned for the driver to press forward.

Within the next hour, things had intensified so much that I was forced to stop under an overpass to protect myself. I called Erin to come get me—things weren't too dangerous for a four-wheel-drive truck, but no doubt they had become too dangerous for a two-wheel-drive bike. We decided to drive a hundred or so miles north, to try to get ahead of the hurricane. (All the towns west of the Carolinas were filled with people who had left the coastal areas.) I got back on my bike outside of Fayetteville but was a worn-out, drowned rat by the end of that long and insane day, and a couple of hours later, I called it quits for the second time that day.

That night, the next day, and the next night, Hurricane Matthew's fury was unleashed on Fayetteville. We came to learn that one thousand rescues happened nearby in those thirty-six-odd hours. I saw firsthand that some hurricanes do turn out to be as potent and destructive as the news makes them out to be. After I'd spent a day and a half holed up in a hotel room in a flooded city, the hurricane ran out of breath, and a window to take off opened up. The storm had knocked me off my plan a bit, but I still had people to see and a finish line in New York to get to, still 650 miles—and only seven days—away.

I didn't cover any ground holed up in the hotel room, but I did find another book participant.

Dr. Meyers

Relationship to cancer: Medical professional

Age: Sixty-two

Family status: Married for twenty-nine years with one adult daughter

Location: New York, New York

First encounter with cancer: Age twenty

Cancer summary: Dr. Meyers is a medical oncologist at NYU Langone Health and its Perlmutter Cancer Center. She has built a busy practice, focusing principally on caring for women with breast cancer.

Cancer specifics: Dr. Meyers treats both female and male breast cancer.

Community involvement: Dr. Meyers is the director of the Perlmutter Cancer Center Survivorship Program. She is also a keynote speaker and is active in the wellness and survivorship communities.

Strongest positive emotion during cancer experience: Gratification

Strongest negative emotion during cancer experience: Helplessness

How we met: I needed a doctor who could speak to the perspective of being the person who delivers bad news, good news, and all the news in between—not just once but nearly every day. I found Dr. Meyers, a seasoned oncologist, while Erin and I were holed up in North Carolina riding out Hurricane Matthew. Erin had done an extensive web search, and Dr. Meyers was one of several candidates she stumbled upon. We discovered Dr. Meyers was a long-practicing medical oncologist at NYU, with a specialty in breast cancer, and that she was active in the survivorship community. We watched some YouTube videos of Dr. Meyers addressing audiences on various care, treatment, and survivorship topics, and we were touched by how she presented herself; she seemed open, honest, approachable, and in tune with the emotions and psychosocial issues related to cancer.

After Erin called her a few times, Dr. Meyers agreed to meet to discuss the project. We couldn't coordinate a face-to-face meeting during my bike ride, but Dr. Meyers and I spoke after I returned home and many times thereafter. Months later, we had the opportunity to meet while she was attending a wellness conference in San Diego. We spoke about issues from the perspective of her patients, such as being diagnosed with cancer as a young mother, balancing care with a career, and encountering fertility issues when seeking treatment. We also spoke about issues from the perspective of a caregiving professional, including how one deals with delivering a terminal diagnosis and how caring for people with cancer can affect the caregiver's perspective on life.

Not only did Dr. Meyers fit the bill of what I was looking for in a medical provider, but her life story was compelling and poignant. In our very first conversation, she opened up about some extremely personal dynamics on the topics I had proposed we discuss. Near the end of our initial conversation, I asked Dr. Meyers who she confides in when dealing with the issues we were going to discuss. Was it her husband?

"No," she said. "We pretty much keep our work at the office."

"Colleagues?"

"Most certainly not." She laughed. "Doctors don't talk to other doctors about things that might make them look weak."

"Your friends, then?"

"No," she replied. "I wouldn't want to burden them with my problems, and they're the same with me. We travel, go see a show, hike, and do things that allow us to sort of 'check out' from our professional lives."

"Who, then?" I pressed. "There must be someone?"

"No. In truth, there isn't," she admitted. "I'd love to talk about these things because I never really have before. You caught me at the right time in my life. It will be interesting to see what we find out."

Dr. Meyers and I spoke many times over the next year, and by the end of our talks, we found out quite a bit.

The Doctor Who Cares

A Home With a Buried Heart

Marleen was born in Queens, New York, in the mid-1950s, at a time when most of America was flourishing. Outlying cities, infrastructure, schools, and churches were being built at a never-before-seen pace. Televisions were in every home. The standard of living was improving across most social classes. The country was in the early stages of a new type of commercialism and convenience, as companies like Disneyland and McDonald's launched. An overall post-WWII boom was in effect—booming information flow, population growth, economic growth, and streams of people moving to the suburbs. It was a vibrant, evolving, auspicious time in the country's history, even with the Cold War lurking in the background.

But both the neighborhood and the circumstances that Marleen was born into were not indicative of the optimism and prosperity of the times. Her family was not moving to the suburbs or partaking in the luxuries of materialism and consumption. Marleen's parents struggled to make ends meet each month; they rarely went out and socialized, they didn't interact with the neighbors, or even talk among themselves; and they had no optimism or eyes toward the future—beyond that which their children might have. They existed *at* that time and not so much *in* that time.

Many families had stay-at-home moms, and Marleen's family was no exception—although it might be more accurate to state that Marleen's mom didn't work than to state she stayed home. Staying home implies there was a sense of family and home life and that she took care of Marleen and her sister and all the things domestic while her dad was at work—or wherever dads went all day and all night. But their household was not centered so much on a traditional sense of family or caring, but rather, it was centered on survival, paying the bills, keeping everyone healthy and, most of all, becoming educated. Neither of Marleen's parents showed attention to, let alone love for, each other. But her mom did pay attention to her girls, especially in pushing them to succeed and in preparing them to venture out in the world. Marleen's dad had nothing to do with his family.

When you grow up in a household where parents just exist, rather than exist *together*, where there is no earnest connection between them and between either of them and the outside world; and where the focus is on just getting by each day, the ties that bind the family can be flimsy and uncertain and susceptible to unraveling, and in Marleen's house, there was no family—even in the loosest sense.

Marleen didn't have friends over, she was too embarassed, and she rarely went over to friends' homes. She didn't participate in social clubs or play sports or engage in many after-school activities beyond the daily afterschool religious studying that she was required to attend. She didn't do most of the things girls born in Queens in the vibrant 1950s and raised in the burgeoning melting pot of Jackson Heights did. Instead, she went to school, she studied most of the afternoon and evening, she read books, she did chores, and she spent her little free time with her sister, mom, and grandmother. Sometimes, she stayed awake late enough to hear her dad come home. And that was that, and it didn't ever vary, and it didn't ever change—until she was thirteen.

One night, she didn't hear her dad come home. He was always sort of never there, and then one day, he wasn't there ever again. He never said good-bye or stormed out as a result of an argument or gave any indication he was going to go MIA. He just left, and neither Marleen nor her mom and sister ever saw or heard from him again.

A Calling Is Formed

After her dad left, Marleen kept even more to herself than before. First, she didn't know what to tell people, and she didn't want her few friends and class-mates to look at her differently or judge her for not having a dad. Second, her mom talked even less than she had in the past—and they *never* talked about what happened or why it happened or what they were going to do without him. Her mom just plain never addressed or allowed her daughters the chance to address the dad's abandonment. As a result, Marleen's trauma never was seen as an open wound that needed tending to. Rather, his leaving was simply another fact in the history of her life.

Marleen's grandmother, a caring and loving, but frail woman, had always lived with them—another sign that their family was not the norm—and like Marleen's mother, she wasn't much of a talker either. The only real discourse that did go on at home was centered around one narrative: Impeccable per-formance at school was the only possible path to a sufficiently stable life. Both Marleen's mom and grandmother were very one-track-minded, and they both constantly pushed Marleen to do more and better.

Years prior, Marleen had skipped the first grade because she was so far ahead of the other students in her class, and after her dad left, she immersed herself even deeper in school. Sure, her mom badgered the 98 percent and seemed gratified with the 100 percent, but Marleen didn't seek perfection at school to appease her mom; she achieved near perfection at school because she was driven and she was *smart*. She liked every subject at school, but she was uncommonly drawn to math and science. Her favorite subject was biology, and when she went with select students from her seventh-grade class on a field trip to a busy hospital, she was absolutely awestruck.

Some girls might have come home after such a field trip and rambled about their day, but Marleen kept her excitement hidden. Her report of the trip was a muted recounting of the day, finished off by the normal "I'm going to go study" exit line. But that day, instead of shuffling off to her room and sitting at the desk that was piled with open textbooks, she lay in her bed and dreamed about becoming a doctor. Thoughts of the day played over and over—nurses measuring patient doses as the drug trolley moved from station to station, doctors reading electrophysiology reports as they measured patients' hearts, and bottles filled with fluid dripping into tubes stuck in people's arms. Lying there, Marleen pretended to breathe in all the chemical smells and imagined hearing all the dialogue filled with medical terms. She knew one day, somehow, she was going to learn everything about medicine. She was going to become a doctor and take care of people. She just *knew* it.

Marleen had the grades and the test scores to apply to several universities, including New York University and other prestigious schools with top premed and science programs. She completed high school two years early and, at sixteen, accepted admission into NYU. Marleen knew that her mom was pleased at her efforts, but the idea of her mom exuberantly expressing pride and joy was just that—an idea. She commuted to NYU daily, and just like that, Marleen plunged herself into a new reality only about eight actual miles away from her strange and desolate Jackson Heights existence but a million psychological miles away.

The Curly-Haired Doctor

Marleen obtained her bachelor of science degree in biology when she turned twenty. The sciences, in particular organic chemistry and molecular and cellular biology, were easy for Marleen. She was able to tutor upperclassmen almost from day one of college, as she self-taught ahead of her intended curriculum. Marleen loved learning, and she loved the thought that the learning of medicine could never be mastered, because applied science was an ever-evolving world. Learning about medicine was going to be a wonderful, never-ending journey.

Medical school at NYU was challenging, but Marleen continued to excel. She was drawn to hematology and oncology but thought she might also want to become a surgeon; the endless possibilities for pursuit multiplied Marleen's enthrallment with her chosen path. All facets of medicine—the cause, research, diagnosis, treatment, and care—fascinated Marleen, and she continued to immerse herself in her studies, effortlessly absorbing the details of whatever complicated subject was at hand. Marleen's education experience couldn't have progressed any better. She had an unending capacity to learn about the human body and then apply the learning.

Much like medical school, residency flew by. The barrage of thirty-six-hour shifts was constant, and Marleen spent a frenzied four-year stint in internal medicine at NYU/Bellevue dealing with every imaginable malady, sickness, and condition possible. Her training and education prepared her in the best possible way to master—or at least deal with—whatever was thrown at her. Well, almost everything. There were two exceptions: First was how to deal emotionally with the horrors she was encountering, which were multiplied being that it was the era of AIDS. Second, none of her teachers had ever acknowledged the rampant sexism against women doctors that existed in the workplace. Gallows humor helped Marleen remain impassive to the carnage and brutality of a world that sometimes seemed intent on revealing how fragile the human body can be, but nobody even bothered to joke about the way women were treated in the workplace. There was no lessening the effects of that anguish. Women were secondary to men, and that was that.

It was maddening to continually be addressed as a nurse, to have to fight to assist on tougher cases, to continually be called on to validate her knowledge or recite potential diagnosis details. After all, not only was Marleen top in her class, but she was a quick thinker. She never folded under pressure, her energy and focus never waned, and she cared only about the actual care—not the politicking and positioning that some of her male peers seemed to care about above all else. But by the end of her residency, Marleen was a *doctor*. And looking back from a decade and a half after the field trip that inspired and solidified her desire her to pursue a life in medicine, she couldn't remember ever wanting to be anything else.

Marleen didn't expect she could ever avoid the sexism, but by the time she was done with her residency, she wanted to be in a field that would have her deliver ongoing care to patients. She applied for and accepted a fellowship in oncology at Memorial Sloan Kettering Hospital for Cancer and Allied Diseases, one of the nation's preeminent hospitals.

In the oncology hospital, there was no relief from the solemnity of each day's events. It was the early 1980s, and cancer was still very much a death sentence. Cancer was serious business; there was no relief from that mind-numbing reality. But it was also an exciting time in the oncology unit; research intensified, which suited Marleen's desire to discover and learn about new drugs and new protocols—and both were advancing at ferocious speeds. In addition, new technologies started to play an increasingly important role in diagnosis and treatment, which allowed Marleen to maintain a forward-thinking mindset, and hoped-for future advancements approached the present at a faster and faster pace.

At first, Marleen's emotions—whether suppressed, undiscovered, unexplored, or just plain undeveloped—didn't stand in her way. She was affected by the sad stories of some of her patients and heartbroken by their diagnoses, but she just wasn't impeded by the weights of her sympathy or the burdens of partiality. At the end of her fellowship, Marleen decided to start her own oncology practice, so she reaffiliated with NYU.

Being back at NYU gave Marleen a balanced environment in which she could both continue learning and gain a leg up on building her practice, since she had so much history within the institution. She was insanely driven and energetic, but more important than those qualities, one aspect of Marleen helped set her apart from her peers: Nothing in her private life attempted to wrest away her attention. Her entire existence revolved around medicine, and she had the makings of becoming a luminary among the younger physicians.

Building a practice was not an easy thing for any new doctor to do, even inside of a prodigious, supportive institution like NYU, but it was *hard* for women because the prevailing environment at the time fostered a distinction between doctors and *women doctors*. One colleague said to Marleen: "How could anybody be expected to refer patients to a woman doctor, especially one with long, curly hair like yours? People don't want a doctor with long, curly hair. If you want me to refer you patients, spend some time at the hairdresser."

Because of the hurdles brought on by being a woman in a near exclusively man's world, Marleen needed to hustle to get patients. She hung out in the ER, she petitioned doctors in the hallways, and she reached out to professors. She did everything she could to get herself in front of enough people who, together, could refer her enough patients to sustain a new practice.

To make matters more difficult, she only had access to an office during the late afternoon and evening and had only limited access to a secretary who worked with a doctor who was in an entirely different office. But the first few years flew by, and Marleen's practice became a viable one—long, curly hair and all.

Learning Compassion

As Marleen's accomplishments became more noticed by her peers, the next generation of medical students became more diverse, and the workplace began to provide slightly more equality and acceptance for women, Marleen's struggle against the narrow-minded, sexist headwinds lessened some. As a result, she settled further into her practice and focused solely on bringing the best care to her patients. Amazing developments in the cancer community—particularly within the specialty of breast cancer—were categorically changing treatment options and protocols. No amount of work dampened Marleen's enthusiasm or her drive to become the best oncologist she could be, and increasing patient loads were handled by working more hours. Her nights and weekends were filled with conferences and peer reviews and doing anything she could do to stay abreast of the advancing knowledge on new procedures and ground-breaking drugs and state-of-the-art technologies. She even managed to start teaching at NYU. Somehow, she was able to squeeze more and more into her days and nights.

But as her professional life flourished, her perspective began to widen. As an oncologist, she interacted with more people in deeper, more personal ways. And although she focused mostly on the clinical aspects of her interactions, it was impossible to avoid the human aspects. As a result, she began to measure her lack of personal fulfillment against the immense professional fulfillment she was enjoying—and when she did, the voids in her personal life began to take on more meaning and more significance.

Marleen wasn't oblivious to the need to have friends, go to parties, date, and relax and dream a little, but those things just didn't come naturally to her. But, eventually, Marleen started to give some real attention to that side of her life, and when she did, she realized she had needs and desires. Where before she'd been somewhat blind to the world around her, she began to notice that friends and people around her in her peer group were getting married and having children, and she began to feel a need for companionship.

Secret Chambers

One day, on a day that was no different from any other, Marleen found herself consumed and practically illuminated by emotions, feelings, and desires she'd never noticed having before. It was as if she'd known exactly where she was and who she was her whole life, and then unexpectedly, she woke up and found herself in a whole different place, with a whole different perception of herself. Certainly, her emotional evolution had taken place over years, but seemingly just like that, with no special or even noticeable provocation, a previously hidden switch had somehow been flipped on, lighting a place inside of Marleen that had never been proactively explored.

She'd gone out with different people over the years, but nothing ever came from it. She hadn't ever been in a place to connect with anyone on any kind of deep, personal level—she had all the connection to work that she'd ever need in her life. Or so she'd thought. But when Marleen met Stanley, she happened to be looking at the world and herself through newly opened eyes, and not unlike the bolt that struck her mind many years before as a school girl at the hospital, she was struck by lightning again—only this time, it hit her square in the heart.

Stanley was a successful tax attorney, and one of Marleen's friends had suggested she consult with him on business matters. When they met, the energy between them was palpable, and Marleen was swept away into a whole new world, one filled with intimacy and passion and vulnerability and expressive exchange. Coincidentally, she and Stanley lived in the same building in New York, which made it easy to see each other without notice or coordination. Stanley was fifteen years older than Marleen and divorced, but they instantly meshed on several levels. It wasn't long before they were married, and soon after, Marleen gave birth to a baby girl.

Motherhood immediately suited Marleen. She didn't carry around the baggage of her own childhood, and thus, nothing dampened or swayed her emotions and feelings. They were true, fresh, and enriching.

As the years raced by, Marleen's relationship with Stanley grew stronger, her oncology practice continued to thrive, and their young daughter was a perfect complement to their lives. The family enjoyed the luxuries of their successes, and with the benefits realized by having a partner and a more balanced life, Marleen allowed herself to scale back her efforts at work a bit. As a result, she was able to *raise* her daughter. She was there to take her to school, take her to piano and dance lessons, help her with her homework, cook, and spend as much quality time as she could hope to spend with her child. Hers was a reality created in stark contrast to her own experiences growing up, and she created her loving, stable, and full home life with the help of a supportive, engaged, loving husband—and while still maintaining her medical practice.

With a broadened perspective and a more balanced life, Marleen's own life experiences grew. Beyond motherhood, she took the time to build deeper friendships. She and Stanley traveled with friends, and she mentored medical students and fellows—especially on how to overcome some of the difficulties she'd encountered. But most of all, Marleen learned to accept the fact that an endless spectrum of enriching feelings and emotions were available to experience and embrace—opportunity, self-worth, contentment, love, gratitude, humility.

By the time her own daughter was off to college, Marleen had a deep recognition of, and appreciation for, how fortunate she'd been in life. At work, she was blessed with the drive to live a productive and distinguished existence caring for others, and she made a positive difference in the lives of people dealing with cancer. At home, she was blessed with a loving spouse and a beautiful, vibrant daughter. The three of them were as close as any family could hope to be. But recognizing and appreciating the scope of her own boundless life experiences had its negative side effects as well.

Caring Hurts

Marleen had always been able to stay cutting edge with regard to her specialty, and she'd always stayed in step with the major changes taking place in the health-care world in general—that never changed after getting married and having her daughter. But Marleen was able to keep her worlds separate; work was work, personal was personal. The two paths she walked on never crossed.

Marleen never stopped working, and even when she'd slowed down while raising her daughter, she still worked full-time hours. But with her daughter out of the house, she had more time to give to her practice. And when she redoubled her efforts, her propensity to increase the meaningfulness of her calling increased. But she was a different Marleen, a more compassionate Marleen. She was *fuller* inside. As a result, when she became reconnected to her work, it was at a much deeper level than before.

Two majorly opposing forces pulled at her. At one end of the spectrum, NYU's medical and oncology centers were feeling the same pressures that all caregiving facilities felt, that of needing to care for more and more patients to try to keep pace with the upwardly spiraling costs of providing medical care in the United States. On a near daily basis, Marleen was pushed to increase the number of people she saw each day, which forced her to spend less and less time with each patient. At the other end of the spectrum, Marleen was overwhelmed with sympathy and compassion for the human experience. Where twenty or thirty years prior, she hadn't had any real or deep understanding of how much was lost by a premature death, it was impossible not to empathize with her patients after all she'd accomplished and all the emotional riches she'd enjoyed over the years.

Back when she was a thirty-year-old, single, career-focused person, she could more readily give a young mother the bleak truth of her diagnosis without *understanding* the human she was caring for. But at fifty-five years old, after making so many soul-enriching memories with her husband of twenty years and her daughter, the daily work of an oncologist became much harder. Giving young mothers, older mothers, fathers, or women who dreamed one day of being mothers the sometimes bleak truths of their diagnosis was an impossible task to do without being deeply affected herself by the harshness and the arbitrary and unjust prognosis that some people were doomed to face. And the magnitude of being an oncologist—of having to be the one to sometimes tell people they wouldn't get to enjoy life's riches, they might not survive long enough to see their babies out of diapers, and they would have no chance to age and gain wisdom and look back at their lives with appreciation and thankfulness—began to hit Marleen every day.

Each of Marleen's patient rooms were steps away from each other, but the walk from one of those rooms, where she might give promising news to one person, to the very next room, where she might have to talk to another person about end-of-life issues, was becoming devastatingly difficult to navigate.

She became run-down and cynical from being pushed harder and harder by the bureaucracy and metrics of the modern world of medicine, but she also became more desperate to bring better care, more resources, and more attention to her patients—and to the growing survivorship population that existed as by-products of that same modern world of medicine. Marleen often left the office both frustrated by all the patients she had to see and satisfied that more of those patients could expect their cancer to be treated successfully, which would give more of them the opportunity to receive life's blessings.

Advancements in cancer research and care not only allowed doctors to have more predictable outcomes for their patients but also allowed patients to live longer lives. The practical applications of this evolving science made caring for people with cancer less of a "practice" and more of an "exactness." But the less obscure aspects of caring for patients freed Marleen to pursue other aspects of the medical world. As a result of expanding her focus—aside from her demanding oncology practice—Marleen became an active advocate in the survivorship and wellness worlds. And as the years passed by and curing cancer became more of a reality, and as posttreatment prognoses were enhanced, the treatment and care of patients were allowed to take on a much longer-term view. As a result, Marleen began to draw a deep line in the sand with her patients when it came to applying all the collective knowledge for her patients' best interests.

Perspectives

Because there are many types of breast cancer—with varying lengths of care, degrees of recurrence, and maintenance and follow-up protocols—Marleen's patient base contained both new patients and patients who'd been with her for many years. And as her practice matured, she became more understanding, sympathetic, and desperate to help her longtime patients, but she also became less open-minded to new patients who didn't wanted to forego known effective treatment for unproven, alternative care.

When she was younger, Marleen was more tolerant when a patient wanted to try everything to treat their cancer—a greens-only diet or supplements or an injection of some magical concoction in Mexico. She'd wait to administer care until the patient came around to the realities of their situation, even if by waiting, the patient had made things worse for themselves. But over the decades, Marleen came to know, all too well, that a "try everything" approach never worked. After forty years of practicing medicine, the reality was that better and better drugs had been developed to successfully combat various cancers; genetic sequencing foretold how some cancers were likely to behave, thus treatment regimens could be better predicted; surgical tactics had improved; and a host of new technologies and new breakthroughs at all phases of the caregiving experience gave physicians the ability to treat more people with better efficacy. Mortality rates had declined, sometimes significantly, and cancer—especially breast cancer—had become more treatable. Magical elixirs and secret diets and miracle shots didn't exist.

Marleen had seen too many people harmed by denying the realities of their prognosis and treatment options. Too many patients delayed or denied traditional treatments, convinced their cancer would abate if only they took charge of making changes in their life. She heard it all: "I'll work out more so I can rid myself of the tumors"; "If I eat better, the cancer will go away"; "Once I reduce the stress in my life, my cancer will disappear."

Marleen believed all those changes *could* help but not at the expense of known effective treatment. Surgery, chemotherapy, and radiation were the main tools that could be used to control cancer, lessen cancer's effects on the body, eradicate cancer, deal with cancer recurrence, and ease end-of-life care.

One day Marleen reached her breaking point when it came to being tolerant with her more myopic patients. Marleen was seeing a new patient, one who had two young toddlers and a husband and a career and friends and family. This patient had been diagnosed with a cancer that, if treated with a very defined regimen of drugs and radiation, had an excellent chance of being cured. The woman, though, was convinced she should "try everything else" first.

"Please," Marleen pleaded, "you have to understand the realities of what we're dealing with. Your cancer is not advanced. Because of such an early diagnosis, I'm extremely confident you'll do well long-term."

"I appreciate that, but I've read so much," the patient said. "There *are* options, right? I mean, people are cured all the time by changing what they eat. I've already gone on an organic, vegan diet. I've also been to a very respected herbalist who is convinced she can help me."

"Look, go ahead and do those things," Marleen said. "Make all the changes in your life that might help your health and mental wellness, but thirty years ago, I'd be telling you that you might die no matter what we did. Now, I can tell you with near certainty you'll live a very normal, cancer-free life *if* you let me treat you. If you don't listen to me and allow the tumors to grow, they'll spread, they might metastasize, and they *will* kill you. But I can treat your cancer so your babies and your husband and your loved ones don't have to go through life without you. This is the reality of what we're dealing with."

"I just don't know," the woman said. "So many people have told me there are other things I can do first."

"But I *do* know. I'm a good doctor. I'm telling you that your cancer can be cured. There's a woman coming to see me today who is certain to die, *to lose her life*. Her cancer is not curable at this point. There is nothing we can do to save her. But we can save you. Do you understand?"

The woman declined treatment. She left, convinced she could cure the cancer herself.

The walk to the adjacent patient room was difficult for Marleen. Thoughts of her daughter raced through her head. She remembered Stanley and her holding her daughter's hand when she was a little girl as they strolled through Central Park on a wintery day. She remembered shopping for a dress for her daughter's first formal and cooking dinners for her and her friends. She remembered seeing how proud Stanley was when he watched her play piano on stage, the look on her face when she was accepted into the college she wanted, and how they both cried when she got on a plane to interview for a job in California.

Marleen knew the woman in the adjacent patient room wouldn't ever get to have any of those memories, and she knew that the woman she'd just seen, the one who was convinced she could cure herself, might deny herself a lifetime of upcoming memories.

The weight of dealing with both patients was heavy. But Marleen loved medicine, and she loved treating people, and she loved the idea that she could help more people navigate their cancer journeys successfully so they could go on to realize the same fortunes she herself was thankful for every single day. She took one last deep, contemplative breath and walked in to talk to the woman who was dying.

The woman smiled at her. "How are you doing, Dr. Meyers?" she asked.

"Me? I'm really great, thank you. Let's talk about you . . ."

Dr. Meyers's Epilogue
· ·

More often than not, I caught Dr. Meyers in the later hours of the evening, after she was done with work and before she was going to head home. Some nights she was more tired than others, but she never begrudged our talks—just the opposite. The more drained she sounded at the beginning of our talks, the fresher and more renewed she sounded by the end. The reason for this, I concluded, was that she cared so immensely for her patients, she bonded with them so emotionally, and she employed all her curative competencies in such a fervent manner. It was almost as if each day wiped her out, but as the night progressed and she reflected on life—either alone while walking home, over tea while reading before bed, or while talking with me—she was renewed again.

I asked her one day whether she thought the weight of everything she went through each day would ever cause her to stop practicing or whether she thought medicine would advance enough to lessen the weight of those realities.

"I don't have much faith in the health-care system," she said. "It's broken, and I don't see it ever being fixed. The pressure to see more patients is overwhelming, the amount of paperwork is maddening, and navigating the world of insurance and just the sheer problems brought on by such a huge and complex system is devastating to patients and caregivers. People aren't cared *about* as much as they're cared *for*. The relationship between the afflicted and the curative resources, whether human or otherwise, has been reduced to a matter of dollars and not of sense. But curing cancer? That's another thing. I don't think it will happen in my lifetime, but it might happen in the lifetime of some of my younger patients. The world of health care is a bleak and dark one, but the light at the end of the tunnel, the curing of diseases like cancer, is starting to glow brighter and brighter every year."

"So, what keeps you going each day?" I asked.

"Knowing I can make the experience a little better for people. That and hoping I can do so long enough to maybe, just once, experience what it will be like to stop telling women they're going to die before they're old, before they have kids or get married or build their careers or do whatever they want to do for the decades and decades they have left to live. That dream is enough to drive me to come back extra early tomorrow and stay just a little later tonight."

Lessons in Reliance

I left the hotel we'd holed up in and started on my route north out of Fayetteville. The storm had subsided, but flood waters were still rising. As a result, some of the highways and roads I'd planned on taking were closed. I rerouted on the fly, but it wasn't easy. Roads were blocked, streetlights were out because the power was down, drivers appeared frustrated and drove erratically, houses were on fire, emergency vehicles were racing by, and rivers all around the area were cresting. Most every low-lying road had turned into a temporary uncontrolled stream. I came to learn that more than fifteen inches of rain had fallen on Fayetteville in the day and a half we were there.

A couple hours behind me, Erin was barely able to get out of town as roads continued to close due to the rising flood waters. When she did get ahead of me, she found a safe route for me to make it to Raleigh, where we planned to meet for lunch. After, I continued on until dark and, once again, called for Erin to pick me up. After yet another monster day—but one that still left me short of my planned end line—we spent the night in South Hill, Virginia.

Day forty was a complicated mess. First, I biked the thirty-odd miles back to where Erin had picked me up the night before. Then she came and picked me up from that same spot and drove me back to the hotel. From there I biked north well into the night. The temperature had turned, and when it got too cold, she picked me up again and drove me all the way back to that same hotel in South Hill.

As I stood in a hot shower thawing out, I thought about all the help Erin had given me throughout the ride, as had Chad, Jerry, Dave, and so many friends and strangers. I'd definitely learned a two-faceted lesson about reliance. When someone was there to help me, I would call for assistance several times. I'd learned how to rely on others, a difficult habit for me to develop, considering I'd spent most of life absent people to turn to for help. I never wanted to stop learning and developing, becoming comfortable with relying on others. Admitting that to myself helped me realize my character was still evolving. On the other hand, when no one was available, I always figured out how to get where I needed to go. Because I'd been self-reliant my whole life, when I didn't have help, I simply figured it out on my own.

Many of the book participants had grappled with issues on both sides of their experience of reliance. Some had nobody to rely on during the toughest stretches of their lives. Some didn't know how or didn't want to rely on the people closest to them. That experience was relatable on its face: Not having anyone to turn to can be just as devastating as not wanting to burden your loved one with hardship.

One book participant in particular, Patricia, had dealt with extremes on both ends of that spectrum. Patricia's story epitomized the essence of so many of life's most extreme themes. It preoccupied me often on the ride, more so as I began to understand for myself the value of both self-reliance and depending on others.

Patricia

Relationship to cancer: Survivor, secondary caregiver

Age: Seventy-one

Family status: Married for thirty-three years with two stepchildren and an elderly mother

Location: Southern California

First encounter with cancer: Thirty-nine years old

Cancer summary: Patricia was diagnosed with various carcinomas and lymphomas. She endured five bouts with cancer over more than three decades. She also helped care for her father, who died of prostate cancer, while she was undergoing treatment for her own cancer. She has been intimately involved in providing support and care for many people battling cancer.

Treatment specifics: Hodgkin's lymphoma, stage IIIA, S; relapse of Hodgkin's lymphoma; melanoma; breast cancer, stage III; thyroid, Hurthle cell carcinoma

Community involvement: Volunteer for three decades at the Cancer Support Community, advocate and speaker for survivorship issues, patient outreach and assistance advocate

Strongest positive emotion during cancer experience: Trust

Strongest negative emotion during cancer experience: Sadness

How we met: I was at Sunday brunch in Calabasas, California, meeting my soon-to-be wife Erin's cousin and his wife for the first time. The Cycle of Lives project had provided a natural icebreaker, and conversation quickly turned in that direction. Tom and Mary kept looking at each other as I explained the premise of the book. I sensed they might have a cancer story of their own. They asked if I'd already secured all the book participants, because I might be interested in talking to Mary's aunt. I responded that I hadn't.

"Her story is very inspiring," Mary said. "She's had cancer five different times, but I think you'll be as interested in her noncancer story as the cancer one. She's amazing. I'd like to talk to her about it and see if she'd be interested."

Patricia was interested, so we scheduled an exploratory phone call.

"I'm happy to talk to you," Patricia said after our introductions. "I'm not sure my story is that interesting, though." Of course, only the most interesting people led with that disclaimer.

One of the real joys of talking with Patricia was that no matter how intense the subject matter got, she was always present and relaxed. She spoke without hesitation or pause, from what appeared to be a genuinely calm mind. At times, we had to work to get her comfortable enough to delve into the heart of an issue, but she was always up to exploring all angles until we made it there.

I Don't Get Colds, I Get Cancer

Patricia awoke to him straddling her, his hands wrapped around her neck, his knees digging into her shoulders. He was raving mad, spewing out spittle as he ranted about some misperceived long-ago slight. Something must have come to his mind in the middle of the night, some imagined wrong that caused him to shatter the calm darkness of sleep and launch into instantaneous full-force rage. Patricia could make no sense of what was happening. His hands were strong, and her breathing was becoming weaker by the second. She only knew she was about to die. Her fitful and panicky struggling was proving useless against him. Consciousness was quickly disappearing, and with it, her will to fight. She felt herself letting go of reality just before he finally loosened his grip and rolled off of her. A pinpoint of vision remained, and as her head fell limply to the side, she could see him saunter out of the bedroom as if he had simply gotten up to fetch a glass of water. Then, as if shocked back by some unknown force, her body convulsed violently, and she struggled to gasp in enough air to refill her lungs. Tears gushed out of her eyes. In a few moments it was over, and she lay there, her head throbbing, holding her knees to her chest, silently crying. A part of her cried because he hadn't killed her.

Patricia was accustomed to sudden acts of violence that came out of nowhere, that were brought on without provocation, notice, or any possible explanation—they were impossible to anticipate and impossible to avoid. The whacko was careful to avoid leaving marks that others could see or that couldn't be hidden by her clothing, but sometimes, Patricia had to stay home from work so that the occasional visible sign of abuse could fade.

She was thirty-three years old and living with a madman, and it was killing her. She had lost weight, she was struggling mentally, physically, and emotionally under the pressure of constant fear and stress, and she was becoming more desperate with each episode. Then came the broken eardrum.

It was the first time he'd sent her to the hospital. The blood had poured out of her ear and down her neck, a nonstop flow, evidence of the escalating force with which he threw his punches. When the whacko drove Patricia to the ER, he didn't say a word. When he parked the car, he turned to her and held up his finger; he pointed it at her with a signature whacko angry glare and then pulled his finger softly to his own closed lips and turned his head slowly from side to side.

The ER doctor saw Patricia alone. He asked probing questions, but Patricia wouldn't dare answer them truthfully. She told him they had been roughhousing and that she'd banged into something. When the doctor urged her to allow him to call the police, she nervously laughed him off, explaining that her injury was the result of a freak accident and nothing more. She knew that she'd be made to pay dearly should she move an inch toward taking help. But as she left the hospital under the quiet, knowing stares of the nurses, Patricia knew that her time was running out. The violence was escalating.

Patricia had imagined that she'd figure out a way to fight back some day, that if she could fight back and live, she'd be the one left standing. The whacko wouldn't know what to do if she finally came out on top, would he? He'd be dead, that fucker. But those thoughts were just that—imagined. The stark truth was that she had to find a way to safely escape before he killed her.

• • •

After the ER visit, as soon as she was able, Patricia called her friend Melinda.

"I think it's time," Patricia said. "He really tried to kill me. I mean *truly*. Do you think we can do this soon? Are we ready?" "This" meant execute the escape plan they'd been making for Patricia for years.

"You know I'm ready whenever. You just have to tell me when," Mel said.

"I need to make sure I didn't make any mistakes. We didn't make any, did we?"

Patricia always had a left-brained knack for lists and details. Her dad, a pragmatic and deliberate man with a private pilot's license, used to talk about the preflight checklists he committed to memory.

"Never take details for granted. I have it all up here," he said and smiled at her while tapping his head. "But I still rely on the list. Miss something and big problems can happen."

She inherited a lot of her dad's qualities, but when plotting to escape from the whacko, none were as important as a deliberate mind.

Miss something and big problems can happen.

When they first met, the whacko wasn't all bad. He was passionate, an accomplished and respected artist. His presence, charisma, and charm were indisputable. But he was brooding and difficult to figure out—mysterious in a way that intrigued her more than frightened her. That intrigue faded as his appetite for restricting her free will increased. Her desire turned into repulsion as rapidly as his charm morphed into dominance. His desirable qualities were just bait for this trap. When she took the bait, the monster came to claim his catch.

In the beginning, they went out in public. But if she looked at another man—or as was more often the case, if he *thought* she'd so much as looked at another man—she'd pay the price. They stopped going out.

He was an authoritative and eloquent creative and professor, able to translate art theory into harnessed skill. His talent sparked ideological debate and drew the adoration of students and peers alike. Peers didn't often receive his attentions, but students—more aptly, female students like Patricia—always merited a special brand of scrutiny. Patricia later learned that he slept with dozens of students over the course of their relationship. He'd leave her bloodied because she had dared talk to someone in passing, then he'd wash her blood off his hands with indifference and go off to satisfy his carnal urges with a wide-eyed, impressionable student.

Patricia took responsibility for making two consequential mistakes. First, she was deficient at picking men, plain and simple. She was unsuccessful, even though she could count the numbers on one hand. She was never attracted to less-than-brilliant men, but at the expense of every other quality. With the whacko, his brilliance was his artistic talent. He was different, though, not one-faceted like the others. Brilliance alone quickly loses its appeal, but he had more: emotion, intensity, passion. He paid attention. Unfortunately, that attention turned into obsession and, ultimately, possession.

Her second mistake was being terrible at moving on from her bad choices. Four years with the whacko was four too many. But in this case, moving on wasn't an option. He scrutinized her every move and forced her to account for every bit of her day. It seemed he could read her intentions and interpret her actions from every angle. He stood over her as she paid the bills. He smelled each piece of her clothing for any proof of some perceived misdeed on her part—that she'd eaten something not contained in her brown bag work lunch, worn perfume, or sweated too much. He checked her for marks he hadn't inflicted. He threw away or burned every photo, note, and trinket he thought reminded her of her life before him. He made certain that none of her prior friends had any access to her.

She knew he studied her while she slept, hoping she'd sleep-talk some confession. No matter that he never uncovered anything—he seemed convinced she had to be plotting against him. She had nowhere to turn for safety or comfort or escape; he was a step ahead of her. The thought to run away would enter her mind, and he'd sense it and tell her that running away was no use. He'd find her if she ever tried. If she resolved not to come home from work one day, he'd show up at her office before quitting time to drive her home. Sometimes, he punched her cold and told her it was for whatever she was thinking about trying to get away with. She'd been strangled, beaten, kicked, punched, broken, pulled, pushed, and attacked constantly and without provocation in one form or another. He would never relent. That was why, when she landed in the ER, she knew her only options were escape or death.

But how? The one time she'd run away, he found her the next night. He'd guessed she would try to escape to her parents' house several hundred miles away. When he showed up, even though she was white as a ghost with fear, she went back with him without a word so she could spare her dad the knowledge of what was going on. If she'd said something, anything, her dad would have jumped in, and the whacko would've probably tried to kill them both. She couldn't bear the thought that someone else, *her own father*, might pay a price for her mistakes.

In a silent, impervious, dark place in her mind, Patricia began to plot. For more than a year, she plotted every detail until the day he sent her to the ER. Then she put her plan of escape in motion.

It was that same safe, inviolable place inside her that she often visited years later, when she was far away from the whacko, fighting for survival in a different way. Cancer would force her to visit that unbreakable life source again and again, drawing as much strength from inside as possible. She was diagnosed with cancer *five* different times over more than three decades. Still, her vigor and fortitude stayed strong, and her ability to overcome endured. Despite the incredible ordeals she endured, Patricia was a survivor, a trait she attributed to various aspects of her childhood experiences.

Beginning Balanced

Patricia was born in 1946 into a Southern California family that was fairly typical of those postwar times. Her father worked at a major aerospace company that had supported the war effort, and continued there until retirement, providing a comfortable living for his family. He met Patricia's mother there when she dropped out of college to help build warplanes. Patricia's mother later pursued a master's degree in education and, once Patricia was in primary school, went on to teach kindergarten in the public school system for thirty-five years.

Patricia experienced counterbalanced influences throughout her childhood, causing her emotional center to develop as a stable, unidealistic place from which to experience life. That grounded center would serve her well through the peaks and valleys of her life.

On one side of the ledger, her mom and dad loved and respected each other. They thought alike on most subjects, especially those affecting their children. They shared the same values on family responsibility, faith, and education. Her parents shared many interests—they were both avid private pilots and would take the family on spur-of-the-moment flights to the local deserts around Palm Springs for picnics or to the Big Bear Mountain area to visit Patricia's grandmother. Her parents gave Patricia a solid foundation by providing a safe home, a mutually respectful environment, and a strong dedication to levelheadedness, commitment, fortitude, a strong work ethic, and pragmatism.

On the other side of the ledger, as with all families, things weren't perfect. Patricia knew her parents loved each other—they were married for fifty years—but she wasn't sure they *liked* each other. Yes, they did things together, but flying planes wasn't done for the love of spending time together, necessarily; it was just something they did. Her dad had an engineer's mind and maintained his own planes, and her mom wasn't about to take a back seat, not even to her husband. They were civil toward each other but didn't seem to enjoy each other much. Patricia didn't remember her parents showing any affection to each other or their children. They lived in an entirely emotionless house.

Patricia *sensed* her father's quiet pride in her, but he didn't show it in action or words. She inferred it through the occasional glance or smile. Her father would sometimes tilt his head toward Patricia and slightly roll his eyes when her mother was being particularly stubborn or when she went on and on with her sometimes less-than-accurate pronouncements. Her mother was tough and unreadable. She seemed to never be pleased or satisfied; she displayed no tenderness. Her mother had no special glance or smile or kind words for Patricia. She was too detached emotionally to foster such displays.

Perhaps it was common in families formed during the baby boom, but feelings weren't conveyed through touch and words. Rather, things like love, respect, adoration, and recognition between parents and children were assumed. Adhering to familial responsibility, maintaining social accountability, and adopting a new standard of American-engineered orderliness were what passed for expressions of emotion.

Because Patricia was raised in a structured, emotionless environment, she had no choice as a young girl but to develop emotional self-reliance. She possessed a strong drive, which helped her complete the things she chose to undertake without the expectation of praise. She learned how to get by without approval. Patricia relied on herself, and she had the tools to accomplish what she wanted to. As a result, she matured early and didn't get rattled in the face of adversity or challenge.

Patricia also learned that consequences stemming from her actions were hers alone to bear. At thirteen, she decided to give up practicing Catholicism. It was just something she didn't want to continue doing. She shared her reasoning with her mother, and that was that. Decisions, important or trivial, were Patricia's to make. There was no lecturing or intense family discussions—she just wasn't interested in organized religion any longer, so she quit. After, her mother often made snide comments and treated her with disdain for her decision. That was to be expected, Patricia knew, because those were practical consequences of her decision.

Much like her father, Patricia's decision-making process was deliberate. Since she didn't dwell on the outcomes, she weighed the known factors that would influence her to go in one direction versus another. On the few times she made quick—even reckless—decisions, she didn't hold it against herself if things didn't turn out well. Patricia didn't dwell on any negative consequences. She lived her life looking forward, not backward. Her proclivity for stability eliminated any quest for adventure. She didn't dream of the future; she existed in the today.

Patricia attended college immediately after high school, but after three semesters, her father was transferred, and the family moved to Northern California. She enrolled in a local college and decided to get a job so that she could save money and one day move back to Southern California.

It wasn't unusual for a teenage girl's first job to be to work for the telephone company, which provided the opportunity to work different shifts, but Patricia wasn't planning to work with the last generation of switchboard operators. Instead, she applied for a position that would exploit her penchant for math and science. The phone company put her on a team in the new Northern California accounting center.

Computers were creating new and dynamically changing career opportunities, and Patricia's timing, work ethic, and smarts led to immediate advancement. She went to classes in the day and worked the swing shift each evening. Before her nineteenth birthday, Patricia was running the phone company's mainframe computer systems for all Northern California.

As much as computers and a degree and finding her way in the world occupied her, there was more inside. Patricia was a left-brained, prosaic, impassive person. She was a controlled thinker. Thus, from the outside, she may have appeared one-dimensional, but she wasn't. She privately yearned to be an artist.

For centuries in the science world, illustrators captured such things as medical procedures, anatomical systems representations, and surgical techniques by hand. In the 1960s, advancements in photographic technology—specifically lighting—were changing the field of medical illustration. But at the time, operating rooms were still rife with medical illustrators, since flash photography was forbidden due to the danger of oxygen explosion.

Patricia had entered college hoping to become a medical illustrator. They needed to possess an uncanny ability to depict the immense detail of the human body. The essence of Patricia's artistic ability was detail. The right side of her brain was also quite left-brained. She enrolled in both drawing and premed classes as a freshman.

The move to Northern California, though, necessitated a redirection of Patricia's energies. Art went to the back burner and became only an occasional indulgence. Her position at the phone company became the primary focus. She ended up completing the first two years of intended undergraduate studies but then turned her attention to computer science. On the balance, that was more practical than art—even than a practical art.

It was the summer of 1967. Patricia's parents were settled in San Jose, her brother was serving in Vietnam, and she was trying to find her way during a dynamic time in America. When she was born just twenty years prior, there was no self-expression-fueled revolution going on. Her upbringing epitomized the post-WWII, put-your-nose-to-the-grindstone mentality. Social conservatism and guarded optimism were the backdrop for her childhood.

But a cultural revolution had begun that year. New and unabashed expressions of peace and love were everywhere. Fighting against the war and racial inequality became the new motivations for a generation of Americans who were a scant decade removed from practicing taking cover under their desks during bomb raids. Patricia didn't get caught up in the cultural change. She was too structured, too sensible to get caught up in the radical changes fueling her generation. She was too busy standing tall at work, expressing herself in the confines of the classroom, and fighting the traffic on the way to Los Angeles to visit her high school boyfriend, whom she'd been dating for five years. She might've been the only nonhippy, nonrevolutionary artist of her generation in the entire San Francisco Bay area.

Becoming Unbalanced

When she was twenty-one, Patricia had saved enough money and moved back to Los Angeles. Shortly after, her boyfriend proposed. He professed that he wasn't capable of love but that he did respect and care for her. He was smart and planning on attending law school after his military service. They had mutual friends and had known each other for years. They were all prudent, sensible reasons to embark on a life together. Marrying him seemed the logical thing to do.

But there was one problem: Their relationship wasn't about love or sharing things or counting on each other. None of those had been important to her parents, and Patricia hadn't believed they would be to her, but as she entered adulthood, she began to want more. Her boyfriend was a default choice, made not out of love but out of convenience and familiarity. Once Patricia opened her eyes to the other side of the spectrum, their relationship was doomed to fail. Soon after the wedding, her husband was shipped out halfway around the world to fight in a war few people could make sense of.

Then, as these things often happen, she met a handsome, mysterious, wayfaring artist. He didn't have his act together as her husband did. He didn't have *anything* together. He was, in every imaginable way, the opposite of what she'd always known, especially his proclamations of being madly in love with Patricia—which was the exact impetus she needed to embrace the changes happening inside of her. A year later, when her husband came home from Vietnam, they amicably ended their marriage, and she jumped into a new one.

It took Patricia a few years to figure it out, but Mr. Didn't Have His Act Together never got his act together. After they married, she quit school so he could have the chance to get his degree. She worked and paid the bills, and he let her. She put all she had, financially and otherwise, into trying to make something out of nothing, even giving up on her own art. They drifted apart, but Patricia allowed the relationship to linger, living together for close to five years as hostile roommates. Once he was done with school and had finally decided to start working, Patricia could walk away more easily. She started attending classes at night so she could finish her own undergraduate degree. She began building new friendships. She started creating art again.

While studying for her degree, Patricia decided to take more art classes. It was time she focused on the things that were important to her. She knew she had remarkable talent; she had just never made art a priority. She was able to transfer her affinity for meticulousness into art in a way that compelled the viewer to lose themselves in her sweeping, intricate drawings. One professor took a particular interest in her work—and in her.

He was exciting, intellectual, and worldly—she was hooked. She left her "roommate," sold her condo, and willingly put the proceeds and her savings into the professor's bank account when she moved in with him. But the curtain hiding the monster soon dropped.

The whacko beat her mercilessly for four years. It was not an exaggeration that she came to believe he'd someday kill her in a jealous rage.

Unhinged

With help from her friend Melinda, Patricia was able to plan and execute her escape. She'd siphoned off unnoticeably small amounts of money here and there and made cash deposits to an account Melinda opened for her. She planned to simultaneously have her car painted, get the license plates changed, and have all communications forwarded to a P.O. box beginning the day she fled. She snuck some clothes out of the house, one article at a time, by double layering her clothes on the way out and stashing the extra pieces in a private cubby at work. Her plan was conceived over years and carried out over months—she was a master of detail—and Patricia waited for the right combination of forces and planning to come together. There could be no trace of her whereabouts. She'd have to walk out of the house and never look back.

At last, that day came. Patricia woke up from a restless sleep and got dressed for work. There was no somber walk around the house, no need to double check for personal mementos, no doubts, no second-guessing. Nothing was as important as escaping, no item worth her life. She drove to work, grabbed the stashed clothes, and told her boss that an emergency had arisen and she was going to take an immediate leave of absence. She provided no information, no forwarding address. Who cared if she had to forgo her final paycheck? She wasn't about to give the whacko a clue about where to look for her when he came around her workplace, which she knew he would do.

She was worried the whacko would be waiting around the corner, in the lobby, or in the parking lot or hiding in the back seat of her car, but her decision was made. Each item on her mental list was checked off. Whatever would come now would come.

It was still morning, but Melinda had reserved a hotel room for Patricia under a fictitious name. Patricia drove an hour out of town, switched the license plates, dropped her car off at the automotive paint mechanic Melinda had arranged an appointment with, and then walked two blocks to the hotel. Of course, she couldn't help thinking *he* was going to drive right up, grab her, and push her into his car.

She made it to the room without a hitch. Just to be safe, she bolted the door and closed the drapes before lying on the twin bed and closing both eyes.

A few hours after falling asleep, Patricia startled awake. It took a second for her to put the pieces together: She was safe in a hotel room and only Mel knew where she was.

Patricia wasn't ready to call her parents. What would she tell them? After all, she'd gone the better part of four years without much communication with them—the whacko had cut her off from family. She was afraid if she did call them, her mom wouldn't believe her story and her dad would be crushed, especially when he realized there'd been an opportunity to save her when she'd run home previously. She might have been able to handle her mom's denial, but there was no way she could have put her dad through that kind of stress. Patricia knew the whacko would stalk every possible person he could think of, including her parents, Melinda, and every person in her world. But she had friends the whacko didn't know about.

Kent and Chris were friends made from odd beginnings. Patricia had met them at a Charlie Brown's restaurant while having a predinner cocktail with her then-husband, a couple of months before enrolling in the night classes that would ultimately trap her in the whacko's web. The hostess that night offered either couple the only table available, a four-top, but since they had met while waiting in the bar, they agreed to share the table and join each other for dinner. Patricia relished the opportunity to share time with people other than her hostile roommate, even if they were complete strangers. As luck would have it, the chance encounter bloomed into an immediate friendship. The two couples spent a lot of time together before she met the whacko and had to fall out of touch. When she thought about a safe haven, it was Kent and Chris who kept coming to mind. The whacko had never heard of them, and she hadn't written their number down in her address book. It had been four years since they'd spoken, but she believed they were her best chance.

Of course, she didn't know if they would or could help her—or if they'd even remember her. Every once in a while at work, Patricia had looked at the scrap of paper she'd written their phone number on. She knew it would have been pointless, even dangerous for them, if she'd stayed in contact. That little note, with just the name "Charlie Brown" and a phone number on it, held all the hope she dared muster in that dark hotel room. She dialed it with shaky hands.

"Hello?" The voice was soft and friendly and faintly familiar.

"Chris?" Patricia squeezed the name out of her dry mouth.

"Yes."

"It's Patricia. It's, well . . . I know it's been a very long time."

The line was silent for a few seconds that seemed an eternity.

"Oh, goodness! Patricia? It's been so long! I'm so happy to hear your voice."

Tears streamed down Patricia's flushed cheeks. She told Chris the story of the previous four years. Everything had been kept inside for so long that when it came out, it sounded like part apology, part confession. But she was able to get it all out in one sobering stream.

"So, you're safe, right?" Chris asked after Patricia finished.

"I'm pretty sure, for now. But I don't want to stay here."

"Can you come to our house? Are you able to do that?"

"Is that okay?" Patricia asked.

"Absolutely. We'll be here until you show up."

Patricia threw her clothes into her bag, picked up her freshly painted and re-plated car, and drove off with hope for the fresh start she'd quietly dreamed of for what seemed an eternity.

Rebalancing

Kent was a pilot with a pilot friend, Dave, who owned a vacant condo unit near them. Kent and Chris arranged things with Dave, and within a few days, Patricia had a new home. She ended up only a couple dozen miles away from the whacko, but it soon seemed a million miles away.

There were nights early on when Patricia hid in the dark, scared out of her wits, too afraid to move toward a window or even turn on a light. It didn't matter that her door was double-bolted or that a locked gate protected the condo building itself. It took weeks before she was able to keep her anxiety at bay. She didn't want to leave anything to chance—the whacko wouldn't simply give up trying to find her.

Those first few weeks, Dave came over to work on the outside of the unit. She would close the drapes, bolt the door, anything to stay hidden. What if she were recognized?

Dave knew Patricia was fragile, as Kent and Chris had spoken frankly with Dave prior to her moving in so he'd know who he was renting his place to and what risks might come with that. After several visits and a few brief exchanges with Dave from the other side of her door, Patricia gathered the nerve to open the drapes, unbolt the door, and open it without holding her breath that someone was hiding out of sight, ready to attack her. She invited Dave in for coffee one day.

Handing the cup to Dave, Patricia's hands trembled slightly, but her gaze and face were calm. She'd forgotten the feeling of physical safety and found it hard to completely relax around others, but she concealed her nervousness well. After all, she knew Dave was no danger to her. She had the feeling somehow that she was safe in his presence.

Patricia didn't so much *watch* Dave as they shared their coffee—she *contemplated* him. Dave's demeanor was hauntingly familiar. Patricia wasn't one for nostalgia, but watching Dave as he talked reminded her of the happiest days of her childhood. The way his eyes wrinkled at the corners when he talked, and the way his head cocked to the side when he listened, reminded her of her dad and an uncle, Bill.

Dave appeared analytical, contemplative, stoic, and somehow unshakable, like someone who'd never panic in a storm. She could read those things in the way he smiled and in the deep creases of his temple, because she'd once been familiar with how those qualities showed themselves in men his age—more so because those qualities were absent from the men she'd known since leaving her girlhood behind almost twenty years before. Dave radiated *goodness*, the kind of unforced, natural goodness that radiates from within. She knew all this about Dave before they'd finished their first cup of coffee together.

• • •

Weeks and months passed by post-whacko, giving way to years of freedom and safety. The bumps in Patricia's life disappeared. She'd found a new, well-paying computer systems analyst job, which filled her closet with suits and her bank account with savings. She navigated a fair amount of the distance between fear and comfort, which helped her regain her confidence and positive outlook on what life might bring. She found herself unafraid to spend time with others, including men—including Dave.

During this stretch of time, Dave was a constant. They learned about themselves with and through each other, and they developed trust. They were both able to shed the weight of the bad times, bad decisions, bad relationships, and wasted years they each carried around, and each had mostly become the person they wanted to be.

Some marriages that start later in life come about because the freshness of life wears off over time and people end up settling, but others come about because life finally begins to feel fresh. Patricia knew that she didn't *need* someone to spend the rest of her life with. When Dave asked her to marry him, though, she recognized that she was in the freshest, lightest, best place she had ever been. Thinking it over with a calm and uncluttered mind, she knew it was okay to need Dave.

Settling into her new life meant she didn't need to settle for less than an ideal existence. The ups and downs of Patricia's life became a thing of the past. She was in a safe, loving relationship, not just living a life she hoped for but living the one she had always yearned for. She thrived at a challenging career, was fulfilled at home, created art, and slept the deep and peaceful sleep of the untroubled. Things were going so well, Patricia decided to undergo surgery to fix a misaligned jaw, then get braces to fix her teeth. She had never liked her smile much, and these days she was smiling much more often.

Dave was flying to Washington, DC, when she went in for surgery. Other than some annoying itching that she disclosed to the doctor, there was nothing to inspire concern on her preprocedural write-up—she was in excellent health. The surgery went well. Several days later, the doctor called her up.

"Is your husband back in town yet?" he asked in an alarmingly measured tone.

"Yes. Why?" Patricia asked.

"We'll discuss the whole situation when you come back in—together, of course."

The next day, Dave and Patricia went to see her doctor, and the untroubled life that had taken decades to achieve threatened to slip away like grains of sand. The doctor had ordered some precautionary blood tests. At thirty-nine, Patricia had cancer. The diagnosis was advanced Hodgkin's disease.

"You'll need to find an oncologist," the doctor said.

• • •

Patricia had cared for people, but she had learned not to *rely* on others for her happiness. Sitting in the doctor's office, it didn't occur to her to panic. But she had found the love she'd waited for, and it shook her as she sat stunned, staring at the doctor. Her chair spun around in circles; her head erupted in chaos. And yet, she couldn't turn to look in Dave's eyes. *What is Dave going to do?* she thought. Life was so good because of Dave. *How could I do this to such a sweet, caring man?*

Patricia tried to pull her gaze away from the doctor. *Look at him. Turn and look. Show him you're okay. Turn your head!* She made the chair stop spinning, calmed the wave of fear crashing against the inside of her skull. The sounds

from the doctor's mouth stopped floating around the room and began to float
into her ears.

"... is very serious. You can't wait even a day to deal with this," the doctor
continued.

Patricia finally turned to Dave. She peered into his eyes. *I'll be okay*, Patricia
thought, but she saw Dave's panic. She *felt* his panic.

"We'll be okay," she told him.

"What do we need to do first, again?" she asked the doctor, though she was
still looking at Dave.

When you have someone who cares about you so much, it just has to be okay,
right?

• • •

Hodgkin's lymphoma is a cancer that attacks the lymphatic system, which is
part of the immune system. Although severe, Patricia's cancer was treatable.
She had a staging laparotomy—a procedure where they cut her open and
examined the extent of the cancer inside her—to determine where the cancer may have spread. The results: stage IIIS, having affected lymph nodes on
both sides of her diaphragm and spread to her spleen. This led the doctors
to remove her spleen. After, because of the advancement of the cancer, they
did total nodal radiation therapy with a linear accelerator over a six-month
period. Once complete, her doctor gave her one drug to help overcome the
effects of radiation on her thyroid and another to make up for its effect on
her ovarian function.

The amount of confusing and incomplete information she was expected to
process during each step of treatment was mind-boggling. More distressing
than that was the sheer volume of questions in Patricia's mind. The doctors
certainly knew more about the cancer than she did, but it was exasperating
that she seemed to know and pay more attention to her body than the physicians did and that too many of her questions about the treatments and their
effects weren't answered.

So Patricia educated herself. She read everything she could find and decided
to start a journal. She wrote down how she felt each day, what she ate, what her
mood was, what surgeries had occurred and the outcome, what medicines she

was taking, and what side effects she was experiencing. She showed up at her doctor's appointments with current articles and copies of pages from relevant books she found at the library. She pressed her caregivers to give her more information. As she began to understand more about what she was going through, she challenged them to better explain her prognosis, treatment options, and outcomes. She wasn't going to leave anything unanswered again if she could help it, and she wasn't going to leave anything to chance.

Of course, her efforts helped her understand and deal with the logistics of her treatment, but the emotional component was another thing altogether. Where her deep-seated, matter-of-fact, businesslike approach helped her better navigate the medically related roads her illness took her on, she had an awakening related to the emotional roads she began traveling down. Cancer quickly enhanced Patricia's view on life, forcing her to look deep within herself. She realized that now more than ever, she needed to determine how she was going to live her life—however much she had left. As a result, she felt a more profound appreciation for each minute of her days, even when they were filled with pain and confusion and uncertainty, because she knew what it felt like to wonder how many days she might have left.

Trying to take back some control over her medical journey didn't prevent the cancer from damaging Patricia, nor did it lessen the severity of her treatment, but it did allow her to become a better informed, more active participant in her recovery.

Her cancer experience also caused Patricia to immediately and purposefully concentrate on making the most of each new opportunity to reshape her thinking. But it didn't make everything better or easier in her interpersonal relationships—especially when it came to her parents.

• • •

When it came to trauma, two recurring dynamics existed in her family. As much as Patricia hoped those dynamics might change, she wasn't optimistic about it when she and Dave decided to tell her parents in person, rather than over the phone, when she was first diagnosed with cancer. First, her mom always checked out when any negative talk happened, as if she either didn't care or wasn't taking the discussion seriously. Second, Patricia was hesitant to share anything too serious or negative because she couldn't stand to see her dad's heart break. She knew she wouldn't have to work to get her dad to believe her, unlike her mother, but she couldn't bring herself to burden him. As a result, in their family, nobody talked candidly about anything serious. And nothing was more serious than cancer.

"You don't need anybody. I feel sorry for you." Patricia had heard her mom say those words many times as a teenager, and she'd seen them again written on her mother's face when she had tried to explain why she'd been out of touch for long periods of time in the past. This time, though, she and Dave were driving to San Jose to tell her parents about the cancer.

Will she feel sorry for me now? I do need people, just not the way she thinks. I need Dave. I need my friends, Dad, and even her. She can't still feel sorry for me, can she?

What her mom didn't care to understand was that just because Patricia wasn't lonely when she was alone, or because she relied on herself when she was in trouble, didn't mean that she preferred solitude to being with people she loved.

She thinks I've exaggerated the bad things in my life, but if she only knew.

Deep down, Patricia knew what to expect, but until she saw her parents' faces, she hoped things might go differently. Instead, Patricia chose not to elaborate on the details of her cancer diagnosis and potential outcomes. As predicted, just sharing her diagnosis and intended treatment regimen gave her mom cause to drift away. Even skimming over things was enough to make her dad struggle to hide his torment.

"If I hadn't wanted to get braces, who knows when they'd have found the cancer," she said, smiling to lighten the atmosphere.

"So, you're not going to get them, of course?" her mom asked.

"No. I'll get them. Why not? I'd love straighter teeth."

"See, it's not so serious, then, right?" her mom replied.

Patricia looked at her dad. "Right. Not that serious," she said.

It was a short and predictably sterile visit.

• • •

Surgery, radiation, and chemotherapy ensued over many months, along with endless testing, poking, and prodding. Throughout it all, Patricia's will to move on stayed strong. She desperately wanted to get back to her life. She was determined to beat the cancer, no matter what.

She was rewarded when her body finally overcame the Hodgkin's and she was able to put the experience behind her. *Right. Not that serious.* After making some last notes on the day she received the results that her cells were cancer-free, she closed the journal for what she thought would be the last time.

After the treatments ended, Patricia decided to go back and get a master's degree in art. The college the whacko taught at happened to be the only logical place to finish her art studies, and she knew running into him was a possibility, but she wasn't going to let that stop her. She could take classes at night, when he rarely taught. Besides, her hair was much shorter and almost seven years had passed, so it was possible he wouldn't notice her if she could avoid running into him face-to-face.

She enrolled and began taking classes. She loved it, and months into the program, she was certain she was on the right path. She and Dave determined they had the means for her to stop working, and she could fill her days with the more gratifying things in her life, such as pursuing art, volunteering, and becoming active in The Wellness Community to help others who were going through cancer diagnoses and treatment.

Thoughts of seeing the whacko continued to run through her mind, although they lessened over time. After all, she had given up thinking about him since the day she opened the drapes and felt unafraid to stand in the daylight. But one night while on a class break, she was walking to the vending machine area, and there he was. *He walked right past me. Keep going. He didn't see you.* Blood flushed her face, and her grip on her bag tightened.

"Patricia! Come here!" came his voice from behind her. Chills ran up the backs of her legs to the top of her skull. *You can turn around and face that monster now. It's your choice.* She turned to face him. He stopped within a couple of feet of her.

"What are you doing here?" he asked. He was smaller than she remembered.

"My master's, but it's really none of your business, is it?"

He narrowed his eyes and snorted. She watched him looking her over and felt sick. His eyes fixed on the ring she wore on her left hand, and his face turned red.

"How?" he asked and pointed his eyes at her ring.

He had long since lost all power over Patricia. Her emotional strength—every bit of it—had returned. She knew she was free of him, completely, and had been for a long time. Standing there, seeing how pathetic and powerless he looked, she knew that a lifetime had passed. She smiled, turned around, and walked away without saying another word. *I don't owe him a thing.* That was that. She never saw him again.

Several more years went by. Patricia volunteered at the Cancer Support Community and created her intricate and detailed artwork. She finished her master's degree, Dave continued to fly, and weekends were spent driving to Arizona to water-ski and enjoy Kent, Chris, and other friends. Aside from her dad having a brief scare with prostate cancer, the roads in Patricia's life were smooth and easy.

But what goes up must come down.

The Teeter-Totter Never Stops

In 1993, seven years after her cancer diagnosis, Patricia's dad's cancer returned in a very aggressive fashion. He wouldn't be expected to live more than several months. She didn't know if she could handle his death emotionally, not because there were unresolved issues between them but because she loved and admired him so much. They weren't going to be able to get the time together that they should have—honestly, that they could have tried better to get for so many years.

Patricia and Dave agreed that she needed to do all she could to see him. She decided she'd drive the nearly four hundred miles north and spend as much time with him as possible, which might help ease her feelings of regret.

Between her first and second trips, Patricia went to her oncologist. She'd felt some suspicious swelling in her chest and insisted on a biopsy. Two days later, she found out she had a tumor in her upper left chest. Her Hodgkin's had relapsed.

Patricia needed to start a ten-cycle regimen of ABVD, the most common combination of drugs used to treat Hodgkin's. But she wasn't going to let cancer keep her from her dad. She wouldn't be able to stay near him, but a plan emerged: She would have the drug infusions on a Friday. For four or five days, she'd become increasingly sicker. When the ill effects waned, she'd drive herself up to Northern California so she could spend time with her dad and help take care of him. Several days after, Patricia would head back to Los Angeles and receive another of her biweekly treatments.

Patricia didn't mind that Dave was flying a lot or that she was driving to her parents' house on her own, because things were easier when Dave was away, and she only had to worry about what she and her dad were going through. Prior to her dad fighting terminal cancer, Patricia knew how hard it was on the caregiver because she'd watched Dave that first time around—but she didn't know how hard. This time, though, the treatment regimen was dramatically more taxing on Patricia. With a better understanding of how much more difficult it was to watch someone you love go through cancer than it was to go through it on your own, she was thankful Dave could get some reprieve from everything by continuing to work.

Everything included a mixed bag of issues to deal with. In addition to hair loss, the side effects of Patricia's chemotherapy included nonstop nausea, vomiting, diarrhea, and unshakable fatigue. Like all chemo patients, she lost her appetite. It was crucial to ingest calories, but the thought of eating was almost always enough to wrench her insides.

"I want something salty, crunchy, and cheap. I'll throw it all up anyway," she told Dave after the first cycle ended and she could even contemplate eating.

He left the house and returned with a bag filled with Taco Bell tacos. *Really? A whole bag full of tacos?* She smiled inside. When she did lean on him to do something for her during her cancer ordeals, he went all the way with it. The tacos worked. Patricia could usually get part of one down, but more importantly, she managed to *keep* it down. If she finished the first, she'd never get much past a bite or two of the second, but Dave never came home with fewer than five or six.

Patricia wasn't going to let Dave hold her head as she threw up, subject him to seeing her at her sickest, or even be too close when she was at her worst if she could help it. It was bad enough he had to see her preparing to lose her dad, but to also watch her battle cancer again was more than Patricia could allow. She had to take care of her dad. She had to get better for Dave.

It didn't come easy, but Patricia managed to gather enough strength during those four and a half months of chemotherapy to see her dad often. Not surprisingly, Patricia and her dad didn't talk much. Just being together was a comfort each could draw from. The idea of seeing him die slowly settled into her psyche. *She* wasn't dying. She was being *treated*, and her prognosis was relatively good. But being helpless to do anything other than just watch her dad die was unbearable. She'd have done anything to make it go away for him—she would have taken it on herself—but the reality was she couldn't do either. He died before her treatments ended.

Speaking at her dad's funeral was out of the question. The dam would have broken, and who knew what damage the emotional flood would cause? It was better to deal with those emotions inside. After all, there was no way she could be open with her mother about her father's death or her own cancer. She knew that denial about the reality of cancer was what her mother needed.

In her own home, though, things were different. Patricia was keenly aware of the weight and stress Dave felt watching her go through chemo, then again when she took in over three thousand rads once the full chemo treatment was completed. She didn't want to see him tortured by what was happening to her physically, but unlike with her parents, they talked openly and often. Their conversations left nothing unsettled or unclear between them—not about her mom and dad, not about her, and not about the cancer. This was her life, and nothing with him was off limits or hidden or left for another day.

Another day might not always come, she'd think. *I won't waste my time sweeping anything under the rug with Dave.* So they didn't. With as much as they dealt with, they continued to live their lives as normally as possible. Patricia tried her best not to allow her cancer experience to rule her life. When she felt up to it during treatment, she and Dave got out of the house and saw friends, took short drives, and enjoyed the fresh air. When she didn't feel up to it, they didn't leave the house.

In June, a few months after her dad died and a few weeks before her final chemo treatment was to be administered, Patricia and Dave went to Lake Mojave with Kent and Chris. The air was filled with rosemary and the kind of dust that lingers in the waves of Arizona summer heat. She and Dave were going for a boat ride. She didn't feel up to water-skiing, but she wanted to be out in the heat, on the water, with the wind on her face, close to their friends. She let go of Dave's hand.

"I'll be back in a minute," she said.

Patricia wore scarves and hats when she wanted, but not having hair didn't bother her. She didn't have the energy or the inclination to worry about what anybody thought. The people who cared about her understood, and that was all that mattered. She unwrapped the scarf on her head and put her hat back on. As she turned to leave, she caught a glimpse of herself in the mirror. She walked over and stood in front of it. *You're quite a sight, Patricia, aren't you?*

She scanned her face. She looked good. She wished she had eyebrows, but she looked good. More importantly, she *felt* incredible—not so perfect physically, but she was enjoying being alive. She smiled at herself, and seeing her straight teeth made her smile more. She knew that if that first diagnosis had been further delayed, if she hadn't wanted to fix her smile, her prognosis could have been far worse. *Everybody has their time in the barrel, don't they? You were just given a few extra turns.*

She pulled herself away from her reflection—and self-reflection—and went out into the warmth.

Turns in the Barrel

A couple of years later, Patricia found a melanoma. The doctors had insisted it was nothing, but she pressed for it to be tested. Malignant. Cancer #3. Fortunately, it was excised before it metastasized.

Not a big deal, again.

In 2007, a decade later and nearly fourteen years after she was treated for her second battle with Hodgkin's, Patricia was diagnosed with cancer yet again. That time, though, she didn't have the luxury of treating her diagnosis in the usual workmanly Patricia manner. She couldn't bring pragmatism to the battle—the cancer was too aggressive. Nor could she bring an optimistic approach either, as there was no room for hope. It was too advanced. The only way to deal with the new diagnosis was an odd combination of desperation, patience, and acceptance of the reality that she was in a fight she couldn't win.

Patricia had been tested every year, at least, after 1986's initial Hodgkin's diagnosis and full nodal radiation: gallium scans; mammograms; MRIs and CT scans of her chest, pelvis, and abdomen; ultrasounds of her thyroid; and more. For what seemed years, she kept feeling a hard lump at the bottom of her sternum, but tests produced no answers. In 2006, she convinced her doctors to dig further, and they did a slew of new tests. Finally, in February of 2007, a chest X-ray showed a mass. They did a biopsy of the sternum lump and it came back positive—a horrible answer, but an answer to what she had felt for years. After a consultation with the Stanford breast tumor board, it became clear that it was stage III breast cancer she'd had for probably eight or nine years. They also discovered an advanced and rare thyroid cancer. Each was a potential death sentence—together, there was little chance for survival.

Because the thyroid cancer was a potentially lethal form of cancer, they would need to remove the entire thyroid. But she immediately needed to start a chemo treatment for the breast cancer. There was a ticking time bomb in her throat, but the thyroid surgery would have to wait.

Patricia spent the better part of 2007 in chemotherapy treatment and recovering from multiple surgeries. By summer of that year, she had a bilateral mastectomy, nine lymph nodes removed—five of which tested positive for cancer—her thyroid taken out, and many other procedures related to both cancers.

In the years since that brutal time in 2007, Patricia has had countless other issues, including heart and lung problems from all the radiation and chemotherapy, a complete hysterectomy, removal of her ovaries, an appendectomy, Barrett's esophagus, and more. She became so used to having surgeries to remove yet another part of her insides that when she encountered cancer, or some collateral issue, she'd tell her doctors: "Just cut out anything I don't need to stay alive—take whatever you need to before it causes problems." And they did.

"You've been at my practice longer than I have," her oncologist joked one day. "I don't know how you've stayed alive, but somehow you have."

"Well, maybe because I've never been sick a day in my life. Besides the cancer, that is. I've often said, 'I don't get colds, I get cancer!'"

Patricia knew she'd been lucky. She'd dealt with cancer for more than thirty years. But she'd also lost friends and doctors in arguments about correct statistics, out-of-date information, and glossed-over side effects. Her journaling definitely helped her know when to seek help. It provided both a roadmap and a record of the monstrous cancer journey she endured over the decades. As a result, she became an active self-advocate, an undeterred, battle-strong warrior.

For certain, she's had her fair share of time in the barrel.

Patricia's Epilogue

No matter how rough things got for Patricia, she brought a constructive, if somewhat narrow, perspective to her life: She wanted to live, enjoy Dave, make a difference with her survivorship work, and most of all, not allow the cancers to define her.

"Keeping my head up and looking forward is the only way I know how to be," she explained to me one day. "When I retired thirty years ago, I put all my suits neatly in the closet. It's doubtful I'll ever take them out again, but I loved working, and I can't make myself get rid of them. You never know what might happen down the road, so be prepared. But you gotta live your life, you know what I mean? Even if it means fighting death and moving on."

When her friend Melinda, whom I had the chance to talk to a few times, mentioned that she didn't know if she could've handled the things Patricia had gone through, I tried to imagine it myself. Could *I*? But there's no imagining Patricia-like epics of diagnosis, treatment, test, surgery—rinse and repeat.

Perhaps what makes Patricia so unique is that she doesn't look at what she's endured as suffering and hardship but rather as issues that needed to be addressed, however they needed to be.

"How does one learn to think like you?" I asked, turning to her for insight and guidance.

"Oh. I don't know about that," she said. "I didn't always get out of the bed every day. Sometimes it got the better of me. But if I got up, I made my bed, went about my day, and never once gave in and went back under the covers. You take control of your life in the ways you can. For me, that meant living my life no matter what I'd had to deal with. You face it, you try to understand it, and you take control when you can. You press doctors to understand what you're going through. You rely on the people who love you. You just make the most of everything you do and live life on purpose."

I still haven't met Patricia in person. I was hoping to see her, along with the four other book participants who are located in the Greater Los Angeles area, on the busy first two days of the bike ride, but she had to cancel our rendezvous because she needed to help her mother with some medical issues. Typical Patricia.

Patricia has spent thousands of hours helping others. In fact, she receives about two dozen calls a month seeking help. Inquiries come from friends, referrals from friends, through the Cancer Support Community she has volunteered with since the mid-1980s, and from sources unknown. She talks to everyone, empathizes, listens, directs them to valuable resources, and is never shy to talk about her strong belief that people need to take charge of their treatment options by learning, asking questions, and being relentless in pursuit of accurate and informed care.

When I described her as a caretaker in the summary I wrote for each of the book participants, she scoffed at the description. Patricia doesn't see her work helping people such as her mother and those she counsels about cancer as caretaking, because to her, caretaking connotes caring for others. Rather, she believes she is attending to herself—*she's* the beneficiary. For Patricia, helping others is a form of self-care.

I asked Patricia what will happen if she receives another diagnosis.

"I don't really think about that," she said. "At this point, I've had all the radiation and chemo one can have, and, well, there's not much more they can cut out. Besides, I don't like to think about how Dave might take it. He's been through so much with me. I guess if cancer comes after me again, I might just ride off into the sunset with it."

Near the end of our talks, Patricia told me that her longtime friend Kent had been diagnosed with an aggressive and terminal form of brain cancer. Chris was having a hard time, and Patricia spent a lot of time with them both while Kent was dying. I detected a small loss of spirit in Patricia's voice. Kent and Chris had been such huge influences in her life. But more than that, I listened with a better understanding of Patricia's true essence as she told me in her stoic, grounded way how she counseled her friends on the reality of their situation, how she was grateful to be able to help them through such tragedy.

There's nothing trite or cliché in Patricia's approach to life, death, and everything in between. When she told me once that she recognized every falling leaf and felt appreciation for every iota of her existence, I didn't understand what that meant until I heard her whole story. *We all have our time in the barrel*, I sometimes think, borrowing her phrase. But as much time as she may have spent there, she's spent so much more in the sunlight.

• • •

Patricia also was not scarred by her parents' absence during her toughest times with the whacko, nor her mother's longstanding dispassion and hard-hearted demeanor, but those very things in my own life have scarred me. My childhood is awash with memories of my mother as a bitter woman whose anger at the world was as intense and overbearing as the Los Angeles summer smog of my youth. I don't always feel the rub of the injury, but when I do, I know there probably won't be any revelation or deliverance, and that is tormenting for me. Patricia is at peace with her parents and the way her life has gone in that regard. I'm not, and talking to Patricia showed me how close to the surface those feelings are.

I thought about my discussions with Patricia many times as I pedaled down long, quiet roads on my journey, and my mind visited many facets of her story, not the least of which was her ability to come to terms with the more difficult times in her life. In my head, I heard and understood what Patricia meant when she told me: "There's nothing to forgive. Things are what they are. Mom is just being Mom." But in my heart, her words were unintelligible. I failed whenever I tried to think of my own mom as "just being Mom." I still had so much to learn, regardless of the self-discoveries or self-healing I had done while biking through Florida.

A Dark and Lonely State of Mind

W ith just days to go, I was fairly certain I'd make it, but the burning in my legs was like nothing I'd ever felt in my life. I had so much accumulated lactic acid buildup that when I began to pedal, my legs instantly lit on fire from ankle to hip. To flush the fire, I'd have to get in my easiest gear, slowly spin my legs against as little resistance as possible, and wait for the pain to subside. Only then could I increase the gearing—and resistance— one gear click at a time until I found a cadence that would move me forward with as little discomfort as possible. Red lights were cruel, as stops and slow starts were excruciating. Climbs were plain insufferable, and Virginia is not a flat state.

Day forty-one, from South Hill to Fredericksburg, was some 111 miles long with more than three thousand feet of rolling hills and dozens and dozens of red lights, traffic jams, and so many stops and starts that my legs felt in flames almost every minute of the eleven-plus hours I rode that day.

Erin surprised me with cookies, candy, and a sandwich in Bowling Green, about twenty miles short of Fredericksburg. She'd gone ahead to check into the hotel but came back to give me those goodies knowing how spent I'd be. After the break, she went ahead to meet up with her friend April, who'd come down from Washington, DC, and left me to navigate the last two hours refreshed and invigorated. Of course, five minutes into biking again, the invigoration subsided and I again felt unrefreshed.

With ten miles to go, I veered off Highway 2—the shoulder was too narrow, and the traffic was too severe—and I rerouted to my destination via side roads. At first, I congratulated myself on a smart decision, but as the large, well-lit neighborhoods near the highway gave way to more rural, unlit ones, I became worried.

Oh, look at that house. Scary looking. Where are all the streetlights? Why are the houses getting further back from the street? That house sounds like it has ten dogs barking. Who needs ten dogs? Really, a chainsaw? At this hour? Why is that car driving with no lights on?

I was convinced I'd entered some *The Blair Witch Project*-like section of rural Virginia, where bad things were going to happen—especially to a stranger who, with all the bags on his bike, must surely be alone, who might not be missed. My imagination got the better of me. I couldn't stop. I couldn't turn around. I just had to get out of there, pedal faster, and avoid the killers lurking in the darkness. I turned my safety lights off. Better not to be seen. I never coasted, because the sound of ball bearings in the rear wheel might empower a faster-moving vehicle to chase me down. I could only pedal fast and hard. My head darted toward every sound. I listened intently after passing every driveway in case the killers were intrigued by the sound of desperate prey. The cold air chilled my fingers and toes, making pedaling and holding the handlebars that much harder, but I dared not stop to put on a jacket. It was only a matter of time; I was certain of it.

A hundred turns, fifteen mini heart attacks, and thirty minutes later, ambient lights from Fredericksburg lit the sky. I was almost safe. I didn't dare look behind me, because I didn't want to see what threat was surely coming after me.

I told Erin and April what had happened as we sat in the warm and safe Capital Ale House enjoying dinner. We laughed at the ridiculousness of my overtired, overactive mind, but I couldn't laugh about the very real feelings of fear, anxiety, and even terror—regardless of how irrational they might've been—that still rumbled in my gut.

It made me think of one of the book participants, Diep, whose fear and anxiety about the health issues she was facing were anything but absurd. They were rational, well-founded, sensible feelings to have about the unknown.

Diep

Relationship to cancer: Patient and medical professional

Age: Fifty-five

Family status: Married with three children

Location: Manhattan Beach, California

First encounter with cancer: At twenty-six, she encountered cancer as a professional while in residency. Her father died from lymphoma in his seventies.

Cancer summary: Diep learned about cancer in medical school. In the past, she's had nonmalignant atypical meningioma tumors removed from her brain. Diep has been forced to give up her career in obstetrics and gynecology due to debilitating migraine headaches and other physical maladies that could have been caused by the tumors.

Treatment specifics: Craniotomy to remove tumor. Radiation therapy to kill any remaining tumor cells. The fear of cancer is ever-present.

Strongest positive emotion during cancer experience: Eagerness

Strongest negative emotion during cancer experience: Distress

How we met: When my twins were six, I put them on the local parks and recreation swim team. I wasn't exceedingly outgoing or interactive with the other parents, who typically just dropped their kids off anyway. One day as I was running laps around the small park surrounding the pool, one of the other parents came running up behind me.

Juan was the spitting image of the Latino musician Marc Anthony, and he smiled as he introduced himself. He shared his happiness at how beautiful the day was, how great it felt to be able to go for a run while his kids did their swim training, and how nice everyone who worked at the pool was. He rattled off one happy observation after another as we made our way around and around the pool's perimeter fence. At first, it was hard for me to swallow that anybody could genuinely be as positive as Juan appeared to be. But in the fifteen years since that day, I don't think I've told anybody about my friend Juan without swearing up and down that he actually *is* the nicest and happiest person I've ever known. As we dried off our kids after practice, Juan made me agree to a casual dinner at his house later that week.

As I drove up to his house for dinner, I became deeply curious—the house was stunning and *huge*. I wouldn't have guessed it because Juan was so humble, unassuming, and down-to-earth. All he had told me about his wife and himself was that they both worked at a hospital.

"I'm so excited to meet you," his wife Diep said, hugging me and my kids at the door. "Juan told me so much about meeting you."

During that first interaction with Diep, she struck me as having a disposition that perfectly complemented Juan's. Her warmth and genuineness were undeniable. By the time my kids and I had removed our shoes in the foyer, I felt as comfortable in their home as if we were old friends.

While Juan and Diep prepared the meal, I pressed the conversation, mixing in questions and probing for more information from these interesting, overly cheerful people. Neither was inclined to talk much about themselves, and it took many subsequent discussions to get a real flavor for their experiences. But it became clear to me that both had overcome harrowing times in their lives. I learned if not for some fortuitous turns of events, they probably would have found themselves in opposite parts of the world, likely immersed in dire circumstances—a far cry from the safe, insulated, upper-middle-class neighborhood of Manhattan Beach where they currently resided.

Over casual BBQs and family vacations together, I discovered that Juan was born and raised in a fatherless household in an exceptionally rough part of Colombia. If it hadn't been for his mother's protection and guidance, he may have ended up dead, in jail, or both, like most of the other boys from the area. But he made it through school, and at eighteen, Juan found his way to the States to live with relatives. There, he went to college and then to medical school. Defying the incredible odds stacked against him, Juan became a pediatrician in Southern California.

Diep was less forthcoming about her childhood, though over the years I learned a tidbit here and there. She opened up more when discussing her creative writing pursuits. Although Diep was a practicing OB/GYN, an entrepreneur, and a mother of three kids, she found time to pursue a master's degree in creative writing at UCLA. But when she got sick, I asked if she'd allow me to talk to her more intimately about her life. We had discussed our various projects, including the *Cycle of Lives* book, and once she was faced with the prospect of having cancer, I pressed her to allow me to include her remarkable story.

Many of the book participants have become friends, but Diep was a friend long before the book project came to be. At times it was difficult going down some of the roads we went down—talking to strangers is sometimes easier than talking to friends and loved ones—but Diep was forthcoming and honest, and her story is every bit as inspiring and thought-provoking as anything else I discovered along the way.

Being Dr. Nguyen

Life Can Be Just Too Hard Sometimes

It could have happened a hundred other times in Diep's life, and at any of those times, it might have made more sense. One night, when she was twenty-six, during the quiet late-night hours of the oncology ward, Diep was in residency watching a mother and her young son cry together. Suddenly, the hard and painful reality of life became too much for her. The proverbial straw had broken her back in that specific, random moment. Sometimes, it seemed as if the straw had been placed there by some cruel-minded, omnipotent spirit, one little strand of tragedy and sadness at a time. This small family scene, late that night, was one strand too much. It overwhelmed her psyche, and Diep collapsed inside—mentally, emotionally, and psychologically.

Diep turned away from the bed and ran out of the room, using every ounce of restraint not to crumple into a heap on the floor. As she raced down the hall, her mind started to darken, blocking out thoughts, feelings, awareness, and control. Her vision began to tunnel. She made it down the two flights of stairs, feeling as if she were stuck in mud, and managed to run out through the doors of the emergency entrance and to her car. She dug for her keys and then collapsed in the driver's seat, sobbing from a place deep inside that she never knew existed.

After a minute struggling to clear away the darkness, she pressed the water from her eyes with the palms of her hands and started the engine. Everything was still out of focus, but she managed to drive off. By the time her breathing returned to normal and she was able to assess what had happened, Diep had driven more than fifty miles north, along Route 2, far into the mountains. She pulled to the side of the road and opened the door, hauling herself up and out of the seat and walking to the back of the car.

"I can't do it," she said aloud. "I cannot do *that* anymore. I can't. I can't." The tears came back then, hot and flowing heavy.

Diep hadn't really cried since she was fourteen—and those tears had been cold, angry, and short-lived—but that night, she stayed leaning against her car for what must have been an hour, crying over a quarter century's worth of straws.

Diep's shift had ended hours before she fled the hospital, but she had continued to do rounds and assist the overburdened nurses and doctors on the oncology floor at the hospital where she was doing her residency. That was Diep—she worked as hard as she could, for as long as she could. She wanted to be of service, to learn, to reduce the burden on others. That's what she had done her whole life, but she wasn't a martyr. She was just accustomed to carrying the load, regardless of the reasons why it existed. She was the one who people relied on. She *handled* things—*everything*.

Diep had thought she wanted to go into oncology. After all, she had yearned to connect with patients, to hold their hands and help them through unimaginable difficulties. There were many areas of medicine she could focus on, but she had been certain that caring for people with cancer was the way she wanted to go. Oncology had to be the most challenging field, so it would make the most sense for her to pursue it. But that night she spent hours crying on the side of the road not only changed the course of her medical career but became the demarcation point for when the true realities of her life finally demanded that she face them. That night it became okay to admit that life was sometimes just too damn hard.

The patient from that night was a thirty-two-year-old female with metastatic stage IV colon cancer. The cancer had spread throughout her body and had overtaken her liver and brain. Although she was lucid and in command of most of her bodily functions, she was approaching the point when both those things would deteriorate at a rapid pace. Over the course of her treatment, the woman had endured several surgeries, multiple rounds of chemotherapy regimens, and targeted radiation therapy. She was not on the oncology floor for further treatment for her cancer—there was nothing left to be done for her cancer. She was there so the doctors who knew her situation best could try to manage the pain from obstructed bowels and care for her while hospice was being arranged.

From what Diep could ascertain, the woman had no siblings, parents, or other close relatives save for an aunt, who appeared to be her primary support, and a sevenish-year-old son, whom the nurses and techs had allowed to stay with his mom despite lack of supervision and the patient's severe limitations with regard to mobility, general awareness, and energy.

Diep had read and reread the woman's chart and notes and knew there was nothing left to be done beyond palliative care in hospice soon.

That night, some unknown force had drawn Diep to spend extra time in the woman's room. She checked and rechecked the woman's pulse and blood pressure, monitored her drip, and talked to her about what they were doing to relieve her pain and manage her overall care.

"Are you going to take more blood?" the woman had asked when Diep first entered the room. "To make me better?" the woman added, noticing her son's intent gaze.

"No. I'm not taking blood. I'm just here to check on you," Diep said, reading the tension on their faces.

"That's good. My son—you remember Riley—he doesn't like to see blood, even if you take it to help me." Riley was lying on the bed next to his mother, spooned onto her as only a child can spoon onto his mother. She stroked his hair. Diep could sense the boy's despondency, confusion, and fear. They were small mirrors of the unconcealable expressions on his mother's face.

"I see you're doing better now after the medication," Diep lied as she moved about the bed, tinkering with the monitors and moving things slightly from one spot to another. Diep's constant checking-in was primarily for show. The woman had to know there was no real point to it. Diep accepted the woman's appreciative nods.

"I am. Much. Always doing better."

Patient to doctor, woman to woman, human to human, they both played their part: The woman fought to hold a steady voice as she asked Diep questions, knowing the questions provided only a diversion from the reality of her situation, a cover to protect her son from that reality. Diep pretended the things she did were necessary, to show that people were trying to make the boy's mother better. They engaged in this subtle dance between them together.

"How's the level of—" Diep said, cutting herself off and nodding to the unit connected to the tube in the woman's wrist in lieu of using the word *pain* in front of the boy.

"Okay," the woman answered with a grimace. After a moment, she smiled at her son. "It's okay, really."

The lengths people will go to to protect their kids, Diep thought. She flashed back to a vision of her own father trying to protect her and her sisters many years before—under very different circumstances.

"I can tell you're a very good mother." Diep said, unsure as to why she allowed herself to make such a personal observation.

"I don't know," the woman replied with a shrug. "It's hard to be when . . . well, you know."

"Can you put that in me?" Riley asked Diep, looking at the tubes in his mother's wrist and then up at the PCA. "I know it makes Mommy hurt, so can you put it in me? It maybe won't hurt *me* so bad."

"The IV?" Diep asked him.

"Yes." He looked at his mother. "You can put it in me, and it won't hurt her anymore."

Diep remembered when she was young and how when her family was in danger, her father had risked his life to save theirs—she remembered how he was helpless, hurt, and bleeding after putting everything at risk for his kids. She thought about how all she'd understood then was that she wanted to help *him*, how she'd have done anything to make it easier for *him*, to take away *his* pain. She understood Riley. She knew how he must feel.

"This tube *helps* Mommy," his mom told him, tears streaming down her cheeks. "It doesn't hurt Mommy. It's to take away pain, not give it."

"Put it in me. It's okay, Mommy. I can take it."

Diep half watched as the woman cried. She knew the boy didn't understand, but he was trying to do something—anything—to help. Diep also saw the desperation and confusion in the eyes of the mom putting up such a strong front. She felt ashamed to be in the middle of such a private and sober moment between them.

"I know you could," the mother said to her son. "You're such a tough boy, so strong."

"That's what all the doctors and nurses always say to me," the boy said and looked up at Diep, forcing her to become part of the exchange. "I tell them I know, but if I could, then maybe Mommy wouldn't die, right?"

Diep didn't know how to answer him. What could she possibly say? *Of course, everyone dies eventually*, she thought. *But eventually is coming too soon for this woman.*

The idea of death was not something they talked much about in medical school. The *reality* of death was, but only in the context of diseases, traumas, and incurable conditions. But the emotions and psychology of death— *impending* death—were confusing for anyone, let alone a small child. Diep didn't have the tools to deal with any of her own hardships; she just buried them deep inside. How could she possibly help him deal with something as unfathomable as watching his mother die? Would lying to him be the right thing to do? Would trying to explain things be the right thing to do? She fumbled for something to say.

"You have such a great mother, Riley—an amazing mother. She'd never *want* to leave you. Look how much she loves you," Diep said. She felt emotions fill up her chest and saw—through her own tears—the woman's uneasiness, gratitude, apprehension, and desolation.

Before anybody could say anything more to Diep, before she'd have to say anything else to those poor people, and before the realities of her own past came welling up to the surface, she ran out of the room—trying not to look as though she was escaping, shattering inside.

The Beginnings of Trouble

Diep learned when she was a little girl that talking about bad things was not something one did. One kept their thoughts and words inside.

Diep's father was the son of a prominent physician. Her mother was the daughter of laborers. Once their relationship was discovered, her parents had been summarily turned away from their families, something traditional values would deem irreversible. The family struggled to find their way in a war-ravaged country—one with little order, let alone opportunity.

Diep's parents lived in Saigon, Vietnam. She was born seven years after the country split, during the height of fighting before American intervention in the early 1960s. Diep was brought into a world of daily bombings; sirens; bleak and dreary days; and deafeningly loud, dark, and frightening nights. She was the first of three girls born to parents who, having been cast out of their families, knew little beyond struggle. Struggles of that sort can knock the shine off even the truest love.

Her mother sometimes found work either selling eggs or fabrics, while her father took on anything he could find, such as working as a freelance photographer or an English or math tutor. Amenities were scarce, and the family often went with little food. Although her mother was uneducated, Diep's father was not, and school was an important constant in Diep's life. Being the oldest, she was expected to help teach her younger sisters, as well as take on the majority of the household tasks. By the time she was six or seven years old, Diep was responsible for both school and chores for her and her sisters.

When she was eight, she took on the added responsibility of following her father around in the afternoons and evenings so she could report back on him to her mother. Her mother suspected that he was keeping company with another woman and sent Diep out with him to deter his dalliances. Diep took instructions from her mother, but her father's persuasive commands prevented her from delivering an accurate accounting of his trysts. Instead, Diep sat outside of the strange house, reading, doing her homework, and waiting for her father to come out. When he did, he reminded her to keep her mind on her own concerns and leave him to address his in privacy.

"People create trouble when they talk, like all this trouble around us," her father said, arms gesturing wide. "No good comes from interfering with private matters. Doing so creates trouble around us, in the family, and at home. Trouble is like a disease—like a cancer that ruins everything around it. You understand? You don't want to be the cause of troubles, do you?"

Perhaps her mother believed her when she swore that her father had only talked to men about work, helped friends, or simply walked around the city doing nothing in particular. Perhaps she didn't, but either way, Diep kept her father's secrets to avoid troubles in the household.

• • •

By the time Diep was a teenager, the country had long since seen all its secrets exposed. The troubles around them were unspeakable. In 1975, when Diep was fourteen, life was measured from one desperate moment to the next. Although her father had found steady work as an interpreter for the Americans, and food and clothing were less scarce, he'd become increasingly convinced they would soon need to flee the country. Her father had asked his many family members for money to buy passage, but they were all unwilling to help. He had long been excised.

As the chaos and unruliness around them intensified, her parents sold everything they could to get enough money to pay a local captain of a small boat to take the family to one of the American ships that were close at sea. The captain took the payment, then disappeared. Desperate, her father ignored the twenty-four-hour curfew and scrounged in the city to find any American contacts who could somehow provide access to passage. He was unsuccessful. The next morning, word came that the president had fled the country. That night, her father told his family they were leaving. He had learned the Americans were not going to be able to maintain the city—or the safety of anyone—any longer. And he was right; it was April twenty-ninth, 1975, one day before the fall of Saigon.

When they got to the harbor, the pandemonium was inconceivable. There were three large barges filling up with families. The desperation was everywhere. People were being either blocked by or guarded by the Americans—Diep couldn't tell which—while endless others were pleading, begging, wailing, and pushing to try to get through. Few made progress against the line of soldiers.

Her father recognized a man who wore a local official's clothing and handed him the small wad of money he had left. He went on to explain to the official that the family had to leave because the Communists would torture him for working for the Americans. The official pushed him back. Her father desperately herded the family down the length of the harbor's access points and found an opening. They rushed through the crowd and the fence and hid on the dock behind one of the barges. Her dad climbed the wall of the barge—it had been fortified with sandbags—and leaned back over and quickly pulled each girl and then his wife up by their arms onto the barge. Diep noticed each let go of or dropped some of what they carried or had hidden under their clothing into the murky water below: a small doll, a handful of photographs, a book. Within an hour, a boat pulled the barge away from the dock, people leaping at it and trying to pull themselves along the ropes that trailed in the water behind the overstuffed rig.

Diep's family sat huddled, having found a small amount of space toward the center of the barge. Diep didn't recognize any of the families, and she wondered how so many people could be on the barge and she didn't know one of them. The firestorms over the Saigon sky cast an orange glow as they whipped plumes of smoke upward. Planes and helicopters filled the skies. The sea was filled with dinghies and small boats and the two other large barges overflowing with people. Diep felt the world was ending in a flurry of chaos and bombs and fire. She watched her father look around, perhaps having the same thought. He then got up, walked around, and came back towards the family. She saw his gaze stop on a group of men huddled close to them. He watched them and then leaned over to whisper to her mother, but Diep could hear him.

"Those guys, look at their language and mannerisms. They are soldiers. They have guns and there are others. They are Communists. I heard them say that they will try to kill us here or pull us back to the harbor. I have to let people know. I have to get help. Don't come after me. You stay here with the kids. Do you hear?"

Her mother blinked in acknowledgment. Her father stood slowly. Diep watched her father. He began to yell.

"Everybody, listen to me! These men are Communists." He pointed at the nearby group. "They are planning to pull us back to the harbor."

The men dispersed into the crowd. Diep's father reached his hands in the air and screamed—no words, just a loud, long scream. He screamed so loudly that Diep saw everyone on the boat look up at him. Then her father ran towards an opening on the side of the barge, still screaming, and jumped off the ship into the dark water.

"Man in water!" someone screamed.

Immediately, Diep's mother jumped up and started running to the side of the boat where her father had jumped from. "Someone help my husband!" she yelled.

Mayhem commenced, and people were screaming all around. People rushed to the edge of the barge. Diep pushed and climbed her way over the frenzied crowd. People barked orders to each other; others quickly tied shirts together to make a rope and then threw one end into the water.

A moment later, they pulled her father back onto the barge. His thighs were gashed from having scraped against the rusted metal on the side of the barge. Diep and her mother and sisters squeezed in close. Her mother wrapped him with a couple of dry shirts handed to them by the women nearby. Four men surrounded her father and led him back to their original spot.

"Those Communist guys are somewhere in this crowd, but they are now separate," one of the men said to her father. "They won't be able to harm you. If they try anything, all us former soldier brothers will attack them."

Her father lowered his head. "I thought I could swim to the American ship. I panicked and misjudged the distance."

"Thanks to your warning, we are all safe now," another of the men said.

Diep and her sisters wrapped themselves around their father as her mother attended to his wounds.

● ● ●

Throughout the night, the soldiers sent SOS signals to the large American vessel in the distance. Finally, in the early morning, a large ship from the Seventh Fleet rescued the nearly three hundred people who had managed to cram aboard that barge.

On the two-day voyage to Subic Bay, in the Philippines, Diep and her family slept sitting up, back-to-back, as they struggled for inches of space alongside thousands of other refugees. Once there, the official processing Diep's family looked over her father's papers. "Interpreter?" he asked.

"Yes, sir."

"Here or the States?" the man asked.

"Please, America. Please, the Communists will retaliate."

The man listened as Diep's dad told him their ordeal. Then the man waved another official over.

"Guam. ASAP."

Hours later, Diep and her family were loaded onto one of the transport planes that was being used to shuttle refugees to Guam. They were among the many tens of thousands of refugees who were then processed there to be disbursed to various refugee camps Stateside and elsewhere around the world.

Diep's family spent three months in a refugee camp at Fort Chaffee in Arkansas before being taken in by a family in Wilmington, Delaware, whose Lutheran church sponsored them. During those three months, Diep attended a makeshift English class at the camp and helped care for her younger sisters. At night, she practiced the new language on her own, listening to the cries and complaints of the families they shared barracks with. They endlessly lamented the country they had been forced to abandon and the troubles that lay ahead of them. Diep's parents didn't partake in such talk. Her father wouldn't have stood for it. Complaining was unacceptable.

Diep's dreams—sounds of rockets and bombs, harrowing visions of death and destruction—woke her up most nights drenched in sweat. She had told her dad in the days leading to their escape that he should teach her how to use a hand grenade so that if he were captured to be tortured, she could assure the family would die at once. She had that nightmare many times over. But she knew to keep her fears to herself.

When her family arrived at their new temporary home, Diep encountered many firsts: rolls of toilet paper, television, carpeting, mattresses raised off the floor, balanced meals, colorful clothes, and candy. The family in Delaware was exceptionally charitable and kind. The wife took the women shopping and tried to introduce them to American life, and the husband secured a job for Diep's dad operating a Xerox machine at his work. Soon thereafter, Diep's family was placed in a temporarily subsidized apartment. Her dad got a job at a print shop, and her mom found work as a seamstress.

Money was tight. So, too, was the lid kept securely closed on open communication and showing emotion. When Diep had to forgo things her parents provided for her younger sisters—newer clothes, extra food, time off from chores, breaks from studying—she kept her thoughts and feelings deep inside.

The responsibilities and sacrifices that came with being the oldest child had been the norm her whole life. A new reality and new way of life would have no effect on how the household ran or which conventions it adhered to. Diep didn't complain and didn't attempt to get her parents to adapt to the norms she was learning about in their new country.

Life was as difficult to reconcile outside of the home as in it. Diep quietly accepted it when the American kids laughed and pointed at her because her clothes were out of style. She turned away when the other kids called her names and made fun of her for being a "boat person" and used racial slurs against her. She kept her head down when kids kicked her and her sisters out of their seats on the school bus and when they stole their lunches. She felt so much shame for the poverty they endured and for her color and her race. One time, to get them to finally stop, she yelled back at the other kids, "*If you touch us, we hit you harder,*" and she even felt shame for her anger. But the embarrassment and fear of disappointing her parents prevented Diep from saying anything. The emotional difficulties of dealing with all sorts of trouble was shoved away, boxed up inside.

Regardless of the many responsibilities her parents put on her and the bullying and discrimination she dealt with on a daily basis, Diep excelled at school. She read assignments and chapters in her books a dozen times over, looking up words in the dictionary, teaching herself how to speak better English. She became a straight-A student.

There wasn't much diversion or fun or relief for Diep, but the one light and joyful experience she was able to enjoy was food shopping.

Food shopping might've been a chore for some, but Diep loved it. She loved the colors, packaging, and endless choices. Her family gave her food stamps and small amounts of money, and Diep became a professional at grocery shopping. But one day, even that became a source of trouble.

Diep had been sent to pick a few things up with some extra food stamps found hidden in a drawer. As she got in line, Diep did the math. She was exceptional at math. There would be enough extra to buy some candy for her little sisters. She eyed the choices and put a few perfect surprises for them on the counter. The checker started to ring the grocery items up. When she came to the candy, she stopped. She crossed her arms and peered down her nose at Diep.

"What do you think you're doing?" she snapped.

Diep shook her head, unsure of the nature of the question.

The woman eyed the candy. "That. Are you stupid?"

Diep looked confused.

"Do you speak English? You just get off the rice boat or what?"

Again, Diep didn't know what she meant or why she was talking to her that way. She started to tear up—cold, angry tears.

"This." The woman grabbed the candy off the counter. "This? You damn stupid rice-eater. You can't buy *candy* with food stamps. You are using stamps, right? Not money? You hear me? Do you have any money? Do you have American dollars and not some fucking handouts? *Do you?*"

Diep shook her head. "I don't have any money. These can buy food." She held out the food stamps to the checker.

The checker threw the candy at Diep, right in her face.

"Put it back, stupid rice-eater. You can't buy candy with food stamps. I mean, seriously. I'm tired of all you people. Bag your shit and get out of here before I call the police on you."

The tears stung her cheeks, but Diep didn't allow them to flow but for a couple of seconds. She didn't want trouble.

Nobody ever heard about the candy. Nobody heard about the boys walking into the girl's bathroom after Diep and threatening to make her do things to them before they laughed it off and pushed her away, either. Nobody heard about Diep's pain when her parents, without explanation, whisked the family away to California after hearing she had been accepted into Bryn Mawr College in Pennsylvania. Diep didn't understand why, but when she begged them to allow her to go, she was told there was no way they'd let her live away from the family. No way.

Nobody heard from Diep when her college boyfriend—she started at UC Irvine after arriving in California—became physical with her. When that boy's mother found out about her son's abuse, Diep didn't tell anybody that she had told Diep to just take it and not cause anybody any trouble. His father was a prominent public figure, and nobody would believe Diep anyway.

That's the way it went, because Diep knew about keeping quiet, not talking about private things, not expressing emotions. But at twenty-six, having had so many traumatic events build up inside of her, one straw at a time, each one a painful reminder not to express her feelings, the poignant, heart-wrenching scene between a dying mother and her little boy broke Diep.

Life Can Be Rewarding

When she finally got back into her car the night she had broken down, she felt as though she'd become a different person. Crying allowed recognition of the things she'd suppressed for so long. The recognition allowed her to assess her life, and that assessment allowed her the freedom to explore the possibility that she had choices. She could forge the kind of life *she* would accept. It gave Diep the confidence to believe she could make the choices in life *she* wanted.

Tears can be cleansing, but Diep's tears were transformative. Once she popped the lid off, she began to explore a new way of doing things: with passion and feeling and self-concern. Diep embarked on a journey of learning how to be comfortable pursuing self-fulfillment, to try to look at the world in new ways. Instead of always doing what she *thought* she should do, she began to do what she *wanted* to do.

In her personal life, Diep committed to pursuing relationships that built her up and helped her develop better relational skills, which meant dropping some people, interacting thoughtfully with others, and redefining the narrow relationships she had with her family. As a result, she found herself emboldened to begin speaking her mind, and she quickly discovered she deserved to pursue happiness, fulfillment, and healthy companionship. Soon, Diep realized she could walk freely without concern that she might cause trouble.

In her professional life, Diep decided to pursue the type of medicine she wanted. Helping people through difficult medical situations had an allure. Relieving burdens was at her core, but she decided she wanted to commit to an area as far away from oncology as there was.

If cancer and death and the ripping of families' hearts out were at one end of the spectrum, Diep posited, then purity and life and helping people form families were at the other. She decided to focus on obstetrics and gynecology, where she could operate from the middle, within arm's reach of new life and end-of-life, and where she could help women deal with diseases and disorders—including cancer—but also with pregnancy, childbirth, and postpartum care. Establishing deep connections with patients, helping them navigate death *and* life issues, would allow her to rely on her inherent strengths while also setting a perfect backdrop for her quest for growth.

Diep's personal journey included a turbulent and brief marriage to a resident physician at a hospital where she first worked. That relationship produced the first of her three children, and although it was unsuccessful, navigating the ups and downs of a relationship helped Diep evolve. She became more confident, developed more insight into what she wanted out of a relationship, and furthered her journey toward remaining self-reliant while learning how to rely on someone else.

A few years later, Diep met her husband-to-be, Juan—a sensitive, happy, optimistic, kind, and personable man. He was a pediatrician who, like herself, had overcome unimaginable circumstances in his youth and young adulthood on the bloody streets of Colombia during the height of the burgeoning violence around the cocaine trade. He'd not only made it safely to America but succeeded at university and medical school so he could become a doctor. After marrying, Diep and Juan had two children together, and over the next twenty-plus years, the family enjoyed a mostly healthy, interactive, communicative, supportive relationship.

Diep became very grateful for the life she and Juan built, not because it was in such contrast to her experience growing up but because she had been given such opportunity and had achieved so much. Diep and Juan owned a beautiful home in one of Southern California's most desired communities. Their professional success allowed them to provide care, housing, and sustenance for various family members. They had no major traumas to deal with and were able to provide a safe, upper-middle-class home for their children. They traveled, lived well, and were all healthy. They even balanced their good fortune with charitable work, often traveling to third-world countries to provide medical care to impoverished communities and expose their kids to other experiences outside of their bubbled lives. Every aspect of their personal lives flourished.

Professionally, Diep's career had progressed with both purpose and passion. Once in practice, she stayed up to date on the most cutting-edge technologies, procedures, and research developments so she could constantly implement changes to enhance the medical care she gave patients. Diep had entered medicine so she could *help people*, and once she found her calling, she worked to develop a rapport that gave her patients an unmatched experience. She never rushed them out of the examination room. She held their hands and listened with purpose so each patient felt they were being heard. She became her patients' trusted physician and *friend*. She loved the excitement, anticipation, and anxiety of helping patients through their pregnancies, and she reveled in the joy that childbirth brought.

At home and at work, Diep had achieved happiness and a sense of self-worth she'd once thought impossible—but she was not without limitations or scars. Fortuity had not eased all her pains. Diep's past had left permanent marks on her psyche that not only affected her but affected those around her.

Diep never fully let go of the past—or embraced it; thus, she remained self-conscious about her journey, the upbringing she endured, the dramatic escaping of a war-ravaged country, the abusive relationships, the lack of confidence, and the passive approach she took in the face of trouble. She had more shame for her past than pride in all she had overcome. Because Diep hesitated to reveal her true self, choosing instead to repress the emotions and experiences she went through, she didn't have deep, open, honest personal relationships, especially outside her family.

Within her family, despite having made a conscious effort to break free of her ingrained tendencies, Diep often avoided dealing proactively with difficult situations. She would choose instead to accept the way things were without question. Her approach only served to perpetuate the often-painful dynamics of her youth. Because she was more comfortable attending to everyone's needs above her own and because she hadn't learned how to express herself or communicate on a real, raw, intimate level about the things she'd gone through, two major difficulties faced her, clouding the mostly beautiful views of her life: First, her kids developed an ever-growing sense of entitlement over the years, growing up in an affluent community, lacking the sense of perspective they should have gained from being taught lessons from her own harrowing experiences. Her kids didn't understand how fortunate they were to have such an insulated, privileged life, and neither Diep nor Juan addressed that dynamic head-on. Second, in addition to not allowing herself to feel comfortable enough in her life to just *be*, Diep and Juan's difficulty in expressing themselves took a toll on their twenty-year marriage. They both had demanding careers as physicians, each experienced the natural lulls that can accompany any long-term relationship, and both were time-tested professionals at avoiding talking about difficult things. When things were good, they were great, but when there was tension or in times when it would have seemed natural for her husband and children to turn to her for solace, and her to them, they did the opposite—turning away from each other, and in her husband's case, even to a brief affair.

Juan's affair was devastating for Diep. She had promised herself her whole life that she wasn't going to allow someone to do the things to her that her father had done to her mother. But Diep tried her hardest to balance that against knowing they and their children had so much to lose if she wasn't able to break that promise to herself and try to find a way to deal with the damage they had both caused to their marriage.

Diep was patient with herself while trying to learn forgiveness, and she was patient with Juan as he faced the harm that his shortcomings and resulting behavior had caused. Diep drew from memories of watching her father express deep regret and try to make amends to his wife and daughters for years after his transgressions, the same way Juan immediately attempted to make amends to her. As the years passed from that horrible time in their own marriage, Juan's betrayal became a more distant dot on the timeline of Diep's memories, and the pain lessened.

It took years for Diep to learn about and feel true forgiveness, for Juan to understand how to express his feelings better and live up to the promises he made, and importantly, for both of them to turn to each other in the face of difficulty instead of away from each other, but they got there. Though there were some trying times, and though Diep struggled to reconcile the past to better control her present, she had enjoyed the best of what the American dream, and life itself, had to offer. She and Juan worked hard to fix their marriage, and they became more in love and closer than they had ever been.

Diep's second quarter century was a journey that saw her reach personal and professional heights and untangle some of the messy emotions of her youth. It was a passage from oppression and disappointment to empowerment and contentment, with just a trickle of trouble muddying the waters below.

But the trickle never disappeared, and one day, it overtook everything.

Life Can Be Cruel

Considering where she was in life in relation to where she started from, Diep's journey had been both intense and remarkable. Each step forward created new challenges, yet she could measure her progression relative to overcoming those challenges. But in her early forties, a challenge came along that not only appeared indomitable but did the opposite of advancing her life.

It began with headaches, the kind that wouldn't go away with rest or common pain relievers. They were bothersome but didn't interfere with her life. But the headaches soon increased in intensity and frequency. Then they began to be accompanied with nausea and dizziness. The headaches did not come from causes such as stress, lack of sleep, changes in the weather, and noise, but rather the headaches were exacerbated by those types of stimuli. And over time, as they continued to become more painful and long-lasting and be accompanied by a variety of symptoms beyond head pain, they started to affect her daily life.

In her midforties, Diep's life was at its fullest and most chaotic point: Her medical practice was flourishing, her eldest daughter was getting ready for college, her two youngest kids were in middle school with full extracurricular schedules, and Juan's pediatrics practice was thriving. Amid all the activity, Diep struggled to command household obligations, provide direction to her kids, and positively interact with a husband who had done so much hard work with her in the recent years to bring their marriage back. Needless to say, suddenly not being able to get out of bed, open her eyes, talk, or do anything but hold a fetal position for days on end while she grappled with the pain of her headaches did more than affect her; it wreaked havoc in every area of her life.

They're just headaches, Diep thought. *There's no reason to think it's more. I'll get up soon.*

But the headaches continued to intensify.

Diep finally went in for testing. Her doctor ordered CT and MRI scans, but the results came back normal. The only diagnosis for her symptoms that made sense was *migraine*, a neurological disorder of unknown cause and for which there is no cure, only potential ways to manage those symptoms.

Manage she did. Diep changed her diet, lightened her load at work, and relied on Juan to do more for the kids. She tried everything: magnesium infusion therapy, Botox for prevention, various antimigraine and antiseizure medicinal cocktails, acupuncture, and even essential oils and meditation to help relieve the pain, but nothing worked. As a result, she had to accept that she sometimes needed to lock herself in a dark bedroom and lie still—sometimes for days at a time.

Even as the migraines became chronic, sometimes lasting for weeks at a time, Diep stubbornly tried to maintain some normalcy. She drove the kids to school when she could. She continued to attend to her practice. Some days, between seeing patients, the nurses gave Diep oxygen and administered injections of Toradol, an anti-inflammatory medication, in attempts to reduce the symptoms.

But things continued to get worse, and Diep's stubbornness almost cost lives. She was driving to work one morning and became extremely dizzy. She swerved into another car on a busy street, causing a mild accident. It might have been much worse had the traffic flow been faster.

Diep was a surgeon. Surgeons can't miss scheduled caesarean sections or operate on their patients when they're dizzy, nauseated, and having trouble standing. Even when she could get out of the house and make it to the office, she couldn't trust herself to be on call or perform procedures at her usual level. She couldn't even hold a scalpel without her hands shaking. She had to face reality: She needed to stop working. That reality was all the more maddening because even though her symptoms were acute and had become near constant, her doctors couldn't find anything to explain what was happening; the MRIs were normal.

Fear, doubt, self-consciousness, and defensiveness flowed through Diep each time she tried to explain to Juan or their kids, doctors, family, or friends—even to herself—that her migraines were real, that her pain was not invented. She could read the skepticism in people's eyes when she explained that her headaches were making her miss work and social events. Juan empathized with her. He certainly saw the helplessness and devastation she was experiencing over her career—and her identity—slipping away, and he con-tinued to care for Diep and the kids, but she could sense a tiny amount of frustration in him as test after test proved negative. As a result of her symp-toms, she was becoming less inclined to get up each day. Her kids were aware of and sensitive to her needs, but Diep could sometimes hear them talking in the next room about how she was being so dramatic, how all she needed to do was get up, move around, and stop being such a victim. They may have been afraid of what was happening to their mom, but Diep saw that they resented her for not being at their sports events or driving them around or cooking for their friends as she always had.

I know it's more. I know I'm not making this up. If I could take charge and handle this, I would. I always have. I'm not the cause of this trouble, Diep thought.

Not Such a Merry Christmas

Six months later, in late December of 2013, Diep's condition worsened. In addition to the other recurrent symptoms she was experiencing, pressure was building in her skull to such an extent that she couldn't move without excru-ciating pain. For days, she stayed in bed, the drapes drawn, unable to move, talk, eat, nothing. Juan had bought a small wooden mallet, and either he or Diep would tap the hammer end of the mallet on Diep's skull, sometimes for literally hours at a time—which either alleviated or masked the pressure—but even that proved mostly fruitless against the pain and pressure. A few days before Christmas, Juan took Diep to the ER. She was nearly catatonic. An MRI of her skull showed a baseball-sized mass on the right side of her brain.

I knew it. Trouble of the worst kind. Cancer.

The doctors performed a craniotomy and found that the mass had extended to Diep's optic canal. Fortunately, the mass had well-defined mar-gins, and the surgeon was able to remove it almost entirely, with no damage to the optic nerve. The pathology showed that she had an atypical meningi-oma, an extremely rare, slow-growing, but more aggressive form of benign meningioma; it grows faster and has a tendency to recur early and may become malignant. If they are benign, as Diep's was, there is a chance that if the tumor reappeared, it could become cancerous. Her doctor suggested that the maximum radiation dose be applied to the tumor area. She had no choice but to proceed with aggressive treatment.

When consulting with her neurosurgeon, Diep, as a doctor, was a little relieved. She knew that catching her tumor before it had metastasized widened the available treatment options and increased her chances for a full recovery. She also knew that her nausea, dizziness, migraines, aversion to light, and other symptoms she had lived with for several years may have been related to the tumor. She also knew how to navigate the system and find the right professionals to care for her. But as a person, Diep thought the worst possible thoughts: The tumors would reappear; they would become malignant; they would spread throughout her brain; she'd have a terrible course of surgeries, with possible surgical and neurological complications; and she was going to die and leave her family alone in the world without her.

$$\bullet \quad \bullet \quad \bullet$$

Within a couple of weeks of finishing her radiation treatments, Diep's life returned to its regularly scheduled chaos. But the very idea of brain tumors—of the fact that she *could have* had cancer—swirled in Diep's mind, and a fear began to creep into her waking thoughts. An inner voice developed. It had begun with a simple *You're in real trouble now* when she first acknowledged the migraines were taking over her life and had progressed to *The trouble is just beginning* when she first heard the words "brain tumor."

Trouble. Trouble, trouble, trouble. That's what you're in for, Diep thought during exhausted moments when her mind wasn't occupied on the tasks of the day—moments that passed like chilling breezes, unsettling her to the core with the thought of more to come.

Nothing but Trouble

Months after the removal of the tumors, after the lingering pain of surgery was gone, after the visions of her shaved and stapled skull had lessened, after most of the irrational fear of cancer had dissipated, after everything about the ordeal was muted by the reality of a full and busy life, as if in homage to the winds in her mind, trouble blew back into Diep's life like a sudden, wicked storm.

The migraines came back. At first, they were manageable, but like before, they soon came more regularly and with mind-shattering force. The dark, cool silence of her bed helped a little, but only in preventing the migraines from worsening from their debilitating level at onset. When she did attempt to seek stimulus such as sitting up, walking, turning on lights—anything but wrapping herself in blankets and folding a pillow over her head, trying not to think of jumping out the window just to stop the pain—she became dizzy, nauseated, and unstable. The only thing that provided even a sliver of relief was striking the wooden mallet all over her head with greater and greater force, over and over and over.

Diep went back to her doctors but to no avail. Another MRI showed no tumors.

One day, Juan drove Diep to the emergency room. She had sudden weakness in her right leg and an unstable gait. She had multiple procedures to make sure she didn't have multiple sclerosis or blood clots. She was diagnosed with hemiplegic migraine, which is a rare form of migraine that causes temporary weakness, numbness and tingling, and paralysis on one side of the body.

A few months later, she woke up to discover the right side of her face drooping, and she had slurred speech. Again, Juan took her to the hospital; she had experienced a minor stroke.

And again, they couldn't find any tumor. They couldn't find *any cancer*. She was otherwise healthy, by all known ways to test and measure—everything that was happening to her was attributed to her migraines.

I know it has to be worse, Diep thought. *Maybe it* is *cancer this time.*

There were good days, sometimes weeks on end, when Diep was able to be herself, laugh, be active, go places, spend unburdened time with her kids and husband, write and do research and even think about going back to her practice, cook elaborate meals, and entertain friends.

But those periods never lasted very long. Each time the migraines came back, and the crushing, throbbing, stabbing pain clouded her mind, and the queasiness overtook her so that all she could do was hide in the quiet, lonely darkness, Diep braced herself.

Yet the doctors had no idea what was going on.

Cancer, she thought. *Maybe cancer is coming down the road.*

Diep's Epilogue
....

Really listening to Diep's story—walking a mile in her shoes, so to speak—was difficult, not just because her experiences were so heart-wrenching but because they were so foreign to anything I could even attempt to relate to. But metaphorically or otherwise, trying to slip into Diep's shoes was an extremely difficult proposition.

How is it even possible to understand what she might've gone through as a teenager, being forced to leave her home and having to start a new life in the face of prejudice like that? I asked myself after learning more about her experiences. *What must it be like to leave everything behind, have no idea where you're going, what you'll do—no idea if you'll even live?*

Going deep with Diep was an exercise in humility, and although time had distanced her from the traumatic events of her youth, the stark brutality she overcame in her life continued to define who she was and how she dealt or didn't deal with the major events in her life. She could explain the events that shaped her life but not the *feelings* behind those events.

"It's like when a patient tells me it hurts," she explained. "I understand where the pain comes from, perhaps what causes it, even how to cure it, but I can't understand what they're *feeling*. I can tell you about my pain, but how can I make you understand how it hurts me inside when I think of being a young girl in Vietnam and everything that came after, how much it hurts that my kids don't always believe my struggles?"

But when it came to Diep's fear of cancer, that I could understand.

There comes a time in life—even in this enlightened stretch of time where we have such long lives, have solved so many of the problems that ail us, and have made unimaginable advancements in technology and science—when the chilling, mysterious, frightening reality of death hits us right between the eyes. One day we hadn't thought of dying, of the reality that one day we'll be gone, then the next, we're knocked down with the thought. Nothing and no one delivers that devastating punch better than cancer. Cancer isn't a force we instinctively understand.

A car accident we understand. Old age makes sense. Heart disease, diabetes, and kidney failure we can comprehend. But cancer is an enigma. We can try to live clean, and then some cancer can swoop in and attack the pancreas, and two months later we're dead. We can quit smoking to avoid lung cancer, and then colon cancer hits us, and we're goners. Beat prostate or breast cancer, and it can come back with a vengeance and take us out. There's no rhyme, no reason, no predictive consistency, no sense to cancer.

Who doesn't know both the model of healthy living who gets cancer and dies, and the smoking, drinking, unhealthiest person ever who lives to be a hundred? Cancer is nothing short of voodoo—*but the fear of cancer is universal, once the reality of death encroaches on our understanding of the human experience.*

Diep was afraid of cancer—not a paralyzing, unable-to-move-or-breathe type of fear but more of a constant, nagging, inescapable fright. Because the doctors couldn't find anything after her meningioma, Diep thought it had to be the great unknown: cancer. Her tumor would recur. They wouldn't be able to radiate it because she'd had the maximum radiation. Surgery would be the only option. Upon second entry, they would injure the delicate structures near her scars, leaving her with facial drooping, blindness, loss of memory, or even loss of intellectual capacity. Maybe they didn't know it yet. They might not know it for years to come, but it was cancer, and those things might happen. *It had to be.*

Dressed in that fear, Diep wears shoes that fit us all—those of us who have lost people to cancer, have had lives affected by cancer, or work to research more about cancer. It may not be rational, it may not ever manifest into reality, but once in our consciousness, the fear of cancer, in some form or fashion, becomes a part of us. You can't see it from day to day, but you can't deny the feelings are there, changing us, changing the way we view the world and time and ourselves. Each of us—well, those who know we'll die one day—have been Diep. We all have walked in those particular shoes.

Diep is still going through the ups and downs of her debilitating migraines. She can't practice medicine, but she can be more of a mother and a wife than she ever allowed herself to be before. She writes, she cooks, she volunteers, she takes vacations, she helps her kids, and she's a caring, involved wife to her husband. Diep's relationship with Juan is the best it has ever been, and her kids have developed more empathy and maturity and humility, because she has allowed them in and embraced their love for her in a way she wasn't able to when her busyness provided cover for a lack of emotional vulnerability.

Diep has fought through depression and thoughts of suicide. She's had to resign herself to the fact that she won't return to being who she was professionally over a nearly twenty-five-year career, that she has lost some of her functions, and that she may have to deal with chronic pain and debilitating symptoms for the rest of her life. But she's also realized that she cannot give up fighting each day. She wants to set the right example for her kids and be everything she can be for Juan. She tries to live for each day, to be her best, to learn, to teach, to heal, to love. To keep handling things the way she always has, as only she knows how to do.

Diep doesn't have cancer. She isn't dying at any faster a rate than the rest of us, but there's a lingering fear that a special brand of trouble might one day show its face. If that happens, if cancer crosses her path, she'll do her best to fight, to rely on Juan and the kids, to take it day by day, and to be more in tune with her emotions, more present for her loved ones, and more appreciative of who she is and where she came from.

Diep can't do anything but be Diep. None of us can.

Ice Cream Cones

Although it was only seventy miles from Fredericksburg to Washington, DC, it was another three-thousand-feet-of-climbing day. I was only a few hundred miles from New York and was noticeably deliberate in my attack. Every day, every mile made a huge dent in the distance between me and Central Park. Day forty-two was a short day, but nothing came easy. I was a 180-odd-pound bag of lactic acid buildup, and each turn of the pedals whacked a stick at the bag—until I joined the Mount Vernon Bike Trail just south of the Reagan Airport Park.

For more than four thousand miles, the roads had been either deserted or filled with flurries of cars and trucks, nothing but quiet wind or the roars of furious machines whizzing by broke the monumental daily efforts. But in a blink of an eye, I found myself immersed in civilization again, where bikers biked, joggers jogged, two-wheeled commuters commuted by with backpacks and briefcases swung over their backs, and I was simply another guy biking on a bike trail, not some sore thumb sticking out where it didn't naturally belong. When I got to the park, I stopped to soak in the sight of people out biking and running—something I hadn't seen since the Strand in Manhattan Beach six weeks prior.

A plane banked to align with the runway and roared overhead seemingly just out of my reach—and then another and another. The shock to my senses of seeing all the activity going on around me, when I hadn't seen anything like it in weeks and weeks, kept me from moving.

So many people flying from all over the world. So many people moving about. So many people with so many stories.

I felt so insignificant once I was just a guy on my bike rather than the central character in an epic and solitary battle against thousands of miles of hot, windy, angry road—immersed in an endless stream of nonstop and unpredictable struggles. With that feeling came a rush of relief, as though my journey had somehow just become less onerous and daunting. Out there on the road, I was Atlas, alone with my stories and the endless thoughts about others' trauma, holding them up as I struggled along my journey. But watching the planes approaching one after the other, knowing the Washington Monument, the White House, the major memorial parks, the National Cemetery, and so many more significant places were only a few short miles ahead, all overrun with countless meaningful and remarkable people with significant and moving stories to tell, I felt much-needed, humbling relief. My story of losing my sister, having such a disjointed past, and wading through life's emotional murk sometimes just trying to keep my footing was just another tale in a book with millions of pages.

The pain in my legs didn't go away once I got going again, but somehow, moving forward required less effort.

That night, Erin, April, and I met a friend of mine, Seong, for dinner at the Old Ebbitt Grill in downtown Washington, DC. Seong's mother was battling the effects of terminal cancer. She was hanging on, but time was short for her. I watched Seong talk about her mom. I saw the love, pain, and fear in her eyes. Seong's anguish was unmistakable; it hung in the middle of every syllable and was visible in every angle of light that shone on her features. A day never passed that I wasn't presented with some moving reminder of people's struggles with the disruptive and traumatic force that is cancer. Listening to her and watching her struggle was like listening to and watching *every* person.

Before embarking on day forty-three, a 109-mile day characterized by more than 4,300 feet of climbing, heavy traffic, and endless construction detours, I was scheduled to meet with one of the two US senators from California to discuss cancer care and research, the young adult cancer community's needs, proton therapy awareness, and other related topics. Erin and I almost didn't make our appointment because we were running late, but the sergeant in charge at the Senate building took us in himself. Once I explained what we were doing—and he was able to confirm that we did, indeed, have an appointment with the senator—he took an interest in helping us get to our appointment with her. He had, just weeks earlier, lost his wife of twenty-five years to breast cancer.

Once out on the road again, I made my way through Maryland, soaking in the character of the little townships along Route 1—such as Mt. Rainier, Hyattsville, College Park, and Hanover—and then made my way through Baltimore and finally to North East, Maryland. Throughout dinner, I felt a bit anxious. So, at about eight o'clock, I put on bike clothes and safety gear and headed out on the next day's route, toward New Jersey. A few hours in, I called Erin to come get me. Two flat tires, frayed nerves, and ongoing construction that made navigating the detours with a bike at nighttime just plain reckless all made my attempt to cut into the next day's ride a useless one. I went to bed frustrated that even after all the days and all the miles, I couldn't master my physical intentions any better than on day one. As in life, no matter the level of experience you might have, you have to be prepared to take each day for what it is; there's no controlling the future.

Day forty-four—from North East, Maryland, to East Brunswick, New Jersey, the penultimate day of the ride—was a 103-mile, eleven-hour whirlwind of varied landscapes and experiences. Early on, I biked through Wilmington, enjoying the rivers and trees that lined the side roads along I-95. About half-way through the day, I made my way through the endless urban sprawl of Philadelphia—maybe the City of Brotherly Love, but not toward cyclists—and then on to Trenton, which made Philadelphia seem a walk in the park. As darkness approached, I rode past the stately, mansion-lined, shoulderless roads around Princeton before finishing up so Erin and I could make it to dinner and drinks with a group of friends who'd gathered to celebrate the (almost) completion of the ride. The stories and laughs were many, but there was no missing the somberness that hung below the surface of our celebrations, especially when talking about the book participants and the very real emotional hardships they had or, in some cases, *were* enduring. My friend Steve, who'd driven up from a suburb of Philadelphia with his wife, asked me what *one* lesson I'd learned above all others during the adventures of my travels.

"I'm not sure," I answered him. "I learned so much."

After expanding on some of the more obvious lessons—overcoming the desire to quit, learning to rely on others, knowing one can push themselves much harder than ever imagined, and a few others—his question still itched my brain.

What had I learned more than anything else?

A few hours later, fighting off sleep, I hadn't found the right answer.

I awoke slowly the next morning and dressed deliberately. It was the last day of my ride—seventy miles of rolling hills from East Brunswick, New Jersey, to New York City. I stared in the mirror for a long time. I looked gaunt, probably about twenty pounds skinnier from the effort, and dark-skinned from long days in the sun. I searched my own weary but deeply self-gratified eyes, seeing if I could will forward the answer to the looming question from the night before. Nothing came to me before it was time to leave.

I made my way along the busy Route 1 and into Newark, then up through Rutherford and Fort Lee, before I rolled up to the entrance of the pedestrian section of the George Washington Bridge. I hadn't routed past that point, and I was running late for my intended finish time. Erin and a group of people were waiting for me at the designated spot, and I didn't want to leave them waiting, so I stopped to ask a fellow cyclist for directions on how to get to Central Park from the end of the bridge.

As she was telling me what to do, I saw her notice the Stupid Cancer logo on the arm of my jersey.

"Where'd you bike from?" she asked.

"Manhattan." I smiled. "Manhattan Beach, California."

"Just now?"

"Yup, this is the finish line," I said.

"You're doing it for a cause?"

"Yeah, to raise awareness and funds for people with cancer." I went on to tell her about Cycle of Lives.

"I lost my dad to liver cancer almost four years ago," she said with a crack in her voice.

Before the Cycle of Lives, my answer would probably have been something like "I'm sorry for your loss." Then I'd have ridden away. That's when it hit me: the answer to Steve's question. What had I learned the most?

"Were you close to him?" I asked.

"Unbelievably."

"What was he like?"

"Oh my God," she said. "He was the best dad ever. We were so close my whole life. When he first got cancer, it was tough, but when it came back and we knew it was going to be terminal, it was devastating. He wouldn't have sat around and moped about his fate, though. He *loved* cycling. Loved it. We spent a good part—months and months altogether—traveling the world, cycling in the most incredible places. Sometimes it was difficult. But it was magical. The perfect thing to do before he had to face the reality of dying."

"Sounds like you're so grateful for that time."

"There's not a day that goes by I don't think of him. Every time I get on my bike, I think about a memory or a story he told me or something he said to make me laugh. I am so grateful we had that time together."

"Thanks for sharing that," I said.

"He knew people were going to be heartbroken at his funeral, but he wanted to leave them with a smile. He asked to be buried in his favorite biking outfit—one covered in little ice cream cones. All different colors. So we did. And everybody laughed so hard when I spoke that day and told them about his plan."

She reached in, and we hugged over our bikes and then rolled away in opposite directions, our paths to assuredly never cross again. I pedaled fast over the bridge, wound my way onto West Drive in the park, and made the final turn onto Center Drive a few hundred feet before the south edge of the park, where a group of people—Erin; my kids, whom Erin had flown out to surprise me; and several friends—were waiting with signs, smiles, and waving arms.

What lesson did I learn more than all others? *Not to be afraid to talk to people about cancer.*

I learned to ask them what they're going through and how they're feeling. Ask them about the people they've lost. Don't just offer sympathy. Invite people—loved ones or strangers—to share their feelings, to express the traumas they've endured as a result of cancer. Ask them to share their stories. Engaging in meaningful, intimate conversation will allow us to learn from what they're going through, what they've gone through, what they've endured, and what they might still be struggling with. Listen to what they've learned or what they're on a journey to figure out. Talk to them about what we've learned from others. If we do these things, maybe one day we will be able to better deal with our emotions, our feelings, our pain, our fears, and our hope as we navigate our own extraordinary human experiences—even the traumatic ones. Thus, the cycle of lives can continue.

• • •

As I have many, many times since that last night of my journey, I imagined how helpful it could be to me if people knew what I had learned. I imagined that instead of asking me questions about how scary the roads were, how hot an Arizona highway can get, how loud big rigs on the interstate really are, or how I found my book subjects, people would ask questions like "What was June like? How did it feel to lose the one person who understood about your childhood? What emotions are you still dealing with after seeing your sister go through what she did? How are *you* doing through it all?" Maybe that would help me deal with it better.

Like you, if you've experienced the trauma of losing a loved one to cancer, I'm not looking for sympathy or pity or puppy-dog eyes. I don't need those things. I'm lucky, fortunate, loved, healthy, grateful, and humbled by so much in life. But probably like you, if you've dealt with some form of cancer-related trauma, I haven't fully processed the emotions and feelings that remain inside. They're still mostly bottled up, waiting for the right time, circumstances, and opportunity to be dealt with properly.

But I've learned that I won't leave them bottled up forever—I won't always want to carry them alone, and I hope you won't either. Don't be afraid to talk to each other, about your experiences, your emotions, and your pain. Because while cancer and other traumas may bring us unimaginable emotional chaos, sharing that burden is what brings us strength, makes us more one with the human experience, and most of all, makes us realize we are not alone.

www.cycleoflives.org

Making a Difference

· ·

The following organizations have been designated by the book partici-pants to receive a portion of the book's profits. In addition, the Cycle of Lives non-profit offers financial support to many additional cancer-related organizations. I invite you to learn more by visiting the www.cycleoflives.org website and any of these outstanding organizations below. Thank you for sup-porting the fight against cancer.

Stupid Cancer

Empowers young adults affected by cancer by ending isolation and building community.

www.stupidcancer.org

Perlmutter Cancer Center

A nationally recognized comprehensive cancer center and part of NYU Langone Health, one of the nation's premier academic medical centers.

www.nyulangone.org

Children's Hospital Los Angeles

A nationally ranked, freestanding acute care children's hospital.

www.chla.org

Moffitt Cancer Center

A nationally recognized comprehensive cancer center focused on treatment and research, located in Tampa, Florida.

www.moffitt.org

American Cancer Society

A nationwide voluntary health organization dedicated to eliminating cancer.
www.cancer.org

California Protons Cancer Therapy Center

At the forefront of medical care, research and biotechnology, utilizing revolutionary cancer-fighting treatments and tools to treat both common and very rare cancers.
www.californiaprotons.com

Cecilia Gonzalez De La Jolla Cancer Center at White Memorial Medical Center

Providing comprehensive cancer care to the community, combining sophisticated technology with a warm, caring touch.
www.adventisthealth.org

Horizons for Youth

A Chicago-based organization dedicated to helping children recognize and achieve their full potential.
www.horizons-for-youth.org

Michelle's Place

Empowering individuals and families impacted by cancer through education and support services.
www.michellesplace.org

Cancer Support Community

Dedicated to ensuring that all people in the Valley/Ventura/Santa Barbara community who are impacted by cancer are empowered by knowledge, strengthened by action, and supported by community.
www.cancersupportvvsb.org

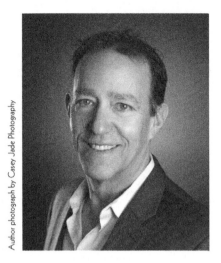

Author photograph by Casey Jade Photography

About the Author

· ·

D avid is an author, endurance athlete, financial services professional, and public speaker. He uses the lessons learned in his life to enrich and inspire others. As a former sedentary, overweight smoker, David discovered that he needed to focus not on what others wanted out of him, but on what he wanted out of life. With his first book, *Winning in the Middle of the Pack: Realizing True Success in Business and in Life*, David discussed how to get more out of ourselves than ever imagined.

Over the last fifteen years, David has completed over fifty triathlons, including fifteen Ironman-distance triathlons (2.4-mile swim, 112-mile bike, 26.2-mile run); more than fifty runs longer than marathon distance, including four consecutive marathons (104 miles) from Santa Barbara to Manhattan Beach; and a forty-five-day, 4,700-mile solo bike ride across the country.

David was raised in Southern California and splits his time between San Diego and Las Vegas. His wife is a successful employment, privacy, and health-care attorney and his college-aged twins are as aspirational as their father.

2016 - Bike Ride

Made in the USA
Coppell, TX
25 February 2021